Manipal Manual of

CLINICAL BIOCHEMISTRY

Manipal Manual of

CLINICAL BIOCHEMISTRY

FIFTH EDITION

Shivananda Nayak B
MSc PhD FAGE (Manipal) NRCC-CC (USA) FACB (USA) FABM PGDHC DSc

Professor of Biochemistry
Department of Preclinical Sciences
Faculty of Medical Sciences
University of the West Indies
Trinidad and Tobago, West Indies
Visiting Professor
Subbaiah Institute of Medical Sciences
Shivamogga, Karnataka
Sri Ramachandra Institute of Higher Education and Research
Chennai, Tamil Nadu, India

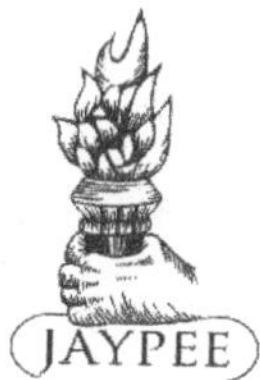

JAYPEE BROTHERS MEDICAL PUBLISHERS
The Health Sciences Publisher
New Delhi | London

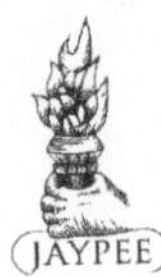

Jaypee Brothers Medical Publishers (P) Ltd

Headquarters
EMCA House
23/23-B, Ansari Road, Daryaganj
New Delhi 110 002, India
Landline: +91-11-23272143,
+91-11-23272703
+91-11-23282021, +91-11-23245672
E-mail: jaypee@jaypeebrothers.com

Overseas Office
JP Medical Ltd.
83, Victoria Street, London
SW1H 0HW (UK)
Phone: +44-20 3170 8910
E-mail: info@jpmedpub.com

Corporate Office
Jaypee Brothers Medical Publishers (P) Ltd.
4838/24, Ansari Road, Daryaganj
New Delhi 110 002, India
Phone: +91-11-43574357
Fax: +91-11-43574314
E-mail: jaypee@jaypeebrothers.com

EU GPSR Authorised Representative
Logos Europe, 9 rue Nicolas Poussin
17000, La Rochelle, France
Phone: +33 (0) 6 67 93 73 78
E-mail: Contact@logoseurope.eu

Inquiries for bulk sales may be solicited at: jaypee@jaypeebrothers.com

Manipal Manual of Clinical Biochemistry

First Edition: 2002

Second Edition: 2005

Third Edition: 2007

Reprint: 2008

Fourth Edition: 2013

Fifth Edition: 2024, Reprint: **2025**

ISBN : 978-93-5696-322-1

Printed in India

Dedicated to

My parents and family

Message

The BMLT program got recognition as a separate entity just twenty years ago. Until then, all the laboratory technology was a part of the biochemistry and other medical subjects. Now, the BMLT program has been well entrenched with the progress in the right path. I am happy to know that Professor Shivananda Nayak has contributed yet again with a Fifth edition of the lucid and comprehensive book entitled *Manipal Manual of Clinical Bichemistry*, which was first published in the year 2002. I was fortunate to be part of the inauguration of the release of this book at that time. From the first edition onwards, the book has become very popular not only because of its content value but also for its simplicity of the presentation in addition to the meticulous organization of the different chapters. Professor Nayak has continued to maintain the same style of presentation by adding and modifying the contents as per the present knowledge. Having all the details for the students of MLT and health science, I am sure the book will be continued to be used by other health sciences students and teachers as well; because, the correct laboratory diagnosis is very crucial in the management of different diseases. Obviously, the correct diagnosis depends on the right laboratory techniques and procedures.

I am very satisfied to see that Professor Nayak has taken meticulous care to bring out a valuable book on Clinical Biochemistry.

I wish him all the success in all his future endeavors.

S Gurumadva Rao MBBS MD
Former Registrar, Manipal Academy of Higer Education, Manipal and Vice Chancellor
RAK Medical and Health Sciences University
Ras Al Khaimah, UAE

Preface to the Fifth Edition

I am happy to bring this fifth edition of the *Manipal Manual of Clinical Biochemistry* for laboratory medicine) (DMLT, BSc MLT, MSc MLT, MSc and MD) in clinical biochemistry and medical students. I sincerely thank all those who warmly received the fourth edition of this title. My aim was to present the new edition of the textbook that covers all the essentials of clinical biochemistry in a simple, narrative form, which meets the present requirements of the students. The good feedback and the suggestions helped me to incorporate interesting diagrams along with self-test and case studies to improve the quality of this title. This edition may help the student community to learn each unit to practice clinical biochemistry. I hope the chapters such as carbohydrates, electrolytes, fluid balance, acid-base balance, liver function test, renal function tests, quality control, special tests and case studies may be useful for the readers. The self-test of each unit will help the readers to check their knowledge in the area of clinical biochemistry.

With the cooperation of the publishers, the printing is done in multicolors. I put my sincere effort to revise the textbook thoroughly. I am always grateful to Dr Sudhakar Nayak, former Head, Department of Biochemistry, and Dr Shivaraj, Professor of Biochemistry, for their excellent support throughout my service. It is my pleasure to thank each and everyone who supported me to bring this fifth edition. I extend my thanks to my niece Mrs Chaithra Nayak for editing the language.

A textbook will be improved only by successive revisions. I tried to keep up my promise of revising this book every two-three years. I always respect the suggestions and constructive criticisms that come from the readers. I would like to have good interaction with the users of this manual to get their timely feedback. Please feel free to communicate at my e-mail address as: *shiv25@gmail.com,* if you have any suggestions. The success of the book was due to the active participation of the publishers.

My special thanks to Shri Jitendar P Vij (Group Chairman), Mr Ankit Vij (Managing Director), Mr MS Mani (Group President), Dr Madhu Choudhary (Director–Educational Publishing), Ms Pooja Bhandari [Director–Production (Books and Journals)], Ms Sunita Katla (Executive Assistant to Group Chairman and Publishing Manager), Ms Samina Khan (Executive Assistant to Director–Educational Publishing), Dr Sangeeta Yadav (Development Editor), Mr Rajesh Sharma (Production Coordinator), Ms Seema Dogra (Cover Visualizer), Mr Vakil Khan (Proofreader), Mr Kulwant Singh (Typesetter), Mr Gopal Kirola (Graphic Designer), and other team members of M/s Jaypee Brothers Medical Publishers (P) Ltd, New Delhi, India, for their encouragement and cooperation given to me for making this book popular both at national and international levels.

Shivananda Nayak B

Preface to the Fifth Edition

Preface to the First Edition

There are very few textbooks, which deal mainly with both theory and practical aspects in clinical biochemistry for students of bachelor in medical laboratory technology. During my experience of more than 10 years in teaching the undergraduates, mainly medical laboratory technology students has compelled to depend on different textbooks during their study of clinical biochemistry. Thinking of these difficulties of students, I have put my effort to include both theory and practical aspects of clinical biochemistry in this book. I have also tried my level best to incorporate several things in a single book that can help even postgraduate students in biochemistry.

This book is written covering the syllabus for bachelors in medical laboratory technology. However, some of the important laboratory procedures are included in almost all the chapters. The presentation of each chapter is made in such a way that it should give some idea about the theoretical and practical aspect. This manual has been written to serve as a workbench reference for the clinical laboratories of India. This book can also be used as a textbook for medical laboratory technology students and for inservice training of fresh technicians in clinical laboratories. The chapters on the instrumentation and techniques, specimen collection and handling, tumor markers, liver function and kidney function tests and diabetes are written in a manner even these technicians can easily grasp. In this book, each chapter is written as unit-wise.

I am grateful to many persons in compiling this valuable book, specially I am obliged to Dr Sudhakar Nayak, Professor and Head, Department of Biochemistry, who always gives me moral support. I am also grateful to Dr B Shivaraj, Professor, Department of Biochemistry, for his support throughout my service. I am thankful to my colleagues Dr Nalini K, Dr Gopalakrishna and Dr Madhukar Mallya for their help during compiling of this title. I am highly indebted to Mr KR Keshavamurthy, Retired Senior Lecturer, Department of Clinical Biochemistry, for having gone through this book. It is my pleasure to thank Mrs Akkayya for excellent secretarial work.

My expectation is to bring out new editions every two years. Suggestions if any, from the teachers and students are most welcome.

Shivananda Nayak B

Contents

UNIT 1 Introduction to Clinical Biochemistry

LEARNING OBJECTIVES

At the end of this unit, the learner should be able to understand:

- How to process the samples for biochemical investigations.
- The different types automation used in the laboratory.
- The hazards from the different chemicals in the clinical laboratory.
- What are the basic laboratory techniques.
- How to prepare the normal, molar and percent solutions.
- How to prepare the different types of buffers with required pH.
- Different types of indicators used in the laboratory.

INTRODUCTION

Clinical Biochemistry mainly deals with the biochemical aspects that are involved in several clinical conditions. The results of qualitative and quantitative analysis of body fluids assist the clinicians in the diagnosis, treatment and prevention of the disease and drug monitoring, tissue and organ transplantation, forensic investigations and so on.

USE OF BIOCHEMICAL TESTS

Biochemical tests are involved, to varying degrees, in every branch of clinical medicine.

- The results of biochemical tests may be of use in diagnosis and in the monitoring of treatment **(Fig. 1.1)**.
- Biochemical tests may also be of value in screening for disease or in assessing the prognosis once a diagnosis has been made.
- The biochemistry laboratory is often involved in research into the biochemical basis of disease and in clinical trials of new drugs.

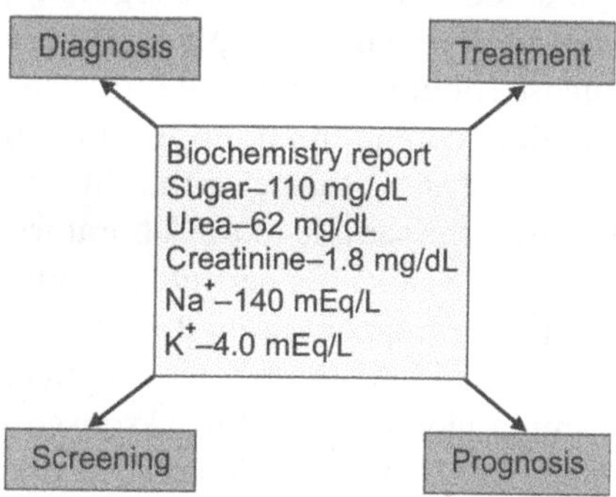

Fig. 1.1: Use of biochemical tests.

Sampling Errors

There are a number of potential errors that may contribute to the success or failure of the laboratory to provide the correct answers to the clinician's question. Some of these problems arise when a clinician first obtains specimens from the patient.

- *Blood sampling technique:* Difficulty in obtaining a blood specimen may lead to hemolysis with consequent release of potassium and other red cells constituents. Results for these will be falsely elevated.

- *Prolonged stasis during venipuncture:* Plasma water diffuses into the interstitial space and the serum or plasma sample obtained will be concentrated. Proteins and protein-bound components of plasma, such as calcium or thyroxine will be falsely elevated.
- *Insufficient specimen:* Each biochemical analysis requires a certain volume of specimen to enable the test to be carried out it may prove to the impossible for the laboratory to measure everything requested on a small volume specimen.
- *Errors in timing:* The biggest source of error in the measurement of any analyte in a 24-hour urine specimen is in the collection of an accurately timed volume of urine.
- *Incorrect specimen container:* For many analyzes the blood must be collected into a container with anticoagulant and preservative. For example, samples for glucose should be collected into a special container containing fluoride which inhibits glycolysis; otherwise the time taken to deliver the sample to the laboratory can affect the result. If a sample is collected into the wrong container, it should never be decanted into another type of tube. For example, blood that has been exposed even briefly to EDTA (an anticoagulant used in sample containers for lipids) will have a markedly reduced calcium concentration, approaching zero.
- *Inappropriate sampling site:* Blood samples should not be taken 'down-stream' from an intravenous drip. It is not unheard of the laboratory to receive a blood glucose request on a specimen taken from an intravenous drip and to receive a blood glucose request on a specimen taken from the same arm into which 5% glucose is being infused. Usually, the results are biochemically incredible but it is just possible that they may be acted upon, with disastrous consequences for the patient.
- *Incorrect specimen storage:* A blood sample stored overnight before being sent to the laboratory will show falsely.

FLOW OF BIOCHEMISTRY SAMPLES

Analyzing the Specimen Collected

Once the form and specimen arrive at the laboratory reception area, they are matched with a unique identifying number or bar code. The average laboratory receives many thousands of requests and samples each day and it is important that all are clearly identified and never mixed up. Samples proceed through the laboratory as shown in **Flowchart 1.1**. All analytical procedures are quality controlled and the laboratory strives for reliability. Once the results are available, they are collated and a report is issued. Cumulative reports allow the clinician to see at a glance how the most recent result(s) compare with those tests performed previously, providing an aid to the monitoring of treatment.

Sensitivity and Specificity

Sensitivity of an assay in a measure of how little of the analyte the method can detect. As new methods are developed, they may offer improved detection limits which may help in the discrimination between normal results and those in patients with the suspected disease. Specificity of an assay related to how good the assay is at discriminating between the requested analyte and potentially interfering substances.

Reference Values

Analytical variation is generally less than that from biological variables. Biochemical test results are usually compared to a reference. Most reference range are chosen arbitrarily to include 95% of the values found in healthy volunteers, and hence, by definition, 5% of the population will have a result out with the

Flowchart 1.1: Circuit diagram of clinical biochemistry process.

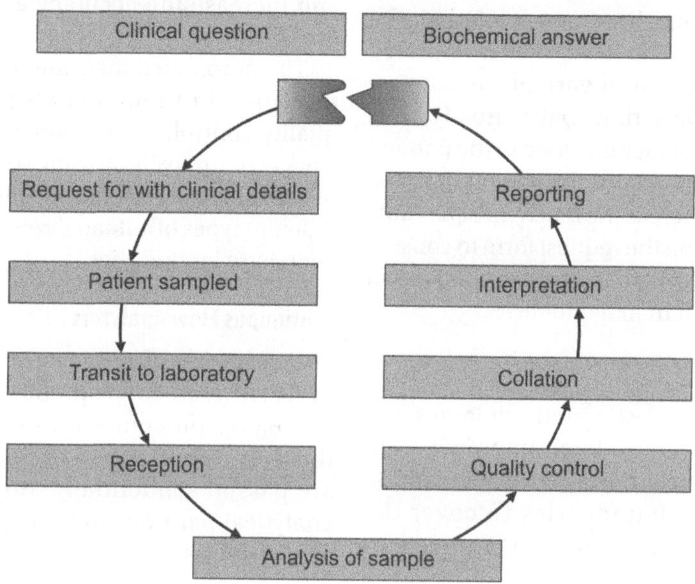

reference range. In practice, there are no rigid limits demarcating the diseased population from the healthy; however, the further result is from the limits of the range, the more likely is to represent pathology. In some situations, it is useful to define 'action limits', where appropriate intervention should be made in response to a biochemical result. There is often a degree of overlap between the disease state and the 'normal value'. A patient with an abnormal result who is found not to have the disease is a *false positive.* A patient who has the disease but has a 'normal' result is a *false negative.*

Biological Factors Affecting the Interpretation of Results

The discrimination between normal and abnormal results is affected by various physiological factors which must be considered when interpreting any given result. These include:

- *Sex of the patient:* Reference ranges for some analytes, such as serum creatinine are different for men and women.
- *Age of the patient:* There may be different reference range for neonates, children, adults and the elderly.
- *Effect of diet:* The sample may be inappropriate if taken when the patient is fasting or after a meal.
- *Time when sample was taken:* There may be variations during the day and night.
- *Stress and anxiety:* They may affect the analyte of interest.
- *Posture of the patient:* Redistribution of fluid may affect the result.
- *Effects of exercise:* Strenuous exercise can release enzymes from tissues.
- *Medical history:* Infection and/or tissue injury can affect biochemical values independently of the disease process being investigated.
- *Pregnancy:* This alters some reference ranges.
- *Menstrual cycle:* Hormone measurements will vary through the menstrual cycle.
- *Drug history:* Drugs may have specific effects on the plasma concentration of some analytes.

Other Factors

When the numbers has been printed on the report form, they still have to be interpreted in the light of a host of variable. Analytical and biological variations have already been considered. Other factors relate to the patient. The clinician can refer to the patient or to the clinical notes, whereas the biochemist has only the information on the request form to consult. The cumulation of biochemistry results is often helpful in patient management.

AUTOMATION

Advances in diagnostic methodologies and instrumentation have been impressive but most of these are deleted in the teaching program. This chapter tries to cover the automation required for the analysis of samples.

When the volume of work increased, there arose a need for work simplification. Monostep methods are introduced to replace multistep, cumbersome and inaccurate methods, such as Folin-Wu's blood sugar determination. The efficiency of monostep methods was further increased by the introduction of automatic dispensers and diluters. For the common test, such as blood glucose, blood urea, etc. However, most large laboratories found this approach still inadequate to deal with work load and instruments designed to handle the whole analytical process in mechanized fashion have become common place in last decade. This procedure is called **automation**. It is a self-regulating process, where the specimen is accurately pipetted by a mechanical probe and mixed with a particular volume of the reagent and results are displayed in digital forms and also printed by a printer. There is an element of feedback, which detects any tendency to malfunction. The function of autoanalyzer is to replace with automated devices the steps of pipetting, preparation of protein-free filtrated, heating the color forming reagents in a water bath and increase the accuracy and precision of the methods.

The automated instruments not only save the labor and time but also allow reliable quality control, reduce subjective errors and work economically by using smaller quantities of samples and reagents. Following are the different types of autoanalyzers used in clinical chemistry laboratories.

Continuous Flow Analyzers

The early form of automation was introduced by Technicon Instrument Corporation. It was based on continuous flow analysis. In these systems, the samples and reagents are passed sequentially through the same analytical pathway and separated by means of air bubbles.

Discrete Analyzers

The various types of discrete autoanalyzers used in the clinical chemistry laboratories are (A) **Batch analyzers** and (B) **'Stat'** (means immediate reporting or emergency determination analyzers).

Batch Analyzers

These are convenient to analyze specimen in batches, such as of sugar, urea creatinine, etc. Stat testing may not be conveniently carried out on these analyzers. The batch analyzers can be further differentiated as- (1) semiautomated and (2) fully automated.

Semiautomated (Batch) Discrete Analyzers

In the case of these analyzers the initial part of the procedure, i.e., pipetting of reagent and specimen, mixing and incubation is carried out by the technician. Rest of the procedure, i.e., setting of incubation temperature (for kinetic determinations), zero setting, photometric readings, result display, automatic printing and data management and processing is carried out by the analyzer.

The semi-autoanalyzers are cheap and compact, compared to other fully automated analyzer.

Specimen analysis is cheap, since volume of reagent used is 0.5 to 1.0 mL.

The enzymatic reagents are not corrosive and involve monostep testing.

Fully Automated Batch Analyzers

These analyzers carry out all the function of a semiautomated analyzer, in addition to the pipetting of specimen and reagents and also the mixing of the reaction mixtures. The basic working stages of these analyzers, after selecting general system parameters are as follows:

1. The specimen cups are placed on the sampler.
2. The required quantity of reagent is dispensed by a reagent probe, in the reaction cups.
3. The respective specimens from the sampler are pipetted into the appropriate reaction cups by another sample probe.
4. The reaction cups are shaken mechanically to mix the contents.
5. After observing the required incubation time (for delay time in the case of kinetic determinations) the reaction mixture is aspirated by a probe for photometric readings.
6. The resulted values are printed and displayed in appropriate units by digital display.

Stat Analyzers (Random Access Analyzers)

In the case of these analyzers, many reagents (8 to 20 or more) can be pipetted one after another, so that various biochemical determinations can be performed on one specimen, according to the number of tests ordered for the patient. Hence, these are patient (or specimen) orientated autoanalyzers. For example, if serum specimen No. 1 requires following tests to be performed:

1. Urea nitrogen
2. Serum creatinine
3. Total proteins
4. Albumin
5. Serum glutamic pyruvic transaminase (SGPT) and serum glutamic-oxaloacetic transaminase (SGOT)

- The analyzer is programed for these tests with respective system parameters.
- The reagents for urea nitrogen, creatinine, total proteins, albumin, SGPT and SGOT are pipetted automatically by a reagent probe in the respective reaction cups.
- The required specific serum quantities are added to the respective reaction cups by a specimen probe.
- The analyzer identifies various reagents and specimen.
- The photometric determinations are carried out by the autoanalyzer.
- The values of the respective tests are displayed on the computer screen as well as printed on a paper, after the specific test incubation periods.

The advantages of a fully automatic 'stat' (or random access) analyzer are as follows:

1. The advantages the various chemistry tests from the file.
2. It performs a single test, a profile, an organ panel or a 'stat' determination.
3. It reduces the cost per test by utilization of micro-volumes of a reagent.
4. It performs automatic monitoring of specimen and reagent volumes.
5. It can perform various methodologies, such as end point, kinetic, initial rate and bichromatic (readings at two different wavelengths) to eliminate errors which may arise due to hemolytic, icteric or lipemic serum.

Various biological fluids subjected to chemical tests and assays include blood, plasma, serum, urine, cerebrospinal fluid (CSF), ascitic fluid, pleural fluid, feces, calculi and tissues.

HAZARDS FROM DANGEROUS CHEMICALS IN THE CLINICAL CHEMISTRY LABORATORY

Persons working in the clinical laboratories are exposed to various potential hazards. Toxic substances in a laboratory can be absorbed either from direct contact through skin or by inhaling vapors or fine powder or may be swallowed by accidentally while pipetting. Injury results from the effect of these chemicals on other tissues, such as bone marrow, liver and kidney. But these can be minimized by information of the general dangers, eliminating hazards where possible, establishing clean, safe work habits, taking proper precautions, and becoming conscious of safety measures.

The main potential physical dangers in a clinical chemistry laboratory include fire, infection, exposure to toxic fumes, being splashed with corrosive chemicals, and exposure to carcinogenic substances.

Precautions to Take to Avoid the Accidents

1. The bottles containing chemicals and reagents should be clearly labeled and the hazard should be noted.
2. Always carry large bottles by holding with both the hands.
3. Keep bottles in use on shelves lower than eye level.
4. Take great care while opening the bottles or pouring from the bottles containing the corrosive chemicals, such as nitric, sulfuric and hydrochloric acids; sodium and potassium hydroxide.
5. Always add contents slowly to water, preferably while cooling and stirring.
6. Never keep acids and alkalis in bottles with ground glass stoppers as they may get stuck.
7. Whenever possible use small measuring cylinders for measuring acids and alkalis. If more accurate measurement is required, use a pipette plugged with non-absorbent cotton wool or with a rubber tube attached.
8. Toxic chemicals, such as cyanide should be kept locked in a cupboard. Mouth pipetting for these should be totally forbidden.
9. Organic solvents may have toxic properties. Thus, benzene is toxic to bone marrow. Carbon tetrachloride and other halogenated hydrocarbons are toxic to the livers. So keep exposure to the minimum. Carry out procedures including distillation in a fume-hood.
10. Many chemicals have the potential to cause cancer and the most commonly carcinogenic chemicals used are aromatic amines, such as benzidine and orthotolidine. Precautions include keeping them in well-closed bottles labeled 'Carcinogenic' and avoiding any contact with skin. When handling carcinogens, rubber or plastic gloves should be used. This must be washed well afterwards under cold running water.
11. Picric acid when dry explodes on percussion. It should not be stored in ground glass stoppered. It should be stored underwater, in a container closed by a rubber stopper.
12. Keep ether always in brown bottles.

Fire

1. Flammable gases, such as hydrogen, propane acetylene stored in cylinders, constitute fire hazards. Keep cylinders, not in use, in a store, which is outside the laboratory.
2. Do not permit smoking in the laboratory.
3. All connections to flammable gases to instruments, such as the flame photometer must be leak proof.
4. Never store flammable solvents in a refrigerator or deep freeze where the thermostat is inside the compartment.

Infection

The hospital is always filled with sick people, some of whom have contagious diseases.

Sometimes laboratory may receive high-risk samples. The infection hazards are viral hepatitis and acquired immunodeficiency syndrome (AIDS).

The infectious hepatitis contracted by entrance of the virus through breaks in the skin or through the entrance of contaminated material into the gastrointestinal tract. The following precautions should be taken to reduce the chances of infection of any type.

1. Mouth pipetting should be avoided.
2. When processing blood sera, serum should not be poured from one tube to another because a drop of the serum may roll down the outside of the tube and contaminate all who handle it. Use always Pasteur pipettes for transferring the serum.
3. No raw blood material should be poured into the sink. It should be autoclaved before washing.
4. Hand washing with an antiseptic soap after handling blood specimens is a good habit to cultivate.

   The AIDS virus can spread through the use of syringes, needles and instruments, which have been in contact with the blood of a person who is carrying the AIDS virus. So, use disposable needles and sterilize the equipment before use. The virus is very fragile and dies at 60°C. Sterilization can be done either by boiling the equipment for 20 minutes or by steam or pressure-cooking, autoclaving or by soaking for 20 minutes.

Corrosive Chemicals

Strong acids and alkalis are the most common corrosive chemicals to which the clinical technologists are exposed. Most of the dangers occur through the splashing of reagents during their preparation.

1. Injury to the eyes is the greatest danger. In case of acid splashes on the eye, wash the eye immediately with large quantities of water or hold the eye under running tap water. After washing, put 4 drops of 2% aqueous sodium bicarbonate solution into the eye, and then contact the doctor.
2. In case of acid splashes on the skin, wash thoroughly and repeatedly with water then apply 5% aqueous sodium carbonate solution with cotton.
3. In case of accidental swallowing of acids while pipetting, contact doctor. Give 5% soap solution immediately to drink or give 2 whites of egg mixed with half liter of water or milk. If both are not available, give ordinary water to drink. Make the person to gargle with soap solution. If lips and tongue are exposed to acid accidentally, rinse then thoroughly with water and then with 2% aqueous sodium bicarbonate solution.
4. In case of alkali splashes on the eye, wash the eye immediately with large quantities of water or hold the eye under running tap water. After washing with water, wash the eye with a saturated solution of boric acid.
5. In case of alkali splashes on the skin, wash thoroughly and repeatedly with water then bath the affected skin with cotton soaked in 5% acetic acid.
6. In case of accidental swallowing of alkali while pipetting, make the person drink at once 5% acetic acid or lemon juice or diluted vinegar (1:4 dilution with water) solution immediately. Make the person to gargle with same acid solution. If lips and tongue are burned by alkali, rinse thoroughly with water and then with 5% acetic acid solution.

Toxic Fumes

In the clinical chemistry laboratory, it may be necessary to prepare extracts with solvents whose vapors are toxic. The chlorinated hydrocarbon chemicals cause a liver damage after a certain amount of exposure.

Other solvents may depress the bone marrow functions. The simple precautions to be taken are:

1. Always work in a fume hood with good ventilation whenever pouring or using organic solvents.
2. Avoid contamination of the skin with the solvents. If they fall on the skin wash off with soap and water.

Broken Glasswares

Beakers and flasks with broken lips are a hazard in the laboratory, particularly to the personnel who wash them. The best remedy is to remove those partially broken glasswares from circulation and destroy.

Burns Caused by Heat

If the victim is splashed with burning ether or other inflammable solvent, roll the victim in a blanket to smother the flame. Victim should be taken to the doctor immediately.

In the case of minor burns, plunge the affected parts into cold water or ice water to sooth the pain. Apply mercurochrome ointment to the burns.

Carcinogens

The danger of contracting cancer by exposure to carcinogenic chemicals in a clinical laboratory is low because most of the known carcinogens are not used there. Do not pipette carcinogenic chemicals through mouth wherever used.

BASICS OF LABORATORY TECHNIQUES

The accuracy of any of the chemical tests is the deciding factor in the usefulness of its implication in the clinical diagnosis and prognosis. Biochemical analysis demands great accuracy as the constituents in biological fluids are in minute quantities. This is attained only when one is well versed with the basic techniques, such as pipetting, weighing, reagent preparation and equipment management.

Methods of Measuring Liquids

The measuring glasswares most frequently used are:

1. Graduated cylinders
2. Volumetric flasks
3. Volumetric and graduated pipettes
4. Micropipettes
5. Ostwald's pipette
6. Microsyringes.

Glasswares are made up of complex silicates containing boron oxide. The dimensions of these glasswares change a bit with temperature (low coefficient of expansion). Boron free glasswares have high resistance to alkali but its thermal resistance is low.

Usually, high-density polyethylene and Teflon plasticwares are recommended for the use under highly acidic and alkaline medium. Since plasticwares are unbreakable and does not release ions as glass does, therefore wherever possible, plastic one should be used in place of glass. But disadvantages of plasticware are its tendency to bind various solutes and back surface bound constituents into subsequent solutions.

Graduated Cylinders

- Graduated cylinders are usually used for the preparation of reagents especially volume above 25 mL.
- Always the surface of the lower meniscus of the liquid is made to coincide with the graduated mark on the cylinder held in the eye level.
- Upper meniscus is considered for colored fluid.

Volumetric Flasks

Volumetric flasks are preferred for the preparation of standard solutions, when it is desired to transfer fixed volumes, such as 25 mL, 100 mL, 250 mL, 500 mL, etc. **(Fig. 1.2)**.

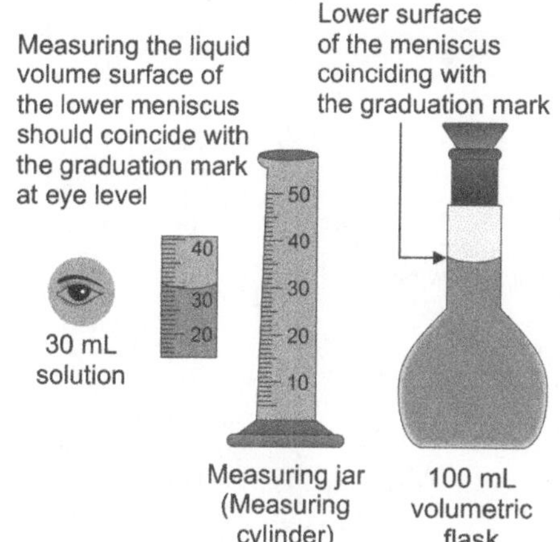

Fig. 1.2: Different volumetric flasks.

Pipettes

The use of pipette is very important in clinical analysis to get accurate results. Various types of pipettes used include (i) serological, (ii) volumetric and graduated pipettes, (iii) micropipettes, (iv) Ostwalds pipette, and (v) microsyringes.

Graduated Pipettes

Graduated pipettes are of two types: (i) completely graduated, and (ii) blow out pipette. For example in completely graduated 10 mL pipette will have markings from 0 to 10. Whereas in a 10 mL blow out pipette graduation is present between 0 to 9 or 9.5 mL. The last portion of the fluid in the pipette must also be delivered into the container **(Fig. 1.3)**.

For transferring opaque solution or blood sample, the upper meniscus of the liquid is considered. In the pipette, only the graduated portion must be used. For example, to pipette 0.5 mL blood, the upper 0.5 mL portion of the 1 mL pipette can be used.

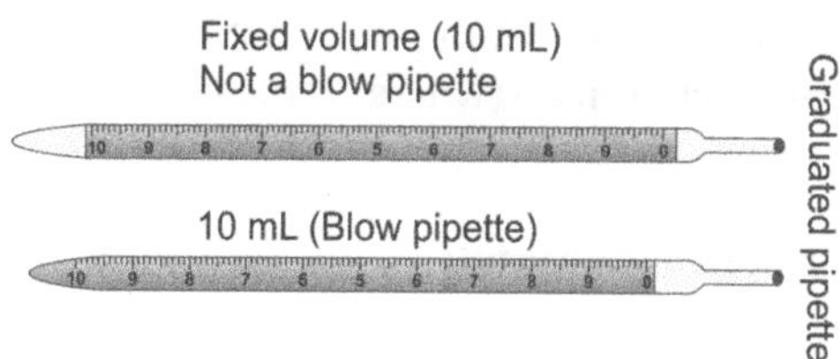

Fig. 1.3: Graduated pipettes..

Micropipettes

Micropipettes labeled 10λ, 25λ, 50λ, 100λ are used to transfer microquantity of samples. (1 λ = 1 μL = 0.001 mL).

Microsyringes

Microsyringes (Hamilton syringes) labeled 10 mL or 25 mL are used to transfer microquantities of sample very accurately **(Fig. 1.4)**.

When using a bulb pipette or volumetric pipette the portion of the fluid remaining in the tip or nozzle is not collected. In these instances, the fluid is allowed to drain by itself with the tip of the pipette touching the bottom or the wall of the container. The volume of volumetric pipette ranges between 2 mL–50 mL **(Fig. 1.4)**.

Ostwald Pipettes

Ostwald pipettes are used to deliver viscous fluids, such as blood, serum or plasma usually in fixed volume (less than 1 mL). In this case, the portion of fluid in the tip is delivered and collected.

In all types of pipetting two steps are to be considered: (i) delivery time, (ii) waiting time. **Delivery time** is the time when the liquid meniscus needs to pass from the calibration mark to stand still at the tip or at the second calibration mark.

Waiting time starts when the liquid meniscus in the tip or at the second calibration mark has come to stop. During the waiting time, "residual liquid" flows downwards from the glasswall. This causes a new rise of the meniscus. After the waiting time, the pipette tip is wiped on the wall of the vessel. A small amount of liquid remains at the narrow section of the tip. But this has been taken into account during calibration. Sufficient delivery time and waiting time must be allocated for the accurate pipetting of the solution.

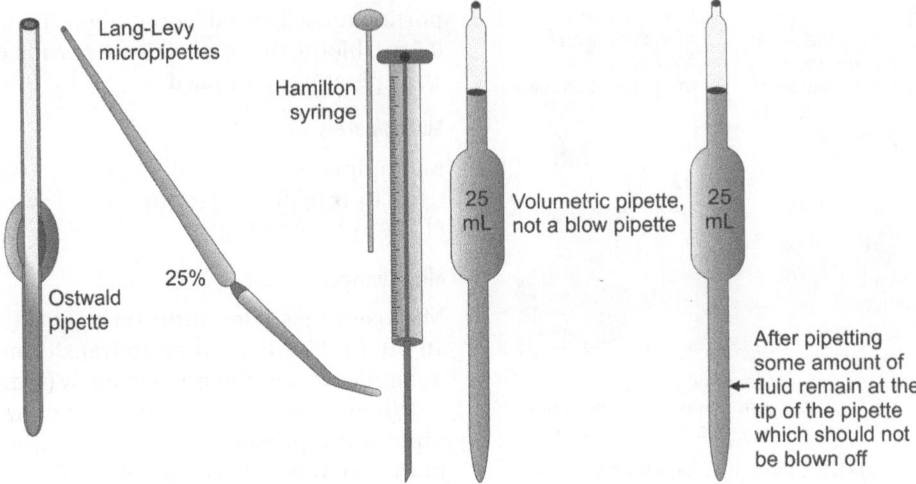

Fig. 1.4: Microsyringes and micropipettes.

Cleaning of Glasswares

Manual Cleaning of Glasswares

- Usually the glasswares are wiped with a cloth or sponge, each of which is impregnated with a cleaning solution.
- The glasswares shall never be treated with abrasive scouring agents, since this would damage the surface.
- In the dipping bath procedure, the laboratory glasses are placed into the cleansing solution at room temperature for 20–30 minutes then rinsed with tap water followed by distilled water.
- Subject the glassware to abrupt changes in temperature and pressure.

Method of Weighing

The ordinary scientific balance is used for weighing chemicals required for the preparation of reagents, which weigh more than 500 mg. The analytical balance is used for weighing standard chemicals, less than 500 mg. Analytical balance is more sensitive.

Points to note during the handling of physical balance:

1. Always handle weights with a pair of forceps.
2. Never add or remove anything off the pans unless the balance is at rest.
3. Do not give a jerky movement to the knob.
4. Do not weigh substances unless it comes to room temperature.
5. Before weighing see that the platform is horizontal as indicated by index.
6. The pointer should perform equal oscillations on either side of *'0' (ZERO) on the scale.* This indicates the pans of weighing machine are balanced.

Nowadays, the majority of the laboratories use digital balance. In that case, the users manual give brief instructions. But one thing should be borne in mind that during weighing of any chemicals the paper or beaker weight should also be considered. If the balance has "T" option (for nullifying the previous or paper weight) just press the button "T" after knowing the weight of paper or beaker which are used to place chemicals (where 'T' means tearing of weight).

Chemicals and Reagents

Chemicals are available in different grades of purity. A Laboratory reagent grade (LR) chemicals are less pure and used for ordinary laboratory reagent preparation. The analar or analytical reagent (AR) and guaranteed reagents (GR) are high purity chemicals. AR and GR grade chemicals are equally pure and used whenever specifically mentioned.

PREPARATION OF SOLUTION

The following types of solutions are prepared in the clinical laboratory:

a. Saturated solution
b. Percent solution
c. Molar solution
d. Molal solution
e. Normal solution
f. Known standard solution.

Saturated Solution

Solvent—it is the liquid in which solute goes into solution.

Solute—solid chemical to be dissolved in a solution.

The crystalline chemical when dissolved in a liquid, the chemical is referred as the solute and the liquid is called as the solvent. A saturated solution is prepared by continuously dissolving the solute in a solvent until a small amount of crystal is visible in the solution.

Ammonium sulfate crystal is added in a small portion to a fixed amount of water with constant stirring. The addition is continued till some crystals are left undissolved. The clear solution obtained is referred as saturated ammonium sulfate solution.

Percent Solution

Percent solution is prepared by dissolving one gram of substance in 100 mL of solvent. Percent solution is expressed as weight by volume (W/V, if a known weight of solute is dissolved in a solvent) or volume by volume (V/V, a known volume of solvent dissolved in another solvent). A percent solution (W/V) is prepared as follows, e.g., preparation of 0.9% sodium chloride solution.

In this case, 0.9 g sodium chloride is dissolved in 100 mL of its solution.

Method: Weigh exactly 0.9 g (900 mg) of sodium chloride and mix with 80 mL of water until it dissolves completely. Then transfer the contents to a 100 mL volumetric flask or a measuring cylinder with stopper. The volume is made up to 100 mL with distilled water. The cylinder is stoppered, and mixed properly. It is then transferred to a reagent bottle and labeled.

A percent solution volume/volume is prepared as follows, e.g., preparation of 2% HCl solution. Please note that stock HCl provided by the chemical company is of 35 to 38%.

$$V_1P_1 = V_2P_2$$

$$? \times 35 = 100 \times 2$$

$$= \frac{100 \times 2}{35} = \frac{200}{35}$$

= 5.71 mL concentrated HCl make up to 100 mL with water.

Method: Approximately 50 mL water is taken in a 100 mL volumetric flask. Concentrated HCl is drawn into the pipette with the help of the rubber bulb. Exactly 5.7 mL HCl is transferred to the flask containing water with constant mixing. Then water is added up to the mark. The flask is stoppered and the solution is mixed properly. It is then transferred to a reagent bottle and labeled.

Note: Always add acid to water with mixing. This is important because if water is added to acid, water spurts generating great quantity of heat causing the acid to splash out. The concentrated sulfuric acid is diluted under cold (in ice chest containing ice cubes). Addition of acid is done in small amounts with constant stirring.

Molar Solution

A molar solution is one in which one gram molecular weight of the substance is dissolved in one liter of its solution. If 1 g molecular weight of the substance is dissolved in one liter of solution it is denoted as '1 M' solution.

Molecular weight of a substance is obtained by adding the atomic weight of the elements in the proportion contained in the compound, e.g., NaCl

Atomic weight of Na = 23
Atomic weight of Cl = 35.5
Molecular weight of NaCl = **58.5**

H_2SO_4

Atomic weight of H = 1
Atomic weight of S = 32
Atomic weight of O = 16
Molecular weight of H_2SO_4 =
$1 \times 2 + 32 \times 1 + 16 \times 4 = 2 + 32 + 64 = \mathbf{98}$

NaOH

Atomic weight of Na = 23
Atomic weight of O = 16
Atomic weight of H = 1
Molecular weight of NaOH = **40.**

If the molecule of a compound is hydrated, the weight of water is also considered.

For example, COOH-COOH.2 H_2O, i.e., $C_2H_2O_4 \cdot 2H_2O$.

Molecular weight =
$12 \times 2 + 1 \times 2 + 16 \times 4 + 2(1 \times 2 + 16)$
$= 24 + 2 + 64 + 36 = \mathbf{126}.$

Molecular weight of oxalic acid = 126.

During the preparation of molar solution, the weight to be taken is calculated according to the following method using the formula

$M \times S \times V$

where

M = Molecular weight
S = Strength of required solution, (e.g., 0.1 M, 0.2 M, etc.)
V = Volume in liters.

To prepare 100 mL of 1 M sodium chloride solution.

Weight = $M \times S \times V$
$= 58.5 \times 1 \times 1/10 = 5.85$ g

Method: Weigh accurately 5.85 g of sodium chloride crystals. Transfer the weighed crystals carefully and completely into a 100 mL standard flask through a funnel using distilled water. Dissolve the crystals completely. Add water up to 3/4th, mix. Then add water up to the mark. Stopper the flask, and mix well. Transfer the solution to a clean reagent bottle, Label it as 1 M sodium chloride with date and initials.

Exercise: Prepare 100 mL of 0.2 M sodium carbonate solution. In all the cases, the molecular weight written on the chemical bottle should be considered.

Using the above stock, 0.1 M and 0.02 M solutions can be prepared as follows:

The 0.2 M solution is diluted 1:1 with water or 1 in 2 with water. The 1:1 dilution is expressed as 1 in 2 dilutions, i.e., 50 mL of 0.2 M solution to 100 mL in a 100 mL volumetric flask with deionized water.

For 0.02 M solution, dilute the stock 1 in 10 with distilled water, i.e., 10 mL of 0.2 M solution is diluted to 100 mL in a 100 mL volumetric flask.

To find out the molarity of the liquids the following formula can be used

$$\frac{\% \text{ of purity} \times \text{specific gravity} \times 10}{\text{Molecular weight}}$$

For example

% of purity for H_2SO_4 = 98
Specific gravity = 1.84
Molecular weight = 98.08

$$\frac{98 \times 1.84 \times 10}{98.08} = 18.38 \text{ M}$$

The molarity of the supplied concentrate H_2SO_4 = 18.38

Molal Solution

A molal solution is one which is prepared by dissolving one gram-molecular weight of a substance in one thousand grams of its solvent. For example, 40.0 g sodium hydroxide is dissolved in 1000 g of water to get 1 molal solution of sodium hydroxide solution. This type of solution is rarely used.

Normal Solutions

One gram equivalent weight of a substance dissolved in one liter of its solution is called 1 normal solution. It is denoted as N, e.g., if the equivalent weight of a substance is 40 then 40 g is the gram equivalent weight. When 40 g of that is dissolved in 400 mL of water and then made up the volume to 1 liter it is 1 N solution. Likewise 80 g of that substance in 1 L is 2 N, 20 g of it in 1 L is 0.5 N and 4 g of it in 1 L 0.1 N solutions.

To prepare a normal solution equivalent weight is calculated as follows:

Equivalent weight of an acid: Acid is one which has ionizable or replaceable hydrogen ions (H). If an acid has one replaceable H^+ it is called a monobasic acid, if 2—it is called a dibasic acid, and 3—it is a tribasic acid. A monobasic acid forms one type of salt, dibasic two types and tribasic acid forms three types of salts on treating with base, e.g., HCl forms only NaCl. So it is monobasic acid.

H_2SO_4 forms $NaHSO_4$ and Na_2SO_4 and so it is dibasic.

Equivalent weight of an acid

$$= \frac{\text{Molecular weight}}{\text{No. of replaceable } H^+}$$

For example, equivalent weight of HCl = 36.5.

For monobasic acids molecular weight = equivalent weight.

Hence 1 M solution = 1 N solution

But, equivalent weight of H_2SO_4

$$= \frac{\text{Molecular weight}}{2}$$

= 98 /2 = 49.

That is 1 M H_2SO_4 = 2 N

Likewise equivalent weight of H_3PO_4

$$= \frac{\text{Molecular weight}}{3}$$

That is 1 M H_3PO_4 = 3 N H_3PO_4

To find out the weight to be taken for a known volume of V liters of acid of strength 'N' of equivalent weight 'E.'

Weight for V liters of N Normal = E × N × V.

The equivalent weight of a base is taken by molecular weight of the particular base divided by the number of replaceable hydroxyl ions. For example, NaOH has one replaceable OH ion and hence, equivalent weight of

NaOH = molecular weight/1= 40/1

Calcium hydroxide $Ca(OH)_2$ has 2 replaceable hydroxyl ions and its equivalent weight

$$\frac{\text{Molecular weight}}{2} = \frac{74}{2} = 37.$$

The, equivalent weight of salts, such as $AgNO_3$ and $KMNO_4$ and $K_2Cr_2O_7$ are determined by the number of electrons which they give or take during a reaction, e.g., $AgNO_3$ gives out 1 electron. Therefore, equivalent weight of $AgNO_3$ is molecular weight divided by 1.

Approximate normality of the liquids can be calculated using the following formula:

$$\frac{\text{\% of purity of the liquid} \times \text{specific gravity} \times 10}{\text{Equivalent weight}}$$

For example, % of purity for HCl = 37
specific gravity = 1.18 kg
equivalent weight = 36.4

$$\frac{37 \times 1.18 \times 10}{} = 11.9 \text{ N}$$
= 36.4

The above example shows that the normality of the concentrated HCl is 11.9.

To get 1 N HCl, 10 mL of concentrated HCl made up to 100 mL with deionized water.

or

12 mL concentrated HCl + 108 mL water gives 1 N.

Equivalent weight of some common chemicals

Compound	Equivalent weight	% w/w
Acetic acid, glacial	60.05	100
Hydrochloric acid	36.461	37
Sulfuric acid	49.039	96
Oxalic acid		63.033
Sodium hydroxide	40.000	
Sodium carbonate	53.000	6
Nitric acid	63.03	70

Note: Molecular weight of the chemicals will be given on reagent bottles.

Preparation of Normal Solution

Exact normal solutions can be prepared only when a chemical is available in its pure state. Moreover, correct weighing is possible if chemical does not absorb or lose water on exposure.

On the other hand, liquids like acids are not pure as supplied commercially and so an exact solution is possible to prepare only after titration and by dilution.

Sodium carbonate and oxalic acid are available in the pure form and it is easy to prepare exact normal solution by weight. These are called primary standards. Sodium hydroxide when exposed it absorbs water and liquefies. Sodium carbonate can be used as a primary base whereas oxalic is a primary acid. For standardization of other normal solutions these acids or bases can be used.

Preparation of primary standard sodium carbonate solution, e.g., to prepare 100 mL 0.1 N sodium carbonate solution.

Molecular weight of sodium carbonate = 106

Equivalent weight of sodium carbonate $= \frac{106}{2}$

$$g/L = E \times N \times V$$

$$\frac{0.1 \times 53 \times 100}{1000} = 0.53\ g$$

Therefore, 0.53 g of sodium carbonate in 100 mL gives 0.1 N solution.

Method: Transfer 530 mg of sodium carbonate crystals into a clean 100 mL standard flask. Use a clean funnel. Mix properly to dissolve the chemical. Add distilled water up to the mark. Stopper the flask mix again. Transfer to a clean reagent bottle and label as 0.1 N sodium carbonate solution.

Exercise: Prepare 100 mL decinormal (0.1 N) oxalic acid solution.

Mol wt of oxalic acid,

COOH-COOH $2H_2O$ = 126.067

Equivalent weight of oxalic acid $= \frac{126.067}{2}$

$= 63.033$

$= ESV/1000$

$= 63.033 \times 0.1 \times 100/1000$

$= 0.6303$

Accurately 0.6303 g oxalic acid crystals are weighed and prepared 100 mL solution as done in the previous experiment and filled in a clean reagent bottle and labeled.

Standard Solutions

Standard solutions refer to the known weight of chemical substance in a solution in which its concentration is expressed in terms of normality or moles or in weights per unit volume. The standard solutions are mainly useful in the biochemical assays.

Uses

1. Preparation of standard calibration graph. Glucose standard solution is used in the estimation of glucose in blood, and urine.
2. A standard (single or in duplicate) can also be used to estimate the unknown concentration by comparing the absorbance of standard and test solutions which is measured by using colorimeter.

   $$\frac{T - B}{S - B} \times \text{Concentration of Std.}$$

   Where S, T and B are the absorbance of standard, test and blank solutions respectively.
3. *Preparation of buffers:* Standard buffer components like acid and its conjugate base are prepared as standard solutions and mixed in different proportion to get different pH.
4. Standard solutions of glucose, urea, creatinine, albumin, total protein, etc., obtained from distributors, are used to calibrate the autoanalyzer.

ACIDS AND BASES

Acids liberate hydrogen ions (H^+) in solution. According to Bronsted theory, acids are proton donors and bases are proton acceptors. Acids change blue litmus paper to red and bases change red litmus to blue.

Strong and Weak Acids

Strong acids dissociate completely (complete ionization) in solution whereas weak acids dissociate partially.

Ionization is the phenomenon of splitting up of molecules into charged particles in solution, e.g., HCl ionizes as H^+ and Cl^-. This is reversible and written as

$$HCl \leftrightarrow H^+ + Cl^-$$

Mineral acids, such as HCl, HNO_3 and H_2SO_4 ionize in solution to 90 to 95% so they are called as strong acids. Whereas organic acids, such as acetic acid and oxalic acid ionize to a less extent.

The same classification holds well with bases also. Sodium hydroxide is a strong base whereas disodium hydrogen phosphate (Na_2HPO_4) is a weak base.

CHEMICAL INDICATORS

There are certain chemicals which are used as indicators in acid-base titration. These chemicals may be weak organic acids or bases or dye stuffs which change color as the hydrogen ion concentrations in solution increase or decrease. The reason for change of color is reversible ionization of these indicator molecules. The ionized particles will have one color and the unionized molecule of it have an entirely different color. Ionization of different indicators takes place at different pH ranges, e.g., phenolphthalein is a colorless molecule; when it ionizes, it is pink. This takes place between a pH of 8.3–10.00. So below pH 8.3, it is colorless. Beyond 8.3 and up to 10 ionization goes on and different shades of pink color are obtained.

Beyond pH 10 no change in pink color is observed. Therefore, the pH 8.3–10.00 is called the effective pH range of phenolphthalein.

pH and pH Scale

Defined as the negative log of hydrogen ion concentration.

The pH scale ranges from 0–14. pH 7.0 is considered as neutral, pH, below 7 is acidic and above 7 is alkaline.

Measurement of pH of Solution

Using the indicator papers, which are available in various pH ranges, the approximate pH of unknown solutions can be determined. For checking the pH of unknown solution a piece of indicator paper is immersed in it and the color change is compared with those given on the book of indicator paper.

List of indicators, their characteristics and preparation

Name	pH range	Color change	Preparation
Thymol blue	1.2 to 2.8	Red-yellow	0.1 g in 4.3 mL of 0.05 N NaOH diluted to 250 mL with water
Topfer's reagent			
(p-Dimethyl-aminobenzene)	2.9 to 4.2	Red-yellow	0.5 g in 100 mL 95% alcohol
Methyl orange	3.0 to 4.4	Red-yellow	0.1 g in 100 mL water
Bromocresol green	3.8 to 5.4	Yellow-green	0.1 g, in 2.9 mL 0.05 N, NaOH diluted to 250 mL with water
Phenolphthalein	8.3 to 10.0	Colorless pink	0.1 g to 1% in 50% alcohol

The accurate pH of the prepared buffer or solution can be measured by using a pH meter. A pH meter consists of a glass electrode. The electrode is always kept immersed in water. The pH is displayed on the board when the electrode is immersed in a buffer and the pH mode button is pressed. The instrument is standardized with the standard buffer of pH nearer to that of unknown. For example, if prepared solution has pH around 4, the instrument is calibrated with the standard buffer of pH 4.0 or any buffer of nearer pH 4.0. If another is around 8, then the instrument is calibrated with standard buffer of pH 9.2 or any other standard buffer of near pH 8.

Procedure: Say, the pH of test solution is around needs modification 7. Put on the switch and wait for 5 minutes. Electrode is taken out from water by moving up the electrode, wash of the electrode with a jet of water. Dip the electrode into the standard buffer of pH 7 taken in a beaker. Press the button 'standardize' and then set it to '7' using the knob. Take out the electrode from the solution. Wash the electrode with a jet of water. Take test solution in a beaker. Dip the electrode into the test solution and press the button to read the pH. Remove the electrode from test solution. Wash the electrode with a jet of water. Keep it dipped in water.

Note:

- Handle the electrode carefully which is made of glass.
- Electrode is always dipped in water when not in use.

TITRATIONS

Principle: A given strength of acid solution completely neutralizes same strength of a base solution in equal volumes. Thus neutralizing ability of acids and bases enable to determine exact normality or molarity of an unknown strength of solutions.

For example, strength of 1 mL HCl solution is equal to 1 N if it is completely neutralized by 1 mL of 1 N NaOH.

Steps in Titration

1. Preparation of primary base
2. Titration
3. Calculation.

Preparation of Primary Base

The 0.53 g of sodium carbonate crystals are dissolved in water and the volume is made up to 100 mL mark in a volumetric flask, mixed and labeled it as 0.1 N Na_2CO_3.

Titration

A burette is first rinsed with standard sodium carbonate solution. Then it is filled to zero mark after the removal of air bubbles at the tip of the burette. Note the initial burette reading *(a-mL)*. Exactly pipette 10 mL of the diluted HCl into a clean dry conical flask. A few drops of methyl orange indicator is added and mixed because the HCl is a strong acid. Now standard base 0.1 N Na_2CO_3 is added from the burette carefully. The flask is kept rotating during the addition. Note the color change. When the color change is fast, drop by drop. The appearance of pale orange color denotes the completion of reaction. It is the end point or neutra on word lization point of titration. Note the burette reading *(b-mL)*.

Titration is repeated till a concordant value is obtained.

Calculation

The values are tabulated as follows: Burette reading			
Trial no.	*Initial reading (a-mL)*	*Final burette (b-mL)*	*Volume of base added (b-a mL)*
1	0	20.1	20.1
2	20	40.0	20.0
3	0	20.0	20.0

Concordant value = 20 mL

Now, $V_1 N_1 = V_2 N_2$

where V_1 = Volume of acid used = 10 mL

N_1 = Normality of acid = ?

V_2 = Volume of base titrated = 20 mL

N_2 = Normality of base = 0.1N

Therefore

$10 \times N_1 = 20 \times 0.1$

$N_1 = 20 \times 0.1 / 10 = 0.2$

Normality of HCl = 0.2

Approximate normality, molarity and percentage strength of commonly using acids:

Acid	Approximately molar	Approximately normal	% w/w
Concentrated HCl	12	12	37
Concentrated H_2SO_4	18	36	96
Glacial acetic acid (CH_3COOH)	17	17	100

Preparation of 100 mL 0.1 N HCl Solution

The approximate normality of concentrated HCl is taken as 11

- A slightly greater than 0.1 N HCl solution is prepared
- Sodium carbonate of 0.1 N solution is prepared
- Titration
- Calculation
- Dilution of the HCl to get exactly 0.1 N HCl.

Preparation of slightly greater than 0.1 N HCl solution: Transfer 1.5 mL of concentrated HCl to a 100 mL standard flask containing 70 mL of distilled water and make up to the mark. Mix properly and label it as 0.1 N HCl solution.

Preparation of a base: Transfer 0.530 g of sodium carbonate crystals to a 100 mL flask through funnel with a jet of water. Dissolve the crystals completely. Make up to 100 mL mark with water. Stopper, mix well and label it as 0.1 N Na_2CO_3 solution.

Titration: Take a clean burette and fill the burette with 0.1 N sodium carbonate solution exactly to zero mark. Note the initial burette reading (*a-mL*). Transfer accurately 20 mL of the HCl into a clean conical flask. Add 3–4 drops of methyl orange indicator. Start the addition of base from burette into the flask carefully till the red color changes to pale orange color. Note the final burette reading (*b-mL*).

Repeat the experiment for concordant values.

Calculations

	Burette reading			
Trial no.	*Initial burette reading (a-mL)*	*Final burette (b-mL)*	*Volume of base added (a-b) mL*	*Volume of acid taken*
1	0	25.2	25.2	20
2	25.2	50.2	25	20
3	0	25	25	20

$$V_1 N_1 = V_2 N_2$$

$$20 \times N_1 = 25 \times 0.1$$

$$N_1 = \frac{25 \times 0.1}{20}$$

Normality of HCl = 0.125.

Dilution: Use the formula $V_1 N_1 = V_2 N_2$ to dilute 0.125 N HCl to get exact 0.1 N:

where, V_1 = Volume of acid

N_1 = Required normality of acid (0.1N)

V_2 = Volume to be taken for dilution

N_2 = Known normality of acid (0.125)

$$100 \times 0.1 = V_2 \times 0.125$$

$$V_2 = 100 \times 0.1/0.125$$

$$= 80 \text{ mL.}$$

Exactly 80 mL of the HCl is diluted to 100 mL, and label as 0.1 N HCl.

Exercise: Prepare 100 mL of 0.1 N sulfuric acid. Using this, prepare 100 mL each of 0.01 N and 0.05 N solution.

Preparation of 1 N Sodium Hydroxide

The NaOH absorbs moisture and liquefies therefore, an exact weight is impossible to make. Therefore, we prepare 1 N sodium hydroxide solution as follows:

1 N sodium hydroxide is prepared through following steps:

Step 1: Preparation of slightly greater than 1 N NaOH.

Step 2: Preparation of primary standard oxalic acid, 1 N.

Step 3: Determination of exact normality

Step 4: Dilute to 1 N.

Preparation of slightly greater than 1 N NaOH: As sodium hydroxide is a corrosive, handle it carefully. Take care when pipetting NaOH.

The equivalent weight of NaOH is 40. If 100 mL water contains 4.0 g of NaOH it makes 1N. However, since we want a solution slightly greater than 1 N we should use about 5 g for 100 mL.

Preparation of 1 N oxalic acid solution: The equivalent weight of oxalic acid, analytical grade, is 63.033. To make 1 N solution of 100 mL, weigh 6.30 g exactly and prepare 100 mL solution. Label it as 1 N oxalic acid.

Determination of exact normality of sodium hydroxide: The following steps are necessary to determine the exact normality of slightly greater than 1 N NaOH.

Titration: Use 1 N oxalic acid as a primary standard. Using a 10 mL pipet, place exactly 10 mL of 1 N oxalic acid in 100 mL flask. Add few drops of phenolphthalein indicator. Fill the burette with NaOH, gently rotate the flask and add the NaOH drop by drop until the solution becomes faint pink. This is the end point. Repeat the titration. Tabulate your values.

Calculation

Volume of oxalic acid used = 10 mL (V_1)
Normality of oxalic acid = 1 N (N_1)
Vol of sodium hydroxide used = V_2 mL (9.0 mL)
Normality of NaOH = (N_2)?

$V_1 N_1 = V_2 N_2$
$10 \times 1 = 9 \times N_2$
$N_2 = 10 \times 1 / 9 = 1.1$

Dilution

$V_1 N_1 = V_2 N_2$
$100 \times 1 = V_2 \times 1.1$
$V_2 = 100 \times 1/1.1$
$V_2 = 90.90$

Dilute 90.9 mL of above NaOH to 100 mL to get exact 1 N NaOH.

BUFFERS

Buffer solutions are needed in some of the experiments which have to be carried out at a particular pH. This is possible because buffer solution resists the changes in pH upon addition of small portion of acid or alkali.

A buffer system consists of two chemicals in solution one of which is weak acid and the other Na or K salt of the same acid, e.g., acetate buffer is prepared by mixing sodium acetate and acetic acid. Buffer solutions are used in various enzymatic and other reactions. There are variety of buffer mixtures, such as phosphate buffer, citrate buffer, carbonate-bicarbonate buffer, etc.

A buffer solution is labeled with the strength and the pH it maintains, such as 0.2 M phosphate buffer, pH 7.8.

Phosphate Buffer

Solution a: 0.2 M KH_2PO_4 or 0.2 M NaH_2PO_4.
Solution b: 0.2 M Na_2HPO_4.

Mix solution 'a' and solution 'b' to get the required pH as shown in the example and adjust the pH with adding acid or base. If the mixed solution shows pH more than the required pH, use acid to decrease the pH, if it is less than the required one, then base is used to increase the pH.

Example 1: Preparation of 0.2 M phosphate buffer of pH 7.0 and 7.4.

Mix solution *a* of 61 mL and *b* of 30 mL and adjust the pH by adding solution *b* to get 0.2 M buffer, pH 7.0.

Example 2: Mix 80 mL 0.2 M monosodium dihydrogen phosphate and 20 mL of disodium hydrogen phosphate and check the pH if it is not 7.4 then adjust with acid or base prepared.

Volume of a and b to take to get a required pH		
pH	*mL of a*	*mL of b*
6.9	44.6	55.4
7.0	38.8	61.2
7.2	28.0	72.0
7.4	19.0	81.0
7.6	13.0	87.0

Acetate Buffer

pK 4.76

Solution a: 0.2 M acetic acid

Solution b: 0.2 M sodium acetate.

Mix solution 'a' with solution 'b' in the volume given below.

Example 1: Preparation of 0.2 M acetate buffer of pH 4.0.

Mix 80 mL of 0.2 M acetic acid and 20 mL of sodium acetate and check the pH. If the pH is less than 4.0 add some more sodium acetate dropwise until pH 4.0 comes. If it is more than the required pH then add 0.2 M acetic acid to adjust the pH to 4.0.

Example 2: Preparation of 0.2 M acetate buffer of pH 5.0.

Mix 30 mL of 0.2 M acetic acid and 70 mL 0.2 M sodium acetate and check the pH.

pH	*a (mL)*	*b (mL)*
4.2	74.0	26.0
4.4	61.0	39.0
4.6	51.0	49.0
4.8	40.0	60.0
5.0	30	70

Tris-HCl Buffer

Solution a: Tris 0.2 M (hydroxymethyl) aminomethane is prepared.

Solution b: 0.2 M HCl.

Take 0.2 M Tris in a beaker and adjust the pH with 0.2 M HCl.

Example 1: Preparation of 0.2 M Tris-HCl buffer, pH 7.6.

Take 100 mL of Tris and adjust the pH to 7.6 with 0.2 M HCl.

Example 2: Preparation of 0.2 M Tris-HCl buffer, pH 8.0.

Take 90 mL of Tris in a beaker and adjust the pH to 8.0 with 0.2 M HCl.

Note: If the volume of the buffer required is more then proportionately take more acid and base solution before adjusting the pH.

SELF TEST

1. Prepare 100 mL of saturated solution of ammonium sulfate.
2. How do you prepare 0.9% saline?
3. Define the terms acids and bases.
4. Explain the following:
   a. pH
   b. Normality
   c. Molarity
   d. Buffer
   e. Indicators
5. Explain the procedure for the preparation of 10% H_2SO_4.
6. Prepare 100 mL of 1 molar sodium carbonate (molecular weight is 106).
7. Prepare 100 mL of 0.2 and 0.1 molar solution of NaOH using 1 normal NaOH.
8. Briefly discuss the precautions to be taken when working in biochemistry laboratory.
9. Mention the step followed when acid splashes on the eye.
10. How do you explain blow and non-blowing pipettes?

MULTIPLE CHOICE QUESTIONS

1. **In case of alkali splashes on the skin after washing with water the bathing of the affected area is done by:**
   a. 1% acid
   b. 5% alkali
   c. 10% NaOH
   d. 5% NaOH
2. **For transferring opaque solution or blood _______ meniscus of the liquid is considered.**
   a. Upper
   b. Lower
   c. Middle
   d. Near.
3. **In case acid splashes on the eye the solution used after washing with water is _______.**
   a. 2% aqueous sodium hydroxide
   b. 2% aqueous sodium bicarbonate
   c. 3% acid
   d. None of the above
4. **If 1 g molecular weight of a substance dissolved in a liter of a solution it is denoted as:**
   a. 1 N solution
   b. 0.1 M solution
   c. 1 M solution
   d. 0.1 M solution

2

UNIT

Specimen Collection and Handling

LEARNING OBJECTIVES

At the end of this unit, the learner should be able to understand:
- How to collect the blood samples from various sites?
- The tubes used to collect the blood samples.
- The anticoagulants and its uses.
- Collection and preservation of urine samples.
- Collection of cerebrospinal fluid samples.

INTRODUCTION

Blood is the most frequent body fluid used for analytical purposes. There are three general procedures available for obtaining blood. They are:

1. Venipuncture
2. Arterial puncture
3. Skin puncture.

- The technique used to obtain the blood specimen is critical in order to maintain its integrity. Even so, arterial and venous blood differs in some important aspects.
- Blood oxygenated by the lungs is pumped from the heart to all organs and tissues to meet metabolic needs.
- Arterial blood is essentially uniform in composition throughout the body.
- The composition of venous blood varies and is dependent on metabolic activity of the perfused organ or tissues.
- Site of collection can affect the venous composition.
- Venous blood is oxygen deficient relative to arterial blood but also differs in pH, carbon dioxide concentration, and packed cell volume.
- Glucose, lactic acid, chloride, and ammonia concentration also may vary.
- Blood obtained by skin puncture (sometimes incorrectly called capillary blood) is a mixture of blood from arterioles, venules, and capillaries.
- Increased pressure in the arterioles yields a specimen enriched in arterial blood.
- Skin puncture blood also contains interstitial and intracellular fluids.
- The finger prick method is less accurate for test of cell number because of dilution of blood with tissue fluid and activation of platelets, etc.
- Blood will clot within few minutes after it is removed from the body unless an 'anticoagulant' (a chemical) is used which stops the process of clotting.
- Anticoagulant blood is also known as 'whole blood.'
- For hematological studies, unclotted whole blood is needed. Plasma (fluid portion

of unclotted blood) is obtained from the anticoagulated blood.

- Plasma is needed in coagulation studies.
- Serum (fluid portion of clotted blood) is obtained from clotted blood, which is collected without any anticoagulant.
- Blood is collected for various aspects of laboratory works, example:
  - Anticoagulated blood for hematology and biochemistry.
  - Serum for biochemistry, serology and blood bank.
  - Whole blood for biochemistry, hematology and microbiology.

BLOOD COLLECTION BY VENIPUNCTURE

- The volume of blood obtained by venipuncture is sufficient to carry out multiple tests.
- Venipuncture can be done either by the syringe method or by the vacuum tube method (using vacutainer).
- Sterilized sharp needles of bore size 18 to 20 gauges (medium 1.2 to 0.9 mm) for adults and 23 gauges (0.5 mm) for children are needed.
- The bevel length should be medium (20 mm) for adults and short (15 mm) for children.
- The use of disposable needles is recommended.

Syringe

- Syringes of different capacities 2 mL, 5 mL, 10 mL and 20 mL are available.
- The selection of the syringe to be used depends on the amount of blood needed.
- All glass syringes should be properly sterilized and perfectly dried.
- The tourniquet, which is a soft rubber tubing of 2 to 5 mm bore, and 30 to 40 cm length.
- A flat elastic rubber strip can also be used.
- The tourniquet is applied to the arm to slow the blood flow and make the veins more prominent. This helps to select the puncture site for blood drawing.
- Disinfectant must be applied on the skin before the puncture is made.
- Methylated spirit or 70% alcohol is put in a swab, which is rubbed on the skin prior to venipuncture.
- Most biochemical and serological tests are done on serum, which is separated from whole blood collected in a clean, dry, sterile test tube and allowed to clot. After sometime, the clot retracts and the serum separates, and can then be removed with the aid of a sterile Pasteur pipette. Centrifugation will hasten the process of separation of the serum.

Procedure

1. Arrange all the things required during blood collection **(Fig. 2.1)**.
2. See carefully the patient's form, and decide the total amount of blood needed for all the tests. For example, if a hemogram is requested, 2 mL of blood in EDTA will be sufficient, whereas if liver function tests and renal function tests are to be done, 10 mL of blood in a plain test tube are required. For lipid profile, the blood should be taken in the fasting state.
3. Select the blood collection containers and label them with the patient's identification (name and hospital number).
4. Ask the patient to sit alongside the table used for taking blood. Lay his arm on the table, palm upwards. For indoor patients lying in bed, lay the patient's arm in an out stretched position. Talk freely with the patient to make him comfortable. Never draw blood from a standing patient or patient sitting on a high stool. The venipuncturist should be prepared for the occasional patient who may faint and

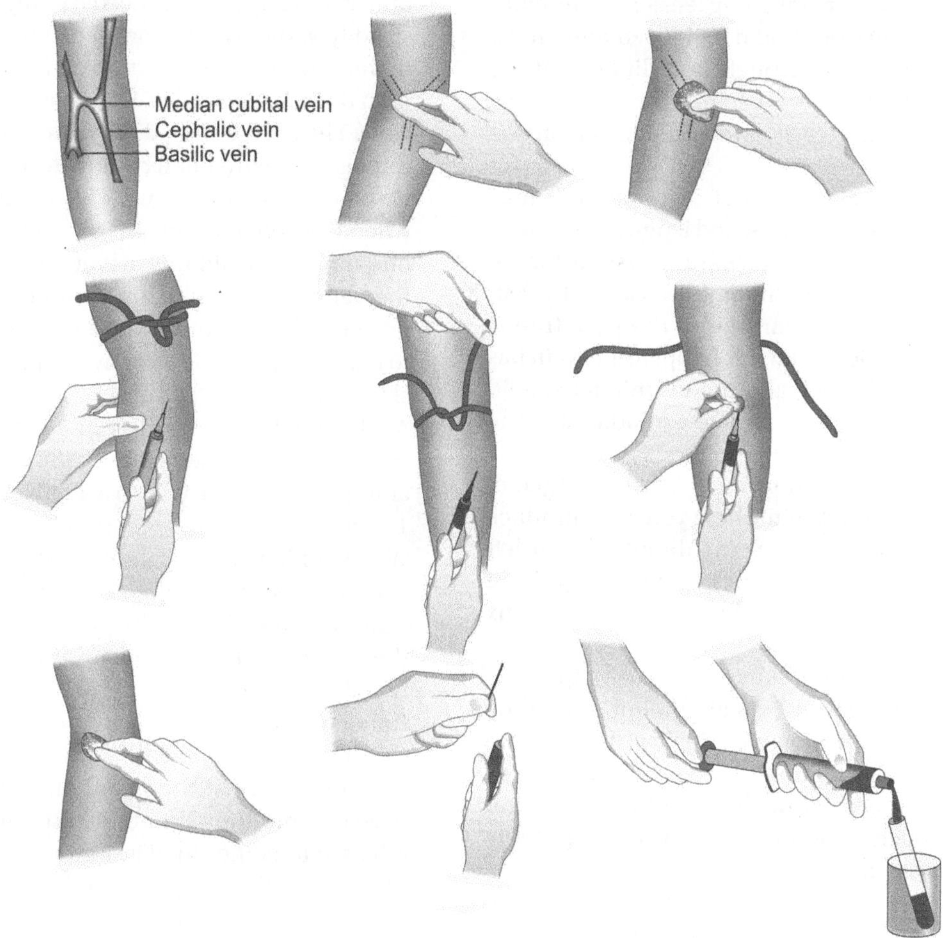

Fig. 2.1: Blood collection by venipuncture.

should be trained to administer first aid techniques if this occurs.

5. Select the puncture site carefully after inspecting both arms. If necessary, apply the tourniquet to select the puncture site and then release the tourniquet to proceed with the next step. Median cubital vein of the forearm is most frequently used for venipuncture. Ask the patient to clench the fist; this brings the vein into prominence by swelling. If necessary, other veins can also be used as alternatives. The cephalic vein is easy to locate, easily palpable and fairly well fixed in place.
6. The following are steps in the application of a tourniquet:
   - Place the tourniquet under the patient's arm just above the bend in the elbow.
   - Grasping the ends of the tourniquet, pull them up so that tension is applied to the tourniquet.
   - With the proper tension, tie a loop in the tourniquet in such a way that it can be easily released when the tourniquet is to be removed.

- While maintaining tension on the ends, one side should be looped and pulled halfway through in a slipknot. If the tourniquet is tied in this manner, it will release easily with a gentle pull on one end.
- If the tourniquet is too tight, it may cause cyanosis, and it pinches the skin, causing unnecessary discomfort to the patient. It may also cause the vein to disappear before the puncture is made. When this happens the vein has collapsed, and the tourniquet should be released for a few minutes and the procedure repeated.

7. Using the index finger of your left hand, feel for the vein where you will introduce the needle. Place the thumb of your left hand over the vein just below the point of entrance and apply a light traction to fix the vein.
8. Disinfect the skin with a swab dipped in methanol or 70% alcohol or 1% iodine saturated swab stick. Begin at the puncture site, and clean outward in a circular motion. Allow the area to dry. Do not touch the swabbed area with any unsterile object.
9. Remove the syringe from the protective wrap or test tube used during sterilization and the needle from the sterilizing vial, assemble them and see that the needle is fixed tightly. Do not touch the tip of the needle or wall of the piston. Check to make sure that the needle is not blocked and there is no air left in the syringe.
10. With patient's cooperation, grasp the elbow with your left hand and hold the arm fully extended. Identify the vein and anchor it with your thumb, drawing the skintight over the vein to prevent the vein from moving. Ask the patient to open and close the fist.
11. Take the syringe in the right hand holding your index finger against the base of the needle. Position the needle with bevel uppermost and push the needle firmly and steadily, without hesitation, into the center of the vein. Try to enter the skin first and then the vein, at a 30° to 40° angle.
    Note: The needle should not pass straight through the vein (counter puncture) or else it will cause a hematoma. This happens when the skin and vein are penetrated at one time. To avoid this, never approach the vein from the side or introduce the needle with the bevel downwards. It is best to make the penetration in two steps—the skin first and then the vein.
12. As the needle enters, the vein there is a sudden loss of resistance. Push the needle along the line of the vein to a depth of 1 to 1.5 cm.
13. With your left hand, slightly pull back the piston. Blood should appear in the barrel. Continue to withdraw the piston and fill the syringe with the requisite amount of blood.
14. Release the tourniquet by pulling on the looped end. Ideally, this should be released once the needle has been inserted into the skin but it can also be released after the blood is drawn.
15. Place a swab of cotton wool over the hidden point of the needle. Withdraw the needle in one rapid movement from under the swab.
    Note: Always remove the tourniquet before taking the needle out of the vein to prevent the formation of hematomata.
16. Ask the patient to press firmly on the cotton wool swab for 3 to 5 minutes. This stops the bleeding from the wound. Do not bend the arm, this may cause a hematomata.
17. Remove the needle from the syringe and gently expel the blood into appropriate pre-labeled container. Avoid foaming or rupture of the cells by using gentle pressure on the plunger of the syringe. Stopper the container and swirl it gently

to mix anticoagulant with the blood, if anticoagulant is used.

Note: If several tubes are to be filled from the amount of blood drawn, the following sequence is recommended:

a. Blood culture tube
b. Plain tube for serum (biochemical analysis)
c. Tube with anticoagulant for plasma and whole blood
d. Other additives.

18. Before the patient leaves, reinspect the venipuncture site to ascertain that the bleeding has stopped. If the bleeding has stopped, apply an adhesive tape over the cotton wool swab on the wound; otherwise continue to apply pressure until the bleeding stops. Check condition of the patient, e.g., whether patient is faint and that bleeding is under control.
19. Initial labels and record the time specimens were drawn. Deliver tubes (with blood) for testing to appropriate laboratory section or central receiving and processing area.
    - If blood must be drawn from a patient who has intravenous equipment attached to one arm, the blood sample should be drawn from a vein in the other arm. If neither arm is free, an ankle vein is the site of choice for the venipuncture.

Complications

- The prolonged application of a tourniquet produces a measurable increase in blood cell concentration (hemoconcentration).
- A missed vein, which may result in hematoma.
- Thrombosis of the vein.
- Infection of the site where blood was drawn.

Failure to obtain blood after two attempts is an indication that another phlebotomist should make an attempt. To avoid unwanted clotted specimens, ensure adequate and prompt tube inversion with mixing of blood and additive.

VACUTAINER

Vacutainer blood collection tube is a sterile glass or plastic tube with a closure that is evacuated to create a vacuum inside the tube facilitating the draw of a predetermined volume of liquid. Most commonly used to draw a blood sample directly from the vein. These tubes may contain additives designed to stabilize and preserve the specimen prior to analytical testing. Tubes are available with or without a safety-engineered closure, with a variety of labeling options and closure colors as well as a range of draw volumes.

Procedure

The vein is first punctured with the hypodermic needle that is carried in a translucent plastic holder. The needle is double ended, the second shorter needle being shrouded for safety by the holder. When a vacutainer test tube is pushed down into the holder, its rubber cap is pierced by the second needle and the pressure difference between the blood volume and the vacuum in the tube forces blood through the needle and into the tube. The filled tube is then removed and another can be inserted and filled the same way. It is important to remove the tube before withdrawing the needle, as there may still be some suction left, causing pain upon withdrawal. The test tubes are covered with a color-coded plastic cap **(Fig. 2.2)**.

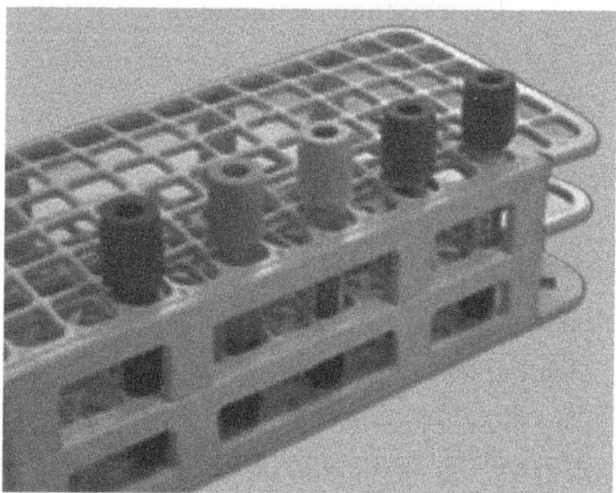

Fig. 2.2: Different vacutainer tubes.

BLOOD SPECIMEN COLLECTION

- *Preparation for blood collection:* The information given on the blood request form should be recorded on the specimen labels essential items include the following:
  a. Patient's complete name and age.
  b. Identification number.
- The specimen containers should be labeled appropriately before the specimen collection.
- Ascertaining whether the patient to fast such care is needed to ensure accurate results.
- The technician must gain the patient's confidence and assure him that, although the venipuncture will be slightly painful, it will be short duration.
- *Positioning the patient:*
  a. The patient should be made to sit comfortably in a chair and should position his arm straight from the shoulder and it should not bend at the elbow.
  b. If the patient wants to lie down, let the patient to lie comfortably on the back, the patient should extent the arm straight from the shoulder.

Equipment for Blood Collection

1. Collection tubes
2. Sterilized syringes and needles
3. Sprit or 70% ethanol
4. Cotton.

Blood Collection

- Compare the requisition form and labeling the tubes
- Selecting vein site
- Applying the tourniquet
- Cleaning the area
- Inspecting the needles and syringes
- Performing the venipuncture.

Separation of Serum

1. Allow the blood to clot
2. Loosen the clot slowly and centrifuge the supernatant fluid
3. By using a pipette, separate the serum from blood cells and store it in a clean and dry test tube.

Blood Collection Tube Top Colors (Fig. 2.3)

White Top

Additive: Potassium Ethylenediaminetetraacetic acid (EDTA)
Mode of action: Forms calcium salts
Uses: Molecular/PCR and bDNA testing.

Order of the Draw

To prevent contamination of tubes with additives from other tubes it is important to draw the tubes in a order called "the order of the draw" (this is very important wen collecting blood sample for various tests). For example, if the additive in the purple stopper tube contaminates the green stopper tube this would cause falsely decreased calcium and increased potassium. The sequence of collection of evacuated tubes in a multi-draw should be in this order:

1. Sterile/blood cultures (yellow top or bottles)
2. Royal blue-red label for trace metal analysis
3. Light-blue coagulation tube—If coagulation tests only are ordered and you are using a butterfly, draw a discard tube to collect the air in the tubing. Failure to do so will result in a short draw which will be rejected by the laboratory.
4. Red—nonadditive
5. Red gel separator tube (speckled or "tiger" top)
6. Green (heparin)
7. Green/gray mottled plasma separator tube (PST) with heparin
8. Lavender/purple top and/or pink (EDTA)
9. Gray top (Oxalate/fluoride tube).

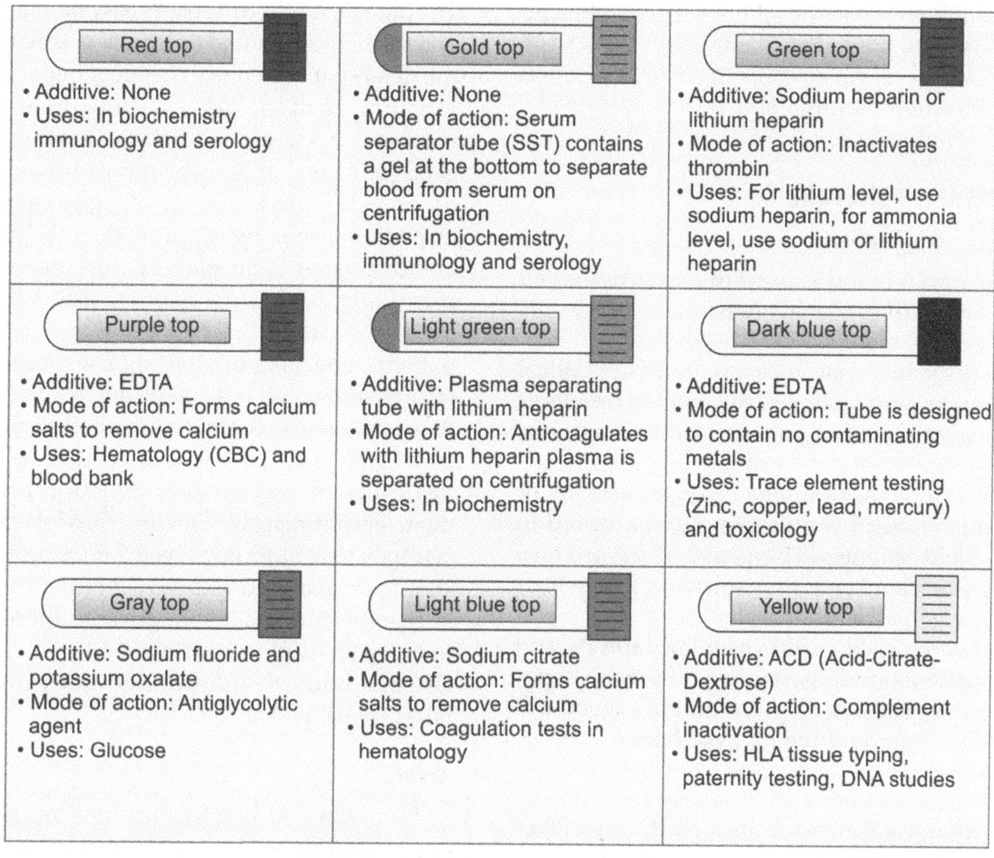

Fig. 2.3: Blood collection tube top colors.

Containers Containing Anticoagulants

- *Red top plastic tubes:* Contains a clot activator and is used when serum is needed.
- Green contains sodium heparin or lithium heparin used for plasma determinations in clinical chemistry (e.g., urea and electrolyte determination).
- *Light-green or green-gray:* For plasma determinations.
- *Purple or lavender:* Contains EDTA (the potassium salt, or K_2EDTA). This is a strong anticoagulant and these tubes are usually used for full blood counts (CBC) and blood films. Lavender top tubes are generally used when whole blood is needed for analysis. Can also be used for some blood bank procedures, such as blood type and screen, but other blood bank procedures, such as crossmatches must be in a pink tube in most facilities.
- *Gray:* These tubes contain fluoride and oxalate. Fluoride prevents enzymes in the blood from working, by preventing the stage called glycolysis so a substrate such as glucose will not be gradually used up during storage. Oxalate is an anticoagulant.
- *Light blue:* Contain a measured amount of citrate. Citrate is a reversible anticoagulant, and these tubes are used for coagulation assays. Because the liquid citrate dilutes the blood, it is important the tube is full so the dilution is properly accounted for.
- *Dark blue:* Contains sodium heparin, an anticoagulant. Also can contain EDTA as an

additive or have no additive. These tubes are used for trace metal analysis.
- *Orange or gray/yellow 'tiger' top:* Contain thrombin, a rapid clot activator, for STAT serum testing.

ARTERIAL PUNCTURE

Uses and Indications

- Arterial blood is used to measure oxygen and carbon dioxide tension, as well as pH arterial blood gases (ABGs).
- These blood gas measurements are critical in the assessment of oxygenation problems encountered in patients with pneumonia, pneumonitis, and pulmonary embolism.
- Patients on prolonged oxygen therapy or mechanical ventilation are monitored to avoid extremes in oxygenation that produce either anoxia with respiratory acidosis or oxygen toxicity.
- Critically-ill cardiovascular patients and patients undergoing major surgery, especially cardiac or pulmonary surgery, are closely monitored for hypoxemia.

Sites

- Increased pressure in the arteries makes it more difficult to stop bleeding with the undesired development of a hematoma.
- Arterial selection includes radial, brachial, and femoral arteries in order of choice.
- Sites not to be selected are irritated, edematous, near a wound, or in an area of an arteriovenous (AV) shunt or fistula.

Specimen Receptacles for Arterial Blood Gases

- The glass syringe, which is particularly better in preserving blood samples with high PO_2. Regular and specialized plastic syringes, vacuum tubes, and capillary tubes should be compared with glass syringes.
- The glass syringe and plunger should be matched for best fit.
- Approximately 1 mL of heparin (1000 or 5000 U/mL, depending on syringe volume) is drawn into the syringe and the barrel lubricated.
- The plunger is tested to ensure easy mobility, and the heparin should be expelled, leaving the dead space filled with residual heparin.
- Advantages of the glass syringe include the most accurate results attainable, a glass plunger that moves upward because of arterial pressure (if 23-gauge or larger needle is used), and reusability. Disadvantages of the glass syringe include relatively high initial cost, need for proper sterilization for reuse between patients, concerns of blood-borne disease transmission, and easy breakage.
- Plastic syringes eliminate the need for resterilization and are low in cost, readily available in any hospital setting, and relatively unbreakable. But the use of plastic syringes may alter PO_2 levels and, if used, should be analyzed within 15 minutes.
- Polypropylene plastic syringes are superior to polystyrene plastic syringes.
- Use of a butterfly infusion set may cause falsely elevated PO_2.

Procedure

1. The radial and brachial arteries are the preferred vessels for arterial puncture. The femoral artery is relatively large and easy to puncture, but care must be taken in older individuals, in whom the femoral artery tends to bleed more than the radial or brachial. The radial artery is more difficult to puncture but exhibits a lower incidence of complications.
2. When using the radial artery, it is essential to assess the collateral circulation (blood supplied from more than one artery, i.e., radial and ulnar arteries) of the hand.
3. The artery to be punctured is identified by its pulsations and cleansed with 70% aqueous isopropanol solution followed by iodine.
4. Prepare the ABG syringe as directed earlier. The needle (18 to 20 gauge for brachial artery) should pierce the skin at an angle of approximately 45° to 60° (90°

for femoral artery) in a slow and deliberate manner. Some degree of dorsiflexion of the wrist is necessary with the radial artery, for which a 23- to 25-gauge needle is used.

5. The pulsations of blood into the syringe confirm that it will fill by arterial pressure alone. If the plunger is pulled and air is aspirated, immediately withdraw the syringe.
6. After the blood specimen is collected, the needle is removed using a needle re-sheather and an airtight cap (Luer tip cap) placed over the tip of the syringe. Gently rotate syringe, mixing blood and heparin. Place in ice water (or other coolant that will maintain a temperature of 1° to 5°C) to minimize leukocyte consumption of oxygen.
7. After the arterial puncture, compression with a sterile gauze pad on the puncture site should be applied for a minimum of 2 minutes and preferably for 5 minutes.

The recommended volume of arterial blood obtained varies, but certainly the greater the specimen volume, the less dilution effect from the heparin. Use of pre-heparinized syringes for blood gas analysis presents a more convenient and rapid method of blood collection. Excess heparin solution must be expelled prior to collection and the prescribed volume of blood (3 mL) must be obtained to minimize dilutional error.

Blood Gas Study Obtained by Skin Puncture

Blood gases obtained by skin puncture may be collected from the finger as a suitable substitute for arterial blood for pH and PCO_2 but may not be acceptable for PO_2. In order for it to be a satisfactory substitute for arterial blood, some estimation of the PO_2 must be available. The recommended site for obtaining arterialized capillary blood is the earlobe because of its vascularity, its slow metabolic requirements, and the ease with which it can be arterialized.

SKIN PUNCTURE

The Usefulness of Skin Puncture

- A capillary is a small blood vessel connecting the small arteries (arterioles) to the small veins (venules).
- The capillary blood is obtained by skin puncture. It provides only small quantities of blood specimens for making a blood smear (differential count), cell count or hematocrit determination. Skin puncture specimen is preferred over venipuncture specimen for the study of a blood smear and a differential count.
- The skin puncture is not preferred for biochemistry or microbiology tests in the normal patients.

1. In pediatric patients: Skin puncture is the method of choice in pediatric patients especially infants because (i) large amount of blood drawn by repeated venipuncture may cause iatrogenic anemia, (ii) accessible veins in sick infants must be reserved exclusively for parental therapy.
2. Adult patients: Skin puncture is useful in adults with: (i) extreme obesity, (ii) severe burns, and (iii) thrombotic tendencies.
3. Geriatric patients: Skin puncture is preferred in these patients because of thinness of skin and loss of elasticity.

Limitations

Provides only small quantities of blood specimen and so it is inadequate for most of the routine tests. Apart from this, other limitations are:

i. Most of the blood counts done by skin puncture are low because blood gets diluted with tissue fluid.
ii. This specimen is not suitable for coagulation study because the specimen is mixed with tissue fluid.

Sites (Fig. 2.4)

1. *Finger tip of the middle or ring finger:* This is recommended for adults and older

children. Specimen collected from this site is a suitable substitute for arterial blood for pH and PCO_2 but may not be acceptable for PO_2.
2. *Ball of the great toe or edge of the heel:* This is suitable for neonates and infants. In infants with respiratory distress syndrome, heel blood deviates significantly from arterial blood in all parameters except base excess and standard bicarbonate.
3. *Earlobe:* This is the recommended site for obtaining arterialized capillary blood in older pediatric or adult patients. Specimen collection from this site is impractical for neonates and infants.

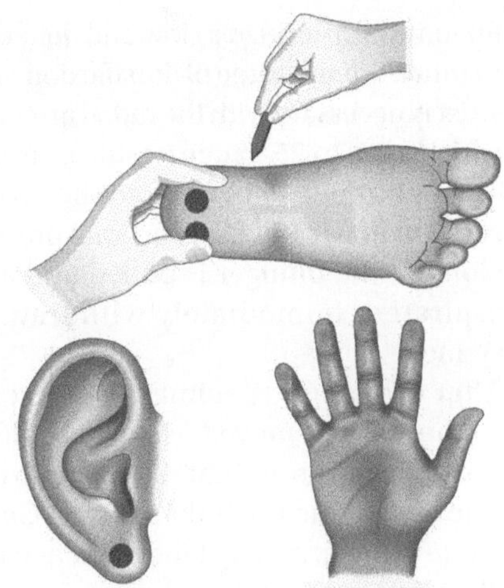

Fig. 2.4: Sites for skin puncture.

Instrument

- The instrument used for the puncture should be carefully selected.
- It is better to use needles with a flat body having a cutting edge.
- Sterile lancet or No. 11 Bard Parker blades pushed through a cork to 3 mm depth are the best.
- The puncture should be 3 to 4 mm in depth. It should be emphasized here that it is important to use a separate lancet, blade or needle for each patient, or to adequately clean and sterilize the instrument between each use.
- Adequate sterilization would include autoclaving, dry heat in a hot air oven for an hour, or even boiling for 15 minutes after careful cleaning.

Procedure

Finger Prick

The site is cleaned thoroughly with alcohol or spirit. This kills bacteria and also removes dirt and oils.

The skin is dried with a piece of sterile cotton wool or gauze before the puncture is made. If the skin is still wet with spirit, the blood will run all over the finger and not collect into a compact drop which is so essential for easy sampling. The excess alcohol will also enter the wound and cause unnecessary pain.

Before making the puncture, raise the skin in the longitudinal axis of the ball of the finger into a small ridge by very gentle pressure on the sides of the finger. The pressure should not obstruct the venous return. With the skin raised into a ridge, the lancet is largely plunged into the crest of the ridge to a depth of about 3 mm and the light pressure on the sides of the finger removed. It is essential to make the prick sharply and quickly, firstly to minimize any pain, and secondly to make a wound from which the blood will flow freely.

When the light pressure is released from the sides of the finger, the ridge of skin subsides, and the wound automatically opens. From the wound the blood should now flow freely and collect as a compact drop on the highest point of the ball of the finger. No pressure is required to accelerate the flow of blood and indeed pressure may have the effect of closing the wound. If the flow of blood is not free enough, tension should be exerted on the skin in an outward direction in order to open the wound more widely. This slight tension is best exerted by placing the thumbs one on each side of the wound and drawing the skin upwards and away from the wound itself. The first drop of blood should be wiped off, and when a sufficiently large drop has again collected, it should be used at once for filling a pipette (experience is required to estimate the size of the drop required in relation to the size of the pipette). No drop should be used which has remained on the finger for more than half a minute, other wise it may contain particles of fibrin. Such a drop should be wiped off with a piece of dry sterile cotton-wool or gauze, and the next drop used. The whole operation of filling the pipettes for blood counts and making three or four smears should occupy no more than a minute. When all the blood that is required has been obtained, the finger should be cleaned with a piece of sterile cotton wool and pressure applied for 30 to 60 seconds over the puncture wound in order to stop the flow **(Fig. 2.5)**.

Ball of the Great Toe or Edge of the Heel

After cleaning the site, a deep heel prick is made at the distal edge of the calcaneal protuberance following a 5 to 10 minutes exposure period with pre-warmed water. The specimen is then handled as described for finger prick method.

Earlobe Prick

The earlobe is arterialized by a paper towel saturated with warm water (39° to 42°C) or by flicking the index finger until definite flushing is observed. The earlobe is cleaned with sterile cotton wool dipped in 70% alcohol and punctured with sterile or disposable lancet. The punctured area should be adequate to obtain a

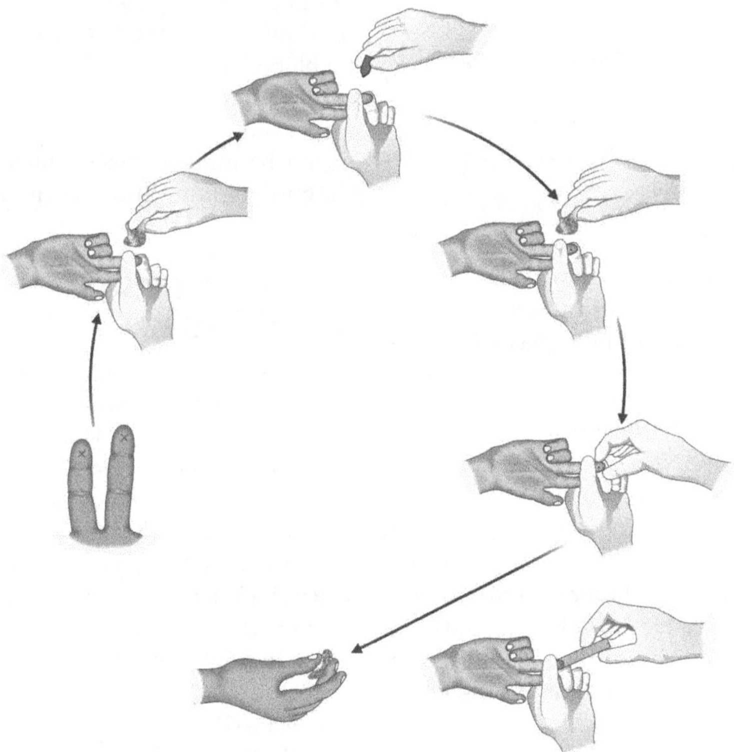

Fig. 2.5: Finger prick technique.

free flow of blood and the specimen collected as described for finger prick method. The earlobe is wiped dry with dry sterile cotton ball.

Routinely Used Anticoagulants

Anticoagulants are substances that prevent the blood from clotting. Anticoagulants are of two types depending upon the mode of action: (i) calcium chelator, and (ii) heparin.

Calcium Chelator

Most of the anticoagulants used in the laboratory act by binding calcium as an insoluble salt which precipitates, or as a soluble but non-ionized salt. This prevents clotting since calcium ions are essential for many of the steps in the coagulation mechanism. Oxalate, citrate, and EDTA chelates the calcium ion. Sodium or potassium salts are not suitable because they interferes with the assay.

Potassium Oxalate

This is used at a concentration of 2 mg/mL of blood. This anticoagulant is most often used for chemical analysis. But the sample added with potassium oxalate should not be used for electrolyte estimation.

Ammonium Oxalate

This is used at a concentration of 2 mg/mL of blood. This anticoagulant causes swelling of the RBC, and is therefore not used for PCV, ESR or blood smears.

Balanced Oxalate, Double Oxalate, or Wintrobe's Mixture

To balance the swelling effect of ammonium oxalate and the shrinking effect of potassium oxalate, these two are combined in a mixture with a ratio of 3 parts of the former (NH_4 oxalate) to 2 parts of the latter (K oxalate). It is used at a concentration of 2 mg/mL of blood. This is usually done by making a solution as follows:

Ammonium oxalate	1.2 g
Potassium oxalate	0.8 g
Distilled water to make	100 mL

Ethylenediaminetetraacetic (EDTA)

This is usually used as the disodium salt of the acid (Na_2 EDTA) or as the dipotassium salt of the acid (K_2 EDTA). These are used in a concentration of 1–2 mg/mL of blood. Usually, a solution containing 10 mg/mL is prepared, and then 0.2 mL solution is placed in the clean dry containers for drying as described for Wintrobe's mixture. EDTA is the most powerful calcium chelating (binding) agent.

Trisodium Citrate

This is most commonly used as a 3.8% solution (3.8 g/dL).

Heparin

Heparin is a highly acidic substance which is normally present in the body in small amounts, and is a natural biological anticoagulant. It is commonly used because chance hemolysis of samples during collection is less. It can be used for some hematological special tests or for blood for biochemical testing of electrolytes or blood gases, or for some blood used in transfusion (for open-heart surgery), but it is expensive and is not used much in the routine diagnostic laboratory or in routine blood banking.

COLLECTION AND RESERVATION OF URINE SPECIMENS

Random urine sample can be used for qualitative tests. However, quantitative determinations, such as urine phosphate, calcium, uric acid, ammonia, etc. A 24-hour-specimen is suitable because the concentrations vary at different times of the day.

The patient completely empties the bladder at 8 o'clock in the morning. This first sample is discarded. Thereafter, start the collection of the urine in a 5 liter bottle till the next morning 8 o'clock. The 8 o'clock morning sample of urine is collected.

If the 8 o'clock sample on the day of starting is collected the next morning 8 o'clock sample is discarded. Thus, a 24-hour-urine specimen is procured.

Preservatives for Urine

- Preservatives commonly used are acetic acid, HCl, thymol, chloroform, toluene, light petroleum and formalin.
- Several changes, such as bacterial action, the precipitation of phosphates (if the urine is in alkaline state) and crystallization of uric acid takes place if the urine kept without any preservative.
- To prevent, these changes concentrated HCl (10 mL) is used as a preservative during the collection of urine for urea, ammonia, total nitrogen, creatinine, uric acid, phosphates, cortisol and calcium estimation.
- The HCl maintains the urine in acidic state and prevents the growth of bacteria and also precipitation of phosphates.
- Ten mL of liquid paraffin, chloroform, toluene, petroleum, thymol and formalin are used as urine preservatives. One of these of about 10 mL is placed in a 5 liter bottle and is given for collecting urine sample for protein, VMA (Vanillylmandelic acid) and HIAA (hydroxyindoleacetic acid). These form a layer over urine and hence prevent entry of bacteria into urine.
- Carefully pipette urine from the bottom to avoid the preservative to enter the pipette. One of the above preservatives mentioned above can be used for the routine investigations.

CEREBROSPINAL FLUID AND ITS COLLECTION

- Cerebrospinal fluid (CSF) is present within the subarachnoid space surrounding the brain in the skull and the spinal cord in the spinal column.
- Its main function is to protect the brain and the spinal cord from injury by acting as a fluid cushion.
- It is the medium through which nutrients and the waste products are transported between brain/spinal cord and the blood.

Formation and Composition of Cerebrospinal Fluid

Cerebrospinal fluid (CSF) is derived by ultrafiltration (of plasma) and by secretion through the choroid plexus located in the ventricles of the brain. It leaves the ventricular system through the medial and lateral foramina to surround the brain and the spinal cord surfaces within the subarachnoid space.

- Reabsorption of CSF occurs at the arachnoid villi which projects into the venous sinuses in the dura mater.
- The CSF is produced at the rate of 500 mL/day.
- Total CSF volume is 90 to 150 mL in adults and 10 to 60 mL in neonates.
- Blood brain barrier maintains the relative homeostasis of CNS environment by tightly regulating the concentration of substances by specific transport systems for H^+, K^+, Ca^{++}, Mg^{++}, HCO_3^-.
- Glucose, urea and creatinine diffuse freely between blood and the CSF.
- Proteins cross freely by passive diffusion along the concentration gradient and is also influenced by molecular weight.

Characteristics of Normal Cerebrospinal Fluid

- Color—colorless
- pH—7.28 to 7.32
- Appearance—clear
- Specific gravity—1.003 to 1.004
- No clot formation on standing
- Total solids—0.85 to 1.70 g/dL
- PO_2 —40 to 44 mm Hg.

Clinical Application of Cerebrospinal Fluid Examination

In the diagnosis of:

a. Bacterial, viral or fungal meningitis.
b. Encephalitis.
c. Malignant infiltrates, such as in acute leukemia, lymphoma.
d. Subarachnoid hemorrhage.
e. Disorders with local immunoglobulin production in the CNS-multiple sclerosis,

subacute sclerosing panencephalitis (SSPE).

f. Spinal canal blockage leading to elevated intracranial tension.

Collection and Handling of Cerebrospinal Fluid

The CSF is usually obtained by lumbar puncture (LP) using an LP needle.

The needle measures 10 to 12 cm in length and is made of platinum or German alloy. It has a needle and the stilette. The stilette of the needle has a pin, which fits into the lot of the head of the needle. The stilette of the needle helps to keep the needle patent **(Fig. 2.6)**.

Uses of the needle: This needle can also be used for cistern puncture, carotid angiography, splenoportogram, and for tapping fluids from the cavities (ascitic, pleural fluid), in addition to the obtaining CSF from lumbar puncture.

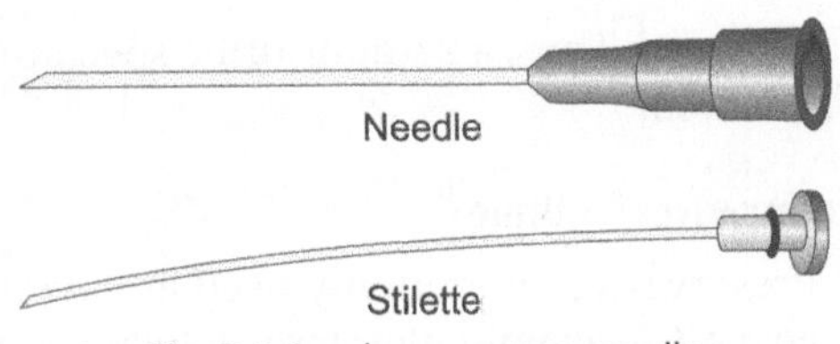

Fig. 2.6: Lumbar puncture needle.

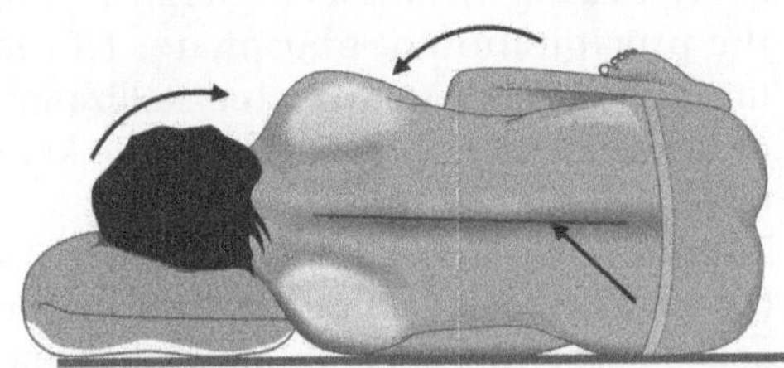

Fig. 2.7: Position for lumbar puncture with patient lying down.

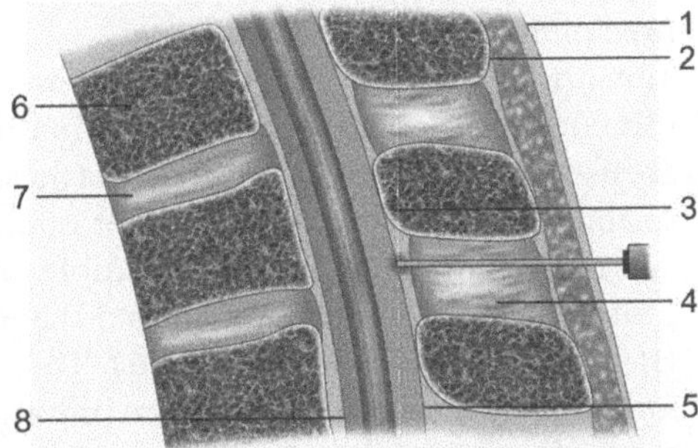

Fig. 2.8: Section of the spinal cord showing the LP needle in the 3rd lumbar space: (1) Skin, (2) Supraspinous ligament, (3) Ligamentum flavum, (4) Interspinous ligament, (5) Dura mater, (6) Vertebral body, (7) Disc, (8) Posterior longitudinal ligament.

Specimen Collection

Procedure for specimen collection by lumbar puncture.

i. *Position:* The patient is placed on his side at the edge of the bed with his knee drawn up and the head flexed as shown in the **Figure 2.7**.
ii. *Site:* In the 3rd lumbar space. This space lies in the plane, which joins the highest points on the iliac crest. The skin over the back from the lower thoracic vertebra to the coccyx is sterilized with cetavlon, ether, iodine and spirit.
iii. *Local anesthesia:* The skin to be punc-tured is infiltrated with 5 mL of 2% lignocaine.
iv. *Puncture:* The LP needle with stilette is introduced after 2 to 3 minutes into the anesthetized space, with the cutting edge of the bevel in the direction parallel to the fibers of the ligamentum flavum. The needle is introduced (slightly upwards and forwards at 5° to avoid injury to the disc) through the supraspinous ligament and interspinous ligament. At about 4 to 7 cm, the firmer resistance of the ligamentum flavum gives way as the needle enters the Dura mater **(Fig. 2.8)**.
v. The stilette is then withdrawn and the fluid, which trickles down is collected in sterile containers but only after recording the CSF pressure (by attaching a manometer to the LP needle).

SELF TEST

1. Describe the procedure for venipuncture.
2. State the use of skin puncture.
3. Briefly explain the procedure for finger prick procedure.
4. Name the anticoagulants used during the collection of blood for various investigations.
5. Write the formation and composition of cerebrospinal fluid (CSF).
6. Mention the characteristics of CSF.

MULTIPLE CHOICE QUESTIONS

1. The fluoride acts as an ______
   a. Preservative
   b. Stimulator
   c. Antiseptic
   d. Competitive inhibitor

2. The preservative used during the urine collection for protein estimation is ______
   a. Toluene
   b. HCl
   c. Chloroform
   d. Sulfuric acid

3. The concentration of oxalate used to prevent clotting is ______
   a. 10 mg
   c. 20 mg
   c. 2 mg
   d. 5 mg.

4. The CSF can be collected by passing the needle between:
   a. L1 and L2
   b. L3 and L4
   c. L5 and L6
   d. L6 and L8

5. All the following are the clinical applications of CSF analysis, *Except*:
   a. Bacterial meningitis
   b. Encephalitis
   c. Viral meningitis
   d. Liver cancer

3

UNIT

Centrifugation Techniques

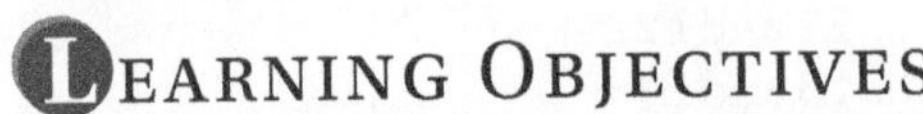

At the end of this unit, the learner should be able to understand:

- Principle of centrifugation.
- Different types and advantages of centrifugation.

INTRODUCTION

Centrifugation is a separation technique commonly used in clinical and research laboratories. It is based on the behavior of particles in an applied centrifugal field.

PRINCIPLE

Particles that differ in density, size or shape, sediment at different rates in a centrifugal field. The particles will tend to sediment under the influence of gravity. If the particles suspended in a liquid are so small or have a density so close to that of the liquid, then the force of gravity fails to sediment the particles into a separate layer. So the basis of centrifugation techniques is to exert a larger force than the gravitational force to enhance the effective sedimentation force for the separating such particles from the liquid.

In centrifugation, the particles are normally suspended in a specific liquid medium, held in tubes, which are located in a rotor. The rotor is positioned centrally on the drive shaft of the centrifuge. Particles that differ in density, shape or size can be separated since they sediment at different rates in the centrifugal field, each particle sedimenting at a rate, which is proportional to the applied centrifugal field.

The rate at which the sedimentation occurs in centrifugation is expressed in terms of sedimentation coefficient and is given by the formula:

$S = V / \omega^2 r$

V = Migration (sedimentation) of the molecule

ω = Rotation of the rotor in radians/sec (angular velocity)

r = Distance in cm, from the center of rotor

The sedimentation coefficient has the units of seconds. It was usually expressed in units of 10–13 seconds, (since several biological macromolecules occur in this range) which is designated as one svedberg unit, i.e., 1 svedberg unit = 10^{-13} seconds. For instance, the sedimentation coefficient of hemoglobin is 4×10^{-13} seconds or 4S; ribonuclease is 2×10^{-13} seconds or 2S. Conventionally, the subcellular organelles are often referred to by their 'S' value, e.g., 70S ribosome.

Centrifuges

The equipment used to perform centrifugation is called "centrifuge". The centrifuge should essentially have a rotor to keep the sample tube. The rotor can be of three types:

1. Fixed angle rotor **(Fig. 3.1)**
2. Vertical tube rotor **(Fig. 3.2)**
3. Swinging bucket rotor **(Fig. 3.3)**

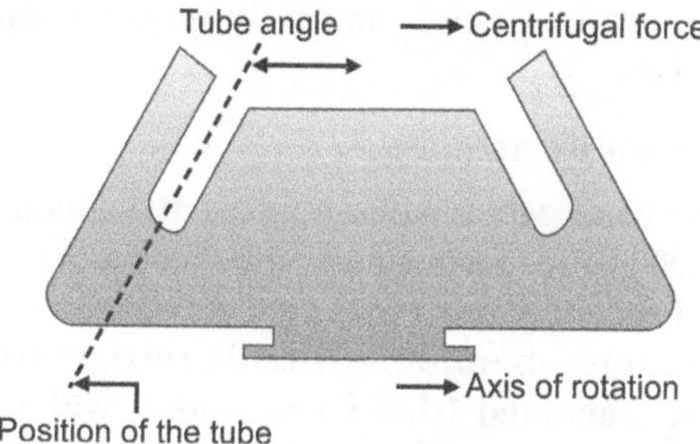

Fig. 3.1: Fixed angle rotor.

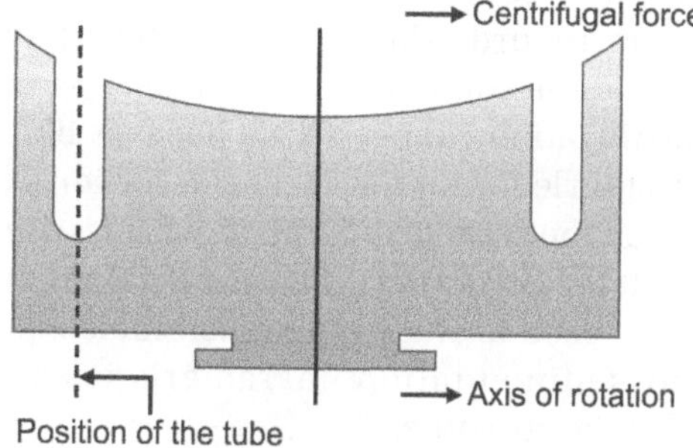

Fig. 3.2: Vertical tube rotor.

Fixed Angle Rotor

In this, tube will be in a fixed position in a specific slanting position throughout the process **(Fig. 3.1)**.

Vertical Tube Rotor

In this, tube will be in a fixed position, but its axis will be parallel to the axis of rotation throughout the process **(Fig. 3.2)**.

Swinging Bucket Rotor

In this type of rotor, at rest the tube axis will remain parallel to axis of rotation. However, during centrifugation the tube swings and will have an angle of 90° with the axis of rotation **(Fig. 3.3)**.

Aluminum alloy or titanium alloys have been used as rotor materials as they can withstand the higher stress force generated during high speed centrifugation. Aluminum alloys rotors, although less expensive, are far more susceptive to corrosion by acids and alkalis. Titanium alloy rotors can withstand nearly twice the centrifugal force of rotors made from aluminum alloy.

Types of Centrifuges

Centrifuges may be classified into four major groups:

1. Small bench centrifuges
2. Large capacity refrigerated centrifuges
3. High speed refrigerated centrifuges
4. Ultracentrifuges—which are of two types—preparative and analytical.

Small Bench Centrifuges

These are simplest and least expensive and available in many designs (may be driven by mechanical force or electrical force). These centrifuges generally will have a maximum speed of 4000-6000 revolutions per minute (RPM) with maximum relative centrifugal field (RCF) of 3000 to 7000 g. They are often used to

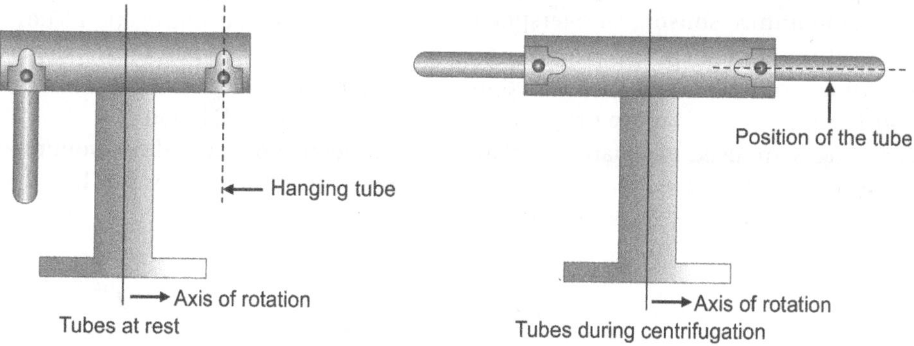

Fig. 3.3: Swinging bucket rotor.

collect small amounts of material that rapidly sediment (yeast cells, erythrocytes, coarse precipitates).

Large Capacity Refrigerated Centrifuges

These have a maximum speed of 6000 RPM and produce a maximum relative centrifugal field approaching 6500 g. These have a refrigerated rotor chambers and vary only in their maximum carrying capacity. These instruments are most often used to collect substances that sediment rapidly, for example, RBCs, bulky precipitates, yeast cells, nuclei and chloroplasts.

High Speed Refrigerated Centrifuges

These are available with maximum rotor speeds in the region 25000 RPM (corresponding to a RCF of 60000 g). These can be used to collect microorganisms, cellular debris and large cellular organelles. But these cannot generate sufficient centrifugal force to sediment viruses or smaller organelles, such as ribosome.

Preparative Ultracentrifuges

These are capable of spinning rotors to a maximum speed of 80000 RPM and can produce a relative centrifugal field of up to 600000 g. The rotor chamber is refrigerated, sealed, evacuated to minimize excessive rotor temperatures generated by friction between air and spinning rotor. The temperature monitoring system is more sophisticated than simpler instruments, employing an infrared temperature sensor. An overspeed control system is also incorporated. For safety reasons, rotor chamber is enclosed in heavy armor plating. And these preparative ultracentrifuges are used to separate, isolate and purify whole cells, subcellular organelles, plasma membranes, polysomes, ribosomes, chromatin, nucleic acids, lipoproteins and viruses.

Analytical Ultracentrifuges

These are capable of operating at a speed of 70,000 RPM (corresponding 500,000 g). These will have a rotor contained in a protective armored chamber, which is refrigerated and evacuated. These instruments will also have a special optical system to observe the sedimenting of material and to determine concentration distributions within the sample at any time during centrifugation. The optical system records the change in refractive index of the solution which will vary as the centrifugation changes. This behaves like a refraction lens resulting in the production of a peak on the photographic plate, which is used as a detector system. These centrifuges are mainly used to study pure macromolecules, their sedimentation characteristics and molecular structure.

Application of Centrifugation

a. Separation of thick precipitates from solution.
b. Separation of serum from clotted blood.
c. Separation of plasma from anticoagulant added blood.
d. Precipitating proteins from serum during colorimetric estimation of serum urea, creatinine. Trichloroacetic acid is added to serum sample, which denatures proteins and precipitates. The precipitate is separated by centrifugation. The protein free filtrate is used for further analysis.
e. Separation of erythrocytes from oxalated (or heparinized) blood.
f. To determine packed cell volume (PCV) or hematocrit values. The oxalated blood is centrifuged in hematocrit

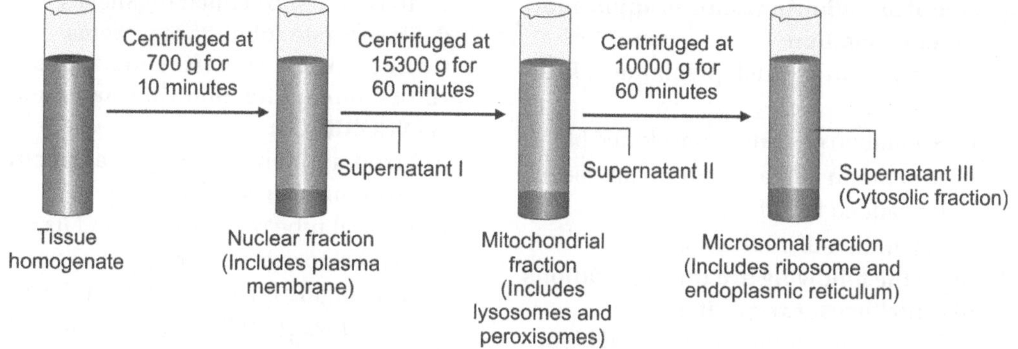

Fig. 3.4: Isolation of subcellular organelles.

tubes (110 mm long and 3 mm in bore diameter) at 3000 RPM for 30 minutes. The proportionate volume of RBCs, settled in the bottom layer below the supernatant layer of clear plasma in the tube, is read from the graduations of the tube as PCV (normally it averages 45% in humans).

g. *Isolation of subcellular organelles:* The cells are subjected to disruption by sonication or by osmotic shock or by the use of homogenizer. This is usually carried out in an isotonic (0.25M) sucrose solution. The subcellular particles can be separated by differential centrifugation **(Fig. 3.4)**.
The purity (or contamination) of the subcellular fraction can be checked by the use of marker enzymes. Example—DNA polymerase is the marker for nucleus, glutamate dehydrogenase for mitochondrion, glucose-6-phosphatase for ribosome, and hexokinase for cytosolic fraction.

h. Determination of molecular weight (in the fields of protein and nucleic acid chemistry) by studying their sedimentation characteristics.

i. Estimation of purity of macromolecules, i.e., purity of DNA preparations, viruses and proteins.

j. Detection of conformational changes in macromolecules, such as DNA and proteins.

SELF TEST

1. Name the different types of centrifuges used in the clinical biochemistry laboratory.
2. Mention the different types of rotors.
3. Mention the application of centrifugation.

MULTIPLE CHOICE QUESTIONS

1. Select the unrelated term in the following:
   a. Rotor
   b. Drive shaft
   c. Monochromatic light
   d. Relative centrifugal field

2. Separation of particles in a centrifuge depends on the following property:
   a. Charge
   b. Density
   c. Fluorescence
   d. Color

3. **One of the following is not an application of centrifugation:**
   a. Separation of thick precipitates from solution
   b. Separation of serum from clotted blood
   c. Separation of plasma from anticoagulant added blood
   d. Separation of inhibitors.
4. **All of the following are the applications of centrifuges, *Except:* It is used:**
   a. To separate serum from clotted blood
   b. To separate erythrocytes from oxalated/heparinized blood
   c. To isolate sub cellular organelles
   d. To separate subunits of proteins.
5. **Concerning the different types of rotors, one of the following statements is INCORRECT:**
   a. Fixed angle rotor fixed in a specific position when swinging
   b. Vertical tube rotor fixed in and its axis parallel to axis of rotation
   c. In swinging bucket rotor, the tube axis will remain parallel to axis of rotation
   d. Horizontal tube rotor remains horizontal during rotation.

4 UNIT Spectrophotometry and Colorimetry

LEARNING OBJECTIVES

At the end of this unit, the learner should be able to understand:
- The principles of spectrophotometry and spectrofluorimetry.
- Advantages of spectrophotometry.

INTRODUCTION

Spectrophotometry and colorimetry are the two common techniques used for the estimation of substance, such as glucose, urea, creatinine, etc., in biological samples after their modification into a colored compound.

SPECTROPHOTOMETRY

Basic Introductory Terms

Light

It is a form of energy. Some of the properties of light can be explained by considering it as a stream of particles, whereas some other properties can be explained by considering it as a wave.

Wavelength of Light (Fig. 4.1A)

When light is considered as a wave the distance between two successive crests or troughs is called the 'wavelength' of that particular type of light. It is designated by 'λ' (Lambda) and expressed in terms of nm (nanometers) or Å (Angstroms).

When ordinary light (white light) is passed through a prism, it is split into seven different components (colors). This property is called 'Dispersion.'

The components from bottom to top will have the following order—Violet (V), Indigo (I), Blue (B), Green (G), Yellow (Y), Orange (O), and Red (R). This visible light will cover a wavelength range from 400 nm to 700 nm **(Fig. 4.1B)**.

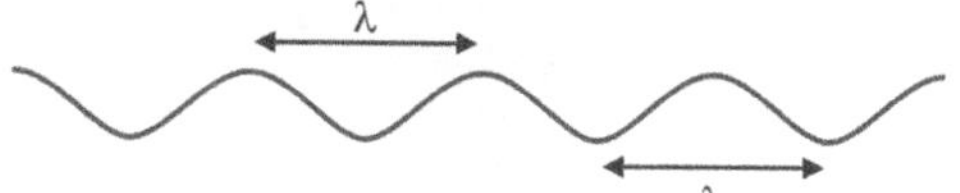

Fig. 4.1A: Wavelength of light.

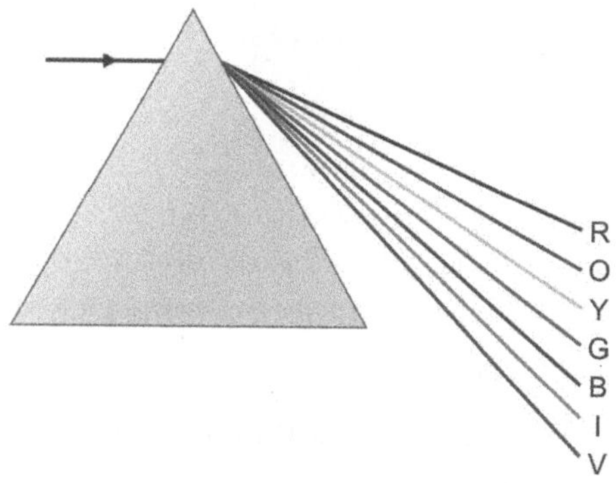

Fig. 4.1B: Dispersion of light.

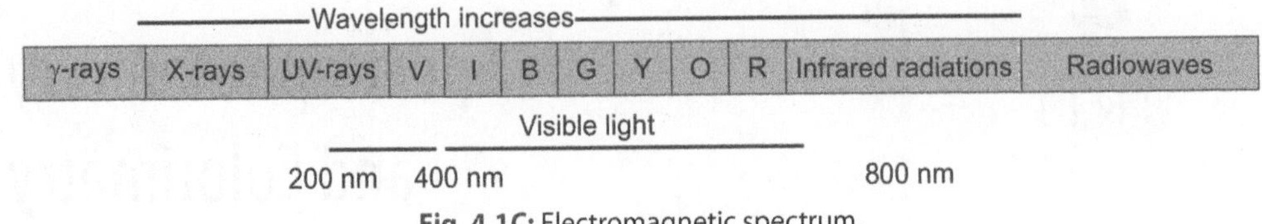

Fig. 4.1C: Electromagnetic spectrum.

Electromagnetic Spectrum

When all the types of radiations are arranged in the increasing order of their wavelengths, it constitutes the electromagnetic spectrum **(Fig. 4.1C)**.

Transmittance (T)

Assume that light, whose intensity is I_o is passed through a solution. Let the intensity of the emergent light be I_e. Then transmittance (T) can be defined as the ratio of intensity of the emergent light to that of the incident original light, i.e., $T = I_e/I_o$ **(Fig. 4.2)**.

Percentage Transmittance (T %)

$T\% = (I_e/I_o) \times 100$

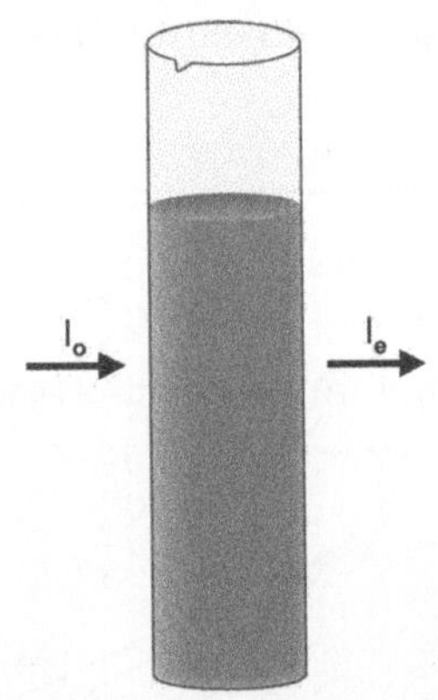

Fig. 4.2: Transmittance $(T) = I_e/I_o$

I_o = Intensity of the original light

I_e = Intensity of the emergent light

Absorbance (A)

It is the negative logarithm of transmittance to the base ten.

$$A = -\log_{10} T$$

Optical Density (OD)

It is the negative logarithm of percentage transmittance to the base ten.

$OD = -\log_{10} T\%$

Principles of Spectrophotometry and Colorimetry

Spectrophotometry and colorimetry techniques are based on the estimation of light absorbing nature of the substances in solution. In colorimetry, only the colored compounds or the compounds capable of forming color complexes by reacting with reagents can be analyzed. In this, the intensity of the color is directly proportional to the concentration of the substance. In spectrophotometry colored and colorless solution can be studied by means of ultraviolet spectral analysis. These techniques are based on two laws:

Beer's Law

"Absorbance of a solution is directly proportional to the concentration of the solution" (i.e., $A \propto C$) or "transmittance of a solution decreases exponentially with the increase in the concentration of the solution" (i.e., $T = e^{-kc}$).

Lambert's Law

"Absorbance of a solution is directly proportional to the thickness of the optical path" (i.e., $A \propto t$) or "Transmittance of a solution decreases exponentially with the increase in the thickness of the optical light path" (i.e., $T = e^{-kt}$).

If both these are combined, the Lambert-Beer's law becomes $A \propto Ct$ or $T = e^{-kct}$ **(Fig. 4.3)**.

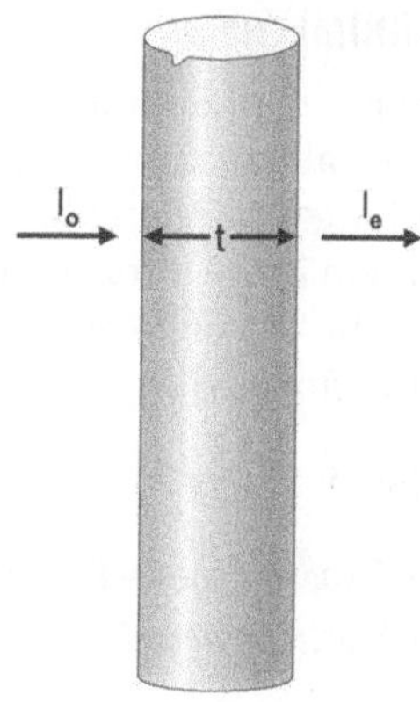

Fig. 4.3: t = Diameter of the container/width of the solution layer/thickness of the optical path

Components of Colorimeter and Spectrophotometer (Fig. 4.4)

Spectrophotometer is more sophisticated compared to colorimeter.

Source of Light

The tungsten lamp is the source of visible light in colorimeters. Spectrophotometers will have two sources of light—a tungsten lamp, which emits visible light (wavelength ranges from 400 nm to 700 nm) and a deuterium lamp which emits ultraviolet (UV) radiations (wavelength range—200 to 400 nm).

Monochromator

A monochromator is an optical system which produces, from a multiwavelength source of radiation, a parallel beam of monochromatic radiation; usually it is by refraction by a prism or diffraction by a grating. In colorimeters, replaceable colored glass filters are used to get the monochromatic light. The multiwavelength radiation from the source passes through the filter and the radiation of a narrow bandwidth comes out.

But in spectrophotometers, monochromators will not be the manually replaceable filters. Instead of this quartz prism or diffraction grating is used to obtain monochromatic light (Diffraction grating is a glass slide like optical hardware consists of a series of ruled lines on a transparent or reflecting base).

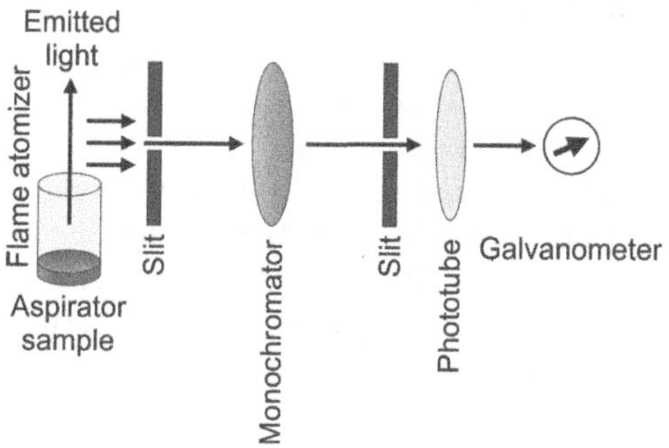

Fig. 4.4: Components of colorimeter.

Color of filter and color of solution are complimentary

Color of filter	*Wavelength*	*Color of solution*
Violet	420	Brown
Blue	470	Yellowish brown
Green	520	Pink
Yellow	580	Purple
Red	680	Green

Slit

This is to allow a narrow beam of selected monochromatic light to pass through the sample solution.

Cuvette

The glass container to keep the test solution, which has to be filled 3/4th of its height. For UV analysis always quartz cuvette is recommended.

Photocells

The photocells convert quanta of radiation to electrical energy, which may be amplified, detected and recorded.

Detector

Usually, photomultiplier tubes (PMT), which are based on "photo ionic effect" used as detectors. (Photonic effect: Light photons impinging on a metal surface in vacuum cause the emission of electrons in proportion to the intensity of the radiation). The light that comes out of the cuvette falls on this and gets converted into an electrical signal.

Recorder

The electrical signal from the PMT is amplified and then recorded by the galvanometer. Usually, the recorders are calibrated in such a way that they directly give the absorbance or transmittance values.

Applications

In clinical diagnostic and research laboratories, these techniques are commonly used for the quantitative estimation of different compounds in various biological fluids. Examples —blood glucose, urea, cholesterol, creatinine, bilirubin and CSF protein, etc.

1. Visible and UV spectra may be used to identify various compounds in both pure state and in biological preparations, e.g., proteins show a maximum light absorption at 280 nm, So we can observe a peak at 280 nm when its absorption spectra is plotted.
2. Similarly nucleic acids show an absorption maximum at 260 nm. So these techniques can be used in the structural analysis of proteins and nucleic acids.
3. Used in the enzyme assay and kinetic studies.
4. *Turbidimetry:* It is a form of spectrophotometry in which very dilute suspensions may be assayed by measuring the extent of turbidity.
5. *Nephelometry:* This technique measures the intensity of radiation scattered by a suspension and is commonly used for estimating concentration of micro-organisms.

SPECTROFLUORIMETRY

Fluorescence is the phenomenon whereby a molecule, after absorption radiation, emits radiation of a longer wavelength. A compound absorbs radiation in the ultraviolet region and emits visible light. This increase in wavelength is known as the stokes shift.

Instrumentation

Advantages and Disadvantages of Fluorimetry over Absorption Spectrophotometry

Advantages

1. Spectrofluorometry is most accurate at very low concentrations when absorption spectrophotometer is least accurate.
2. The sensitivity of fluorimeters is usually easily adjusted over a large range by amplification of the current produced in the photocell circuit.
3. It enables the utilization of great spectral selectivity.

Disadvantages

1. The susceptibility to environmental conditions and the virtual impossibility of predicting whether a compound will fluoresce.
2. The other major problem is quenching, whereby the energy, which could be emitted as fluorescence, transferred to the other molecules.

Applications

1. For the chemical modifications, such as oxidation, reduction, hydrolysis, coupling and self-condensation.
2. The determination and comparison of both excitation and fluorescence spectra of a compound may help to identify it.
3. The assay of vitamin B_1 in foodstuffs, NADH in mitochondria, microorganisms,

hormones, such as cortisol, estradiol, drugs, cholesterol and porphyrins.
4. Enzyme assays and kinetic analysis.
5. Study of protein structure.

FLAME PHOTOMETRY

It is a device for measuring the concentration of metals in solution by measuring the intensities of light emitted by the same metals when their solutions are sprayed into a gas flame. The chemical procedures for measuring sodium and potassium are tedious and costly also. The flame photometry forms a simple, accurate and speedy method for determining the Na^+ and K^+ concentrations in body fluids.

Principle

A standard solution of Na^+ or K^+ or diluted serum is sprayed by means of an automizer into a Bunsen flame. Yellow color or violet color is produced with Na^+ and K^+ respectively. The emitted rays pass through a monochromator, filtered rays fall on phototube and produce a current, which deflects the galvanometer.

Applications

It is mainly used to measure electrolytes and lithium in body fluids.

SELF TEST

1. Explain the following terms:
   a. Wavelength
   b. Transmittance
   c. Lambert's law
   d. Beer's law
2. Write the principle of spectrophotometry.
3. Add a note on monochromator.
4. Mention the applications of spectrofluorimetry.

MULTIPLE CHOICE QUESTIONS

1. Light is a form of ______
a. Energy
b. Transmittance
c. Force
d. Movement

2. Absorbance of the solution is directly proportional to ______
a. Concentration of the solution
b. Concentration of the solute
c. Concentration of the liquid
d. Concentration of the mixture

3. The wavelength of 520 used usually to read ______ color of solution.
a. Red
b. Pink
c. Yellow
d. Orange

4. The wavelength range of visible light is:
a. 400 to 700 nm
b. 450 to 650 nm
c. 700 to 1000 nm
d. 200 to 400 nm

5. The splitting of white light into seven colors is known as
a. Disruption
b. Dispersion
c. Distribution
d. Disturbance

6. The source of UV light in a spectrophotometer is:
a. Tungsten lamp
b. Deuterium lamp
c. Helium lamp
d. Neon lamp

5

UNIT

Electrophoresis

LEARNING OBJECTIVES

At the end of this unit, the learner should be able to understand:
- General principles of electrophoresis.
- The types of electrophoresis.
- Procedures and advantages of electrophoresis.

INTRODUCTION

Electrophoresis is the popular technique used in the clinical and research laboratories for the separation of closely-related compounds, such as mixture of proteins, amino acid and enzymes.

General Principle of Electrophoresis

This technique is used for the separation of charged particles.

Biological materials, such as amino acids, peptides, proteins, nucleic acids possess ionizable groups and hence exist as charged molecules in solutions, either as cations (positively charged) or anions (negatively charged) depending upon the pH of the medium used. The nonpolar substances such as carbohydrates can be given charges by derivatization, e.g., as borate or phosphates.

These charged particles, such as cations move towards cathode (negatively charged electrode) and anions towards anode (positively charged electrode) in an electric field. So it is obvious that the molecules having similar charges move in the same direction. But there is a difference in the movement due to their different molecular weight. Therefore, the difference in Charge/Mass ratio (C/M) forms the basis for the differential migration of particles in an applied electric field. This forms the general principle of electrophoresis.

Forces Acting in an Electrophoresis System

The rate at which the charged particles migrate depends on the balance between three different forces:

1. *Force of electric field:* Which is the impelling force
2. Frictional force, and
3. *Electrostatic force of attraction between the sample component and the supporting medium:* Which are the retarding forces.

Factors Affecting the Electrophoresis

The Electric Field

Voltage: The rate of migration (movement) is directly proportional to the voltage applied between two electrodes. As the voltage increases the migration may fastens but very high voltage is also not suggestive.

Current: The rate of migration is proportional to current.

Resistance: Migration rate of the sample ions decreases when there is increased resistance.

The Sample

The movement of the sample ions in an electric field mainly depends on the charge, size as well as shape of the sample molecules.

Charge: The rate of migration increases with an increase in the net charge on the component.

Size: The rate of migration decreases when there is increase in the size of the molecule which is to be separated and movement of the molecule increases when the size of the molecule decreases.

Shape: Molecules of similar size, but different shapes, such as fibrous and globular proteins exhibit different migration characteristics because of the differential effect of frictional and electrophoretic forces.

The Buffer

This determines and stabilizes the pH of the supporting medium and hence affects the migration rate of compounds in a number of ways.

Composition: The buffer should be such that it does not bind with the compounds to be separated as this may alter the rates of migration. Therefore, the barbitone buffer is always preferred for the separation of proteins or lipoproteins.

Concentration: As the ionic strength of the buffer increases, the proportion of current carried by the buffer will increase and the share of the current carried by the sample will decrease, thus slowing down the rate of migration. Therefore, ionic strength of 0.05 M is preferred for the separation of proteins, or lipoproteins in an electric field.

pH: For organic compounds pH determines the extent of ionization and therefore degree and direction of migration are pH dependent.

The following example of an amino acid shows how the extent of ionization and direction of migration is dependent on pH.

$$H_3\overset{+}{N}-\underset{}{\overset{R}{\overset{|}{C}}}H-COOH \underset{H^+}{\overset{OH^-}{\rightleftharpoons}} H_3\overset{+}{N}-\overset{R}{\overset{|}{C}}H-COO^- \underset{H^+}{\overset{OH^-}{\rightleftharpoons}} H_2N-\overset{R}{\overset{|}{C}}H-COO^-$$

pH	Acidic	Isoionic point	Alkaline
Ionic form	cation	Zwitter ion	anion
Migration	towards cathode	stationary	towards anode

The Supporting Medium

The composition of supporting medium may cause adsorption, electro-osmosis and molecular sieving, which may influence the rate of migration of compounds. The commonly using supporting medium in the laboratory are agarose, polyacrylamide and cellulose acetate membrane.

Types of Electrophoresis

1. *Depending upon the nature of supporting medium:*
   a. Agar gel electrophoresis (AGE)—where agar gel is used as supporting medium.
   b. Polyacrylamide gel electrophoresis (PAGE).
      Acrylamide and methylene bis-acrylamide forms a polymer in this case.
   c. Cellulose acetate electrophoresis (paper strip electrophoresis)
      Cellulose acetate membrane serves as the supporting medium.
2. *Depending upon the mode of technique:*
   a. Slide gel electrophoresis
   b. Tube gel electrophoresis
   c. Disc electrophoresis
   d. Low and high voltage electrophoresis.

Applications

The electrophoresis is useful in:

1. Separating serum proteins for diagnostic purposes
2. Hemoglobin separation
3. Lipoprotein separation and identification
4. Isoenzyme separation and their analysis
5. Nucleic acid studies
6. Determination of molecular weight of the proteins.

Serum Protein Separation by Agar Gel Electrophoresis

Procedure

Steps involved are:

Slide Preparation

About 1.4 mL of warm (60°C) agar solution (100 mg/10 mL of barbitone buffer) is delivered on a slide uniformly at room temperature and allowed to solidify.

Chamber Saturation

Twenty minutes before starting the experiment, both the buffer tanks of the electrophoretic chamber **(Fig. 5.1)** are filled with equal volume of 0.05 M barbitone buffer (pH-8.6) and kept closed to saturate the chamber with solvent vapors.

Sample Application

Small filter paper strip (Whatman No.1, 1 × 5 mm) soaked in the serum sample is kept on the slide perpendicular to the length of the slide close towards the cathode and the chamber is closed.

Slide Projection and Wick Connection

The slide prepared is kept in the chamber and connected to buffer by means of filter paper strips (Wicks) as shown in the **Figure 5.1**.

Application of Electric Field

The electrophoretic chamber is connected to a power pack (equipment used to alter or adjust the required current or voltage values). The power pack is switched on and current is adjusted so that 4 m ampere current flows through each slide. The process has to be carried out for about 90 to 120 minutes.

Fixing of Proteins

The slides are kept immersed in the absolute alcohol for about 20 minutes to prevent the diffusion of separated proteins.

Staining

The slides are dried and kept immersed in the Amido Schwartz 10B dye for about 5 minutes.

Destaining

The stained slides are washed with 3% acetic acid to clear the background and to see the protein bands clearly.

The dried slides can be preserved for a long time. Since the electrophoretic pattern of serum proteins in certain diseases vary markedly from a normal pattern. It is of great diagnostic significance in several conditions, such as nephrosis, liver disease, multiple myeloma, gamma globulinemia and others. The electrophoretic pattern of normal serum and serum samples from patients are shown in **Figure 10.1 of Unit 10.**

Sodium Dodecyl Sulfate Polyacrylamide Gel Electrophoresis (SDS-PAGE)

It is a technique widely used in biochemistry, forensics, genetics and molecular biology

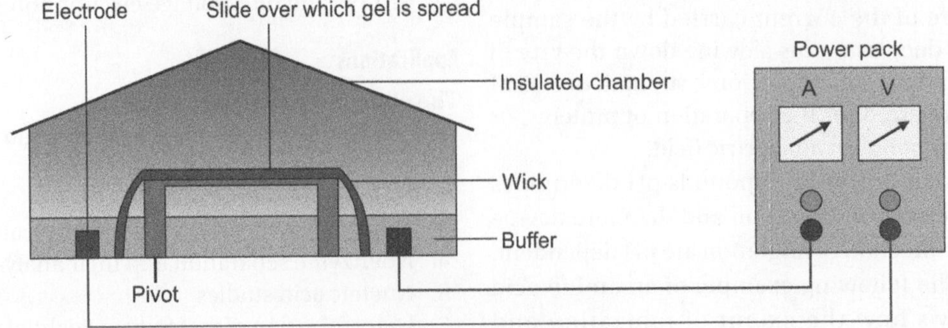

Fig. 5.1: Electrophoresis.

to separate proteins according to their electrophoretic mobility. SDS is an anionic detergent applied to protein sample to linearize proteins and to impart a negative charge to linearized proteins. In most proteins, the binding of SDS to the polypeptide chain imparts an even distribution of charge per unit mass, thereby resulting in a fractionation by approximate size during electrophoresis.

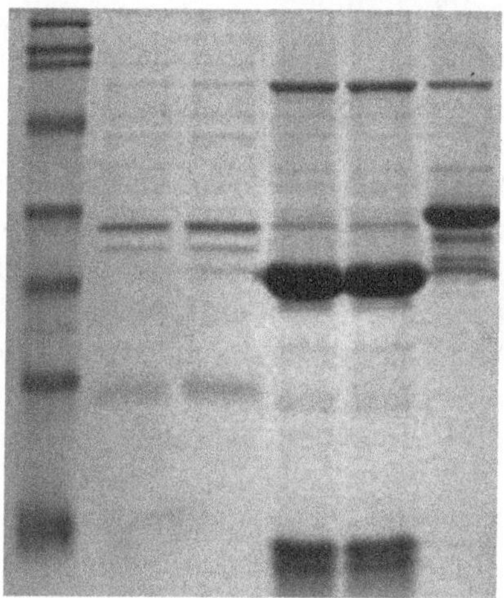

Procedure

Sample Preparation

Samples may be any material-containing proteins, e.g., prokaryotic or eukaryotic cells, tissues, viruses, environmental samples, or purified proteins. In the case of solid tissues, these are often first broken down mechanically using a homogenizer, sonicator or by using cycling of high pressure. Cells may also be broken open by one of the above mechanical methods.

In the case of tissues or cells, a combination of biochemical and mechanical techniques —including various types of filtration and centrifugation—may be used to separate different cell compartments and organelles prior to electrophoresis.

The sample to be analyzed is mixed with SDS, an anionic detergent which denatures secondary and non-disulfide-linked tertiary structures, and applies a negative charge to each protein in proportion to its mass. Heating the samples to at least 60°C further promotes protein denaturation, helping SDS to bind.

1. Mix 50 μL of each sample with an equal volume of one of the denaturing buffers given below.
2. Heat in a boiling water bath for one minute. In most cases, brief boiling (1 to 2 min) improves denaturation, but it may also cause the protein to precipitate.

Preparation of Denaturing Buffer

Tris-HCl	0.25 M
SDS	2%
β-Mercaptoethanol	2% (V/V)
Urea	8 M
Glycerol	0
Bromophenol blue	0.001%
pH	6.2

Running Buffer

Glycine	1.92 M (144g/L)
Tris base	0.25 M (36.3g/L)
SDS	1% (10 g/L)

Dilute 10-fold before use. Replace if the final pH is not within 0.1 pH units of pH 8.3.

Staining Solution: Dissolve 20 mg of CPTS in 1 L of 6 mm HCl. This solution is stable at room temperature.

Wash solution: 6 mm HCl in 20% (v/v) methanol (0.5 mL concentrated HCl in 799.5 mL deionized water, 200 mL methanol). This solution is stable forever at room temperature.

Preparing Acrylamide Gels

The gels typically consist of acrylamide, bisacrylamide, SDS, and a buffer with an adjusted pH. The solution may be degassed under a vacuum to prevent the formation of air bubbles during polymerization. Alternatively, butanol may be added to the resolving gel after it is poured, as butanol removes bubbles and makes the surface smooth. A source of free radicals and a stabilizer, such as ammonium persulfate and TEMED are added to initiate polymerization. The polymerization reaction results in a gel because of the added bisacrylamide, generally about 1 part in 35 relative to acrylamide, which can form cross-links between two polyacrylamide molecules. The ratio of acrylamide to bisacrylamide can be varied for special purposes. The acrylamide concentration of the gel can also be varied, generally in the range from 5 to 25%. Lower percentage gels are better for resolving very high molecular weight proteins, while much higher percentages are needed to resolve smaller proteins. Gels are usually polymerized between two glass plates in a gel caster, with a comb inserted at the top to create the sample wells. After the gel is polymerized, the comb can be removed and the gel is ready for electrophoresis.

Procedure

1. Remove the comb and clamp the gel to the electrophoretic apparatus.
2. Fill the top electrolyte compartment with running buffer.
3. Check for leaks from the top into the bottom compartment. If there are no leaks, fill the bottom compartment.
4. With a plastic Pasteur pipette, thoroughly rinse each well in the stacking gel with running buffer.
5. Apply the sample by using a micropipette to carefully add up to ~25 µL of protein in DB1 or DB2 to the bottom of a well. The volume and protein concentration of the sample should be sufficient to give at least 10 µg of each protein. If possible, avoid using the end wells.
6. Apply 15 µL of the molecular weight standards to one or two wells, preferably in an asymmetric position, to allow the front and back of the gel to be identified later.
7. Carefully record the contents of each well.
8. Replace the cover of the electrophoretic cell, with the (+) symbol on the cover connected to the (+) on the cell, so that the anode (+) is the bottom electrode.
9. Check the electrical connections on the cell to ensure that solution is not in contact with either banana plug, and connect the anode to the (+) terminal on the power supply, and the cathode to the negative terminal. (Notice the convention inversion for electrodes: + is the anode, and - the cathode).
10. Apply 15 mA/gel until the proteins are well into the stacking gel, then 35 mA/gel until the tracking dye reaches the bottom of the gel (about 45 minutes in this system).
11. A tracking dye may be added to the protein solution. This typically has a higher electrophoretic mobility than the proteins.

Electrophoresis

Various buffer systems are used in SDS-PAGE depending on the nature of the sample and the experimental objective. The buffers used at the anode and cathode may be the same or different.

An electric field is applied across the gel, causing the negatively-charged proteins to migrate across the gel towards the positive (+) electrode (anode). Depending on their size, each protein will move differently through the gel matrix—short proteins will more easily fit through the pores in the gel, while larger ones will have more difficulty. After a set amount of time the proteins will have differentially migrated based on their size, smaller proteins will have traveled farther down the gel, while larger ones will have remained closer to the point of origin. Proteins may therefore be separated roughly according to size (and thus molecular weight); however, certain glycoproteins behave anomalously on SDS gels.

Following electrophoresis, the gel may be stained (most commonly with Coomassie Brilliant Blue R-250 or silver stain), allowing visualization of the separated proteins, or processed further. After staining, different proteins will appear as distinct bands within the gel. It is common to run molecular weight size markers of known molecular weight in a separate lane in the gel, in order to calibrate the gel and determine the approximate molecular mass of unknown proteins by comparing the distance traveled relative to the marker.

Add enough staining solution to cover the gel.

Stain for an hour or until adequately stained remove the staining solution and replace with 100 mL wash solution (**Fig. 5.2**).

Swirl the wash over the gel by rocking the (covered) container for several minutes/hours, or until excess stain is removed and unstained areas are completely clear.

The SDS-PAGE is usually the first choice as an assay of protein purity due to its reliability and ease. The presence of SDS and the denaturing step causes proteins to be separated approximately based on size, but aberrant migration of some proteins may occur. PAGE may also be used as a preparative technique for the purification of proteins.

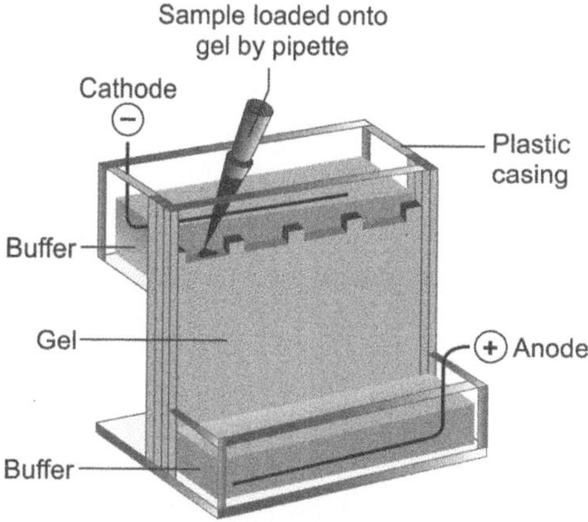

Fig. 5.2: Polyacrylamide gel electrophoresis

SELF TEST

1. Give the general principle of electrophoresis.
2. Enumerate the application of electrophoretic techniques.
3. Explain the various factors affecting electrophoretic mobility of the sample.
4. Discuss the procedure used in the separation of serum protein electrophoresis and mention its diagnostic importance.

MULTIPLE CHOICE QUESTIONS

1. **The extent of ionization of the compounds is determined by:**
   a. Ionic strength of the buffer
   b. pH of the buffer
   c. Voltage
   d. Volume of the buffer
2. **Amido Schwartz 10B is used for the following purpose in electrophoresis:**
   a. Staining hemoglobin
   b. For fixing
   c. For washing
   d. For staining proteins
3. **The pH of the buffer used in serum protein electrophoresis on agar gel is:**
   a. 8.6
   b. 7.6
   c. 9.6
   d. 6.6
4. **All the following are the applications of electrophoresis, *Except***
   a. Separating serum proteins
   b. Separating cellular organelles
   c. Hemoglobin separation
   d. Lipoprotein separation and identification
5. **The basic principle of electrophoresis depends on:**
   a. Charge/Mass ratio
   b. Weight
   c. Number of ions
   d. Volume of the buffer

6. **Concerning electrophoresis, one of the following statements is INCORRECT:**
   a. The cations move towards cathode
   b. The rate of migration decreases with an increase in the net charge of the component
   c. Charge/Mass ratio forms the basis for the differential migration of particles in an applied electric field
   d. Rate of migration is directly proportional to the voltage
7. **Concerning the applications of electrophoresis, one of the following statements is INCORRECT:**
   a. It is used to separating serum proteins
   b. It is used to hemoglobin variants
   c. It is used to separate subcellular organelles
   d. It is used to isoenzymes

6

UNIT

Chromatography

LEARNING OBJECTIVES

At the end of this unit, the learner should be able to understand:

- General principle of chromatography.
- The types of chromatography.
- Procedures and advantages of different types of chromatography.

INTRODUCTION

Chromatography is the technique used for the separation of a number of similar components in a mixture. These closely related compounds include proteins, peptides, amino acids, lipids, carbohydrates, vitamins and drugs. This technique is based on the principle of adsorption, partition, ion exchange and exclusion properties. The selection of a particular type of chromatography to separate the components depends on the material to be isolated.

GENERAL PRINCIPLE

Chromatography consists of a mobile and a stationary phase. The mobile phase refers to the mixture of substance to be separated in a liquid or a gas. The stationary phase is a porous or solid matrix through which the sample contained in the mobile phase enters. The interaction between the stationary and the mobile phase causes the separation of compounds from the mixture. These interactions include adsorption, partition, ion exchange and exclusion type of physicochemical properties.

CLASSIFICATION OF CHROMATOGRAPHY

The type of interaction medium used for stationary phase and mobile phase is the basis of classification of chromatography.

1. *Column chromatography:* In which the stationary phase is packed into glass or metal columns. There are several types of column chromatography, which are as follows:
   a. Partition chromatography
   b. Adsorption chromatography
   c. Ion-exchange chromatography
   d. Gel filtration chromatography
   e. Affinity chromatography
   f. High pressure liquid chromatography (HPLC).
2. *Paper chromatography:* In which the stationary phase is supported by the cellulose fibers of a paper sheet. There are two types:
   a. Ascending
   b. Descending.
3. *Thin layer chromatography:* The stationary phase is thinly coated onto glass, plastic or foil plates.
4. Gas-liquid chromatography.

Principle of Partition Chromatography

The molecules, which are to be separated undergo continuous redistribution between two immiscible phases (stationary phase and a mobile phase). The separation depends on the relative tendencies of the molecule in a mixture to associate more strongly with one or the other phases. Since partitioning process is repeated hundreds or thousand times, small difference in partition ratio permit excellent separation.

For a compound distributing itself between two given solvents the value for this coefficient is a constant at a given temperature and can be defined as follows:

$$\frac{\text{The concentration in solvent A}}{\text{The concentration in solvent B}} = \text{Constant}$$

In paper chromatography, paper serves as a solid support to hold the stationary phase. The solvent system provides both stationary phase and mobile phase. For amino acid chromatography, butanol, acetic acid, water in the proportion of 4:1:5 V/V is used as solvent system. Butanol with a little acetic acid acts as the mobile phase and water-acetic acid forms the stationary phase, which will be held to the paper.

Procedure

- Add the solvent mixture (18 mL n-butanol + 4.5 mL glacial acetic acid + 7.5 mL reagent (grade water) to solvent trough, which is placed in the chromatography chamber and close the chamber.
- Draw a line about one inch from the bottom of the special filter paper (Whatman No 1).
- Mark the spots 1 cm apart along this line.
- Label the spots as indicated in **Figure 6.1**.
- Place small amount of the 0.5% of standard or unknown onto the labeled spot of the paper using Hamilton Oxford pipette or Hamilton syringe.
- Dry the spots.
- Then the marked end of the paper which is added with the sample, dipped in the solvent system so that solvent moves by capillary action and by gravitational forces **(Fig. 6.1)**.
- After 4 hours or when the solvent reaches lower end remove the paper immediately and accurately draw a pencil line across the paper at the solvent front.
- Paper is completely dried and sprayed with 0.2% ninhydrin solution.
- Again dry the paper under fan.
- Next dry the paper in the oven at 80°C for 5 to 10 minutes or until the amino acid spots appear. Mark the spots and calculate the Rf values for each and identify the unknowns.

The separation of the solute depends on the partition coefficient (Kd) of each solute. It is written as follows:

$$\text{Kd} = \frac{\text{Concentration of solute in the stationary phase}}{\text{Concentration of solute in the mobile phase}}$$

The similar compounds with different Kd will move to different extents. For the identification of separation of different solutes, Rf value is considered. Rf value is given as:

$$\text{Rf} = \frac{\text{Distance traveled by the solute (a - cm)}}{\text{Distance traveled by the solvent (A - cm)}}$$

Other Chromatographic Techniques

Adsorption Chromatography (Fig. 6.2)

This was the original chromatographic technique employed by Tswett to separate colored pigments. In this technique, separation of components depends on the difference both in their degree of adsorption on the surface of a solid stationary medium, such as silica gel or alumina and solubility in the solvent used for separation. During the elution, weekly held substances move fast. Strongly held substances are eluted by changing pH and salt concentrations. There are various adsorbent, such as silicic acid, aluminum oxide, calcium carbonate, zinc carbonate and magnesium oxide available commercially. The adsorbent used for column, paper and

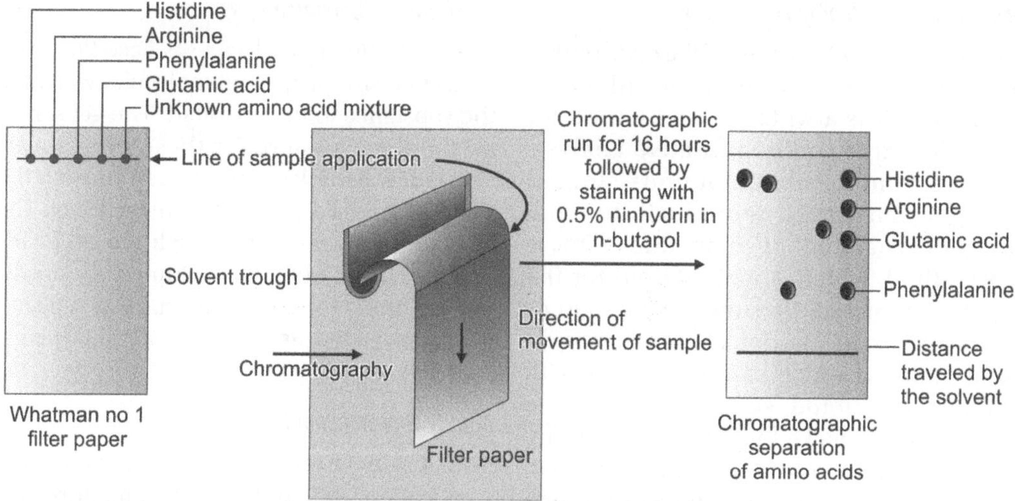

Fig. 6.1: Descending type of paper chromatography.

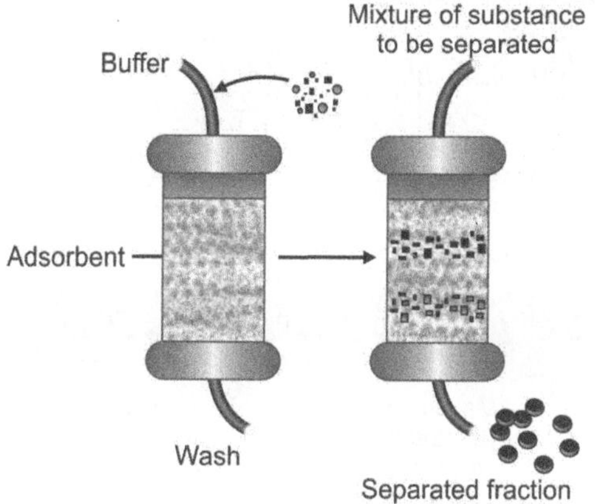

Fig. 6.2: Adsorption chromatography.

thin layer chromatography are composed of irregular-shaped porous particles **(Fig. 6.3)**.

Thin Layer Chromatography

The principle is same as paper chromatography (partition chromatography). The slurry of the stationary phase, such as cellulose, generally in water, is applied to a glass, plastic or foils plate as a uniform thin layer by means of a plate spreader starting at one end of the plate and moving progressively to the other. For analytical separations, the layer is of the order of 0.5 mm and for the preparative separations, it is up to 5 mm. After the stationary phase is coated, the drying can be done in an oven at 100° to 120°C. The sample and the standard mixture are applied with the help of a microsyringe at the one edge of the plate. For the separation, the plate is kept in a tank, which contains developing solvent. The plate is removed after one hour from the tank and it is sprayed with ninhydrin solution if the materials to be separated are amino acids. Compare with the standard to identify the unknown compound or the Rf value of the each spot is calculated and the value is compared with known set of amino acids. Chromatographic separation is faster in this method.

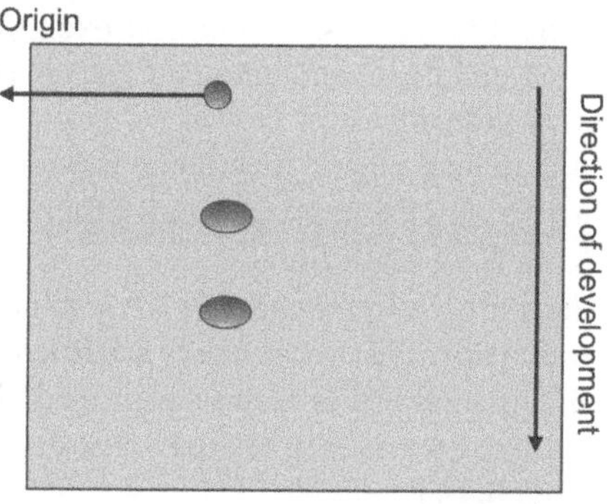

Fig. 6.3: Descending chromatography.

Gas-liquid Chromatography

This technique is based upon the distribution of compounds between a liquid and a gas phase. It is a widely used method for the qualitative and quantitative analysis of large number of compounds since it has high sensitivity, reproducibility and speed of separation of compounds. This is the method, which is mainly used for the separation of volatile substances, such as lipids and drugs. Stationary phase is inert solid material which is impregnated with a nonvolatile liquid, such as polyethylene glycol. This is packed in a narrow column. Under proper condition, volatile material, which is to be separated is passed through column with the help of an inert gas (Argon). Separation of individual substance is based on partition of components.

Ion-exchange Chromatography

In this technique, there is attraction between oppositely charged molecules. Therefore, the separation of molecules is based on their charges. The biological materials, such as amino acids and proteins have ionizable groups that they carry a net positive or negative charge can be utilized in separating mixtures of such compounds. The net charge exhibited by those compounds is purely dependent on the pH of the solution and the isoionic point of the compound. These ion exchange separations are mainly carried out in columns packed with ion exchange resins. Ion-exchange resins used for this purpose are cation exchanger (e.g., CM-cellulose) and anion exchanger (e.g., DEAE-cellulose).

a. *Anion exchanger:* Anion exchanger R^+A^- exchanges its anion (A^-) with other anion (e.g., B) in a solution.
b. Similarly cation exchanger R^-A^+ exchanges its cation (A^+) with other cation (e.g., B^+) ion, which is to be separated. This technique is highly pH dependent **(Fig. 6.4A)**.

Gel Filtration Chromatography

The separation of molecules is based on their molecular size, shape and molecular weight of the substance to be separated. The gel serves as a molecular sieve for these substances. The larger particles cannot pass through the pores of the gel and therefore move faster. The smaller particles enter through the gel beads and they come out of the column very slowly. For example, for gel filtration, materials are Sephadex G-100, Sephadex G-200 and Bio gel P-10 **(Fig. 6.4B)**.

Affinity Chromatography

The affinity chromatography gives absolute purification, even from complex mixture, in a

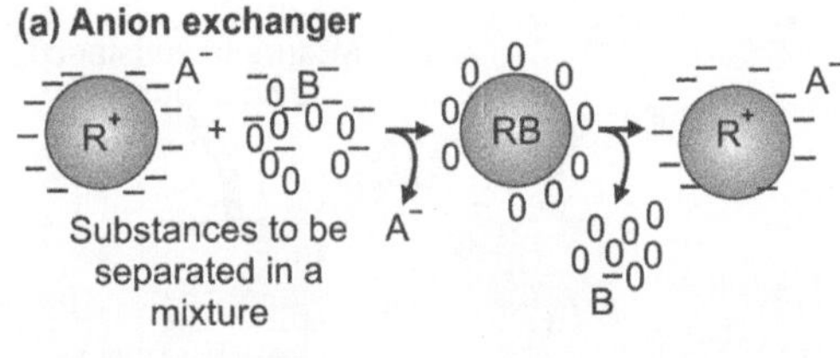

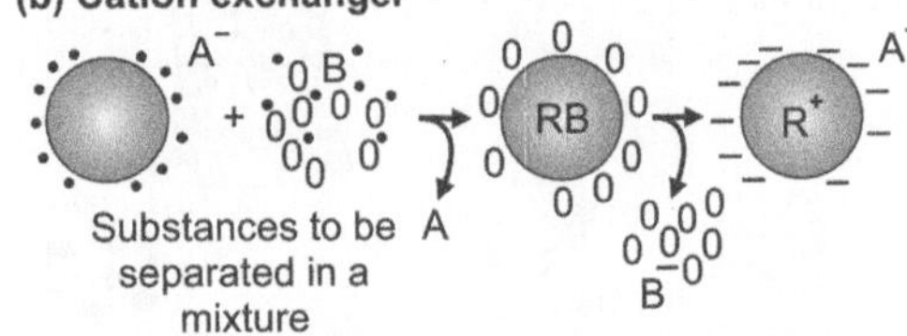

Fig. 6.4A: Ion-exchange chromatography.

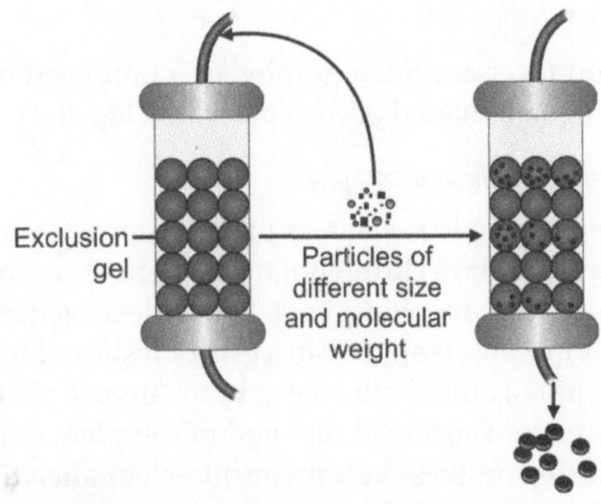

Fig. 6.4B: Gel filtration chromatography.

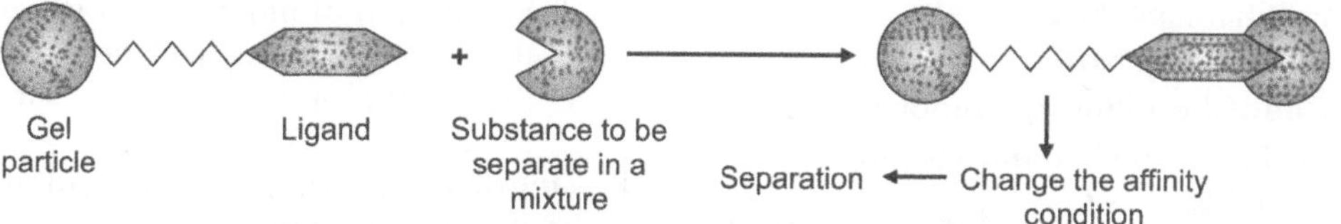

Fig. 6.5: Affinity chromatography.

single process. This was originally developed for the purification of enzymes, now it has been extended for the purification of nucleic acids, immunoglobulin and membrane receptors. The principle is based on the specific and noncovalent binding of substances (such as proteins and enzymes) to a specific ligand (cofactor or substrates) attached to the gel matrix. For example, separation of lactate dehydrogenase from RBC using NAD^+ ligand linked to an affinity gel **(Fig. 6.5)**.

High Performance Liquid Chromatography (HPLC)

The chromatographic techniques explained above are slow and time consuming. So the separation can be greatly improved by applying high pressure in the range of 5000–10000 psi (pounds per square inch). HPLC requires non-compressible resin materials and strong metal column generally made of stainless steel and are manufactured in such a way that they can withstand pressures up to 8000 psi. The column may be packed with one of the materials for adsorption, partition, ion exchange or gel filtration chromatography.

Applications of Chromatography

1. The chromatographic technique is used for the separation of amino acids, proteins and carbohydrates.
2. It is also used for the analysis of drugs, hormones, vitamins and brain amines.
3. Helpful for the qualitative and quantitative analysis of complex mixtures.
4. The technique is also useful for the determination of molecular weight of proteins.
5. The technique is used to separate and identify the phytochemical constituents present in plant extracts.

SELF TEST

1. Define the term chromatography.
2. What are the different types of chromatography techniques?
3. Explain the principle of partition chromatography.
4. Write the steps involved in paper chromatography of amino acids.
5. Name the solvent system required for the paper chromatography of amino acids.
6. Define the Rf-value. Give its use.

MULTIPLE CHOICE QUESTIONS

1. **The compounds get separated from each other on the basis of their molecular weight in the following technique:**
   a. Ion-exchange chromatography
   b. Thin layer chromatography
   c. Affinity chromatography
   d. Gel filtration chromatography
2. **The chromatography technique is used to:**
   a. Purify salts
   b. Purify proteins
   c. Determining the nature of carbohydrates
   d. None of the above
3. **The filter paper used in the paper chromatography to separate amino acid is:**
   a. Whatman No 8
   b. Whatman No 1

c. Whatman No 5
d. Whatman No 6

4. One of the following cannot be separated by thin layer chromatography:
a. Lipids
b. Amino acids
c. Cell organelles
d. Phytochemical constituents of plants

5. Concerning chromatography, one of the following is incorrect:
a. Separation of molecules is based on their volume
b. Separation of molecules is based on their molecular size of the substance
c. Separation of molecules is based on the shape of the substance
d. Separation of molecules is based on their molecular weight of the substance
e. Separation of molecules is based on their charge

6. One of the following is not an application of chromatography:
a. It is used for the separation of amino acids and carbohydrates
b. It is used for the qualitative and quantitative analysis of complex mixtures
c. It is used for the identification nucleic acids
d. Is useful for the determination of molecular weight of proteins

7

UNIT

Immunochemical Techniques (RIA and ELISA)

LEARNING OBJECTIVES

At the end of this unit, the learner should be able to understand:

- The principle procedure and significance of radioimmunoassay.
- The principle procedure and significance of enzyme-linked immunosorbent assay.
- The Principle of Electrochemiluminescent assay.

INTRODUCTION

Immunology is the study of the immune responses, by which the animal defends itself against invasion by foreign organisms. Immune response can be divided into two general types; the antibody mediated response and cell mediated response. The immunochemical techniques employ the antibodies involved in humoral immunity. The substance, which is produced in response to foreign body invasion, is called the antibody and the foreign organisms are considered as antigen. The immunochemical techniques are available to detect or to quantitate the antigen or antibody. They are:

Radioimmunoassay (RIA) and enzyme-linked immunosorbent assay (ELISA) are the two important sophisticated immunoassay techniques available, which are used to measure hormones, drugs, tumor markers and antigens in biological samples.

RADIOIMMUNOASSAY

Radioimmunoassay (RIA) is one of the most important techniques used in the clinical and biochemical field for the quantitative analysis of hormones, steroids and drugs.

Any immunoassay technique involves the reaction between an antigen and its specific antibody.

This immunoassay technique utilizes radioactive isotopes.

ISOTOPES

Atoms of a given element with same atomic number (i.e., no. of protons) but with different atomic mass (i.e., no. of neutrons is different) are called isotopes, e.g., carbon

1. ${}^{14}_{6}C$ is an isotope of carbon (${}^{12}C$) which is written as ${}^{14}C$.
2. ${}^{2}H$ and ${}^{3}H$ (Tritium) are isotopes of hydrogen (${}^{1}H$)
3. ${}^{125}I$, ${}^{131}I$ are isotopes of Iodine (${}^{127}I$).

Radioactive Isotopes

Radioactive isotopes are unstable isotopes which emit particles or electromagnetic radiation, For example,

${}^{14}C$, ${}^{3}H$, etc., emit beta (β) particles.

${}^{125}I$ and ${}^{131}I$ emit gamma (γ) rays.

The instruments, which measure the radioactivity are called scintillation counters—β-emissions are measured in a liquid scintillation counter and γ rays in a γ counter.

The radioactivity is measured as counts per minute. Unit of expression of radioactivity is Curie, millicurie, microcurie, etc.

Half-life

Half-life of a radioactive element is defined as the time taken for the activity to fall from its original value to half of that value. Half-lives of some commonly used isotopes are as follows:

Isotope	Half-life
• ^{3}H	120 days
• ^{14}C	120 days
• ^{125}I	60 days
• ^{131}I	8 days

Antibody

Antibody is a protective protein, which is produced in an animal's body in response to a foreign substance, and it is capable of binding with that of foreign substance.

Antigen

Antigen is a foreign substance that stimulates the production of specific antibody molecules when introduced into the animal's body.

Principle of Radioimmunoassay

This technique is based on the competition between unlabeled antigen and labeled antigen for a limited number of antibodies. At the end of the reaction time, the reaction tube would contain both antigen-antibody complex as well as free antigens (labeled and unlabeled). Under standard conditions, the amount of labeled antigen bound to the antibody will decrease as the amount of unlabeled antigen (antigen in the patient sample) increases. This is explained by the example given below:

4 Ag* + 4 Ab→ 4 Ag* Ab

4 Ag + 4 Ag* + 4 Ab→ 2Ag*Ab + 2Ag Ab + 2Ag* + 2Ag

10Ag + 4Ag* + 4Ab → Ag*Ab + 3AgAb + 3Ag* + 7Ag

Ab = antibody, Ag = antigen (unlabeled)

Ag* = labeled antigen, AgAb = antigen-antibody complex.

The radioactivity of the bound labeled antigen (Ag* Ab) is measured. Therefore, the radioactivity count is inversely proportional to the unlabeled antigen concentration.

In the example given above, number of the antibody and the labeled antigen is kept constant. Only the number of the unlabeled antigen is increased. The same principle is followed in the assay system. A standard curve is constructed by performing the assay with different concentrations of the standard antigen solution taken in different tubes. A graph is plotted by taking the standard antigen concentration on x-axis and counts per minute (cpm) values on y-axis **(Fig. 7.1)**.

Using this standard graph, the amount of antigen (unlabeled) in the patient sample is estimated. Applications of RIA:

A variety of compounds, which are present in serum or other biological fluids in very small amounts, can be estimated by this technique, For example,

1. Hormones like Thyroxin (T4), tri-iodothyronine (T3), insulin, cortisol, renin, aldosterone, follicular stimulating hormone, luteinizing hormone, etc.

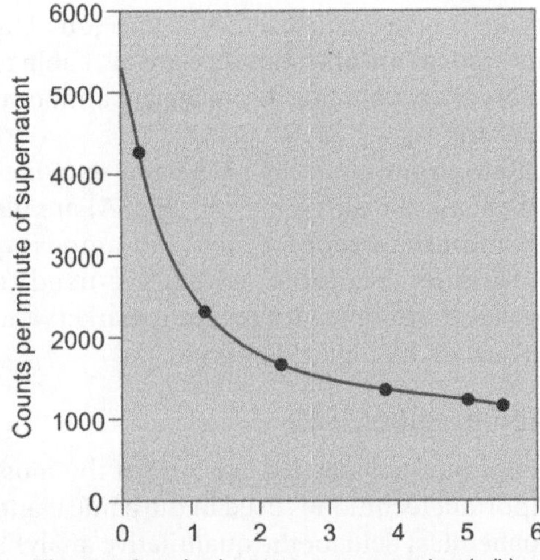

Fig. 7.1: Standard antigen concentration (μ/L).

2. Tumor markers like prostate specific antigen (PSA), alpha fetoprotein (AFP), etc.
3. Vitamins.
4. Drugs like digoxin.

Advantages and Disadvantages of Radioimmunoassay

Advantages

1. The method is highly sensitive—very small concentrations even up to the picogram level of the antigen can be measured.
2. It is a highly specific method.

Disadvantages

1. High cost of the equipments and the reagents.
2. The shelf life of the reagents ^{125}I, ^{131}I is quite short due to their short half-life. Hence, the reagents cannot be stored for long.
3. *Radiological hazards:* Proper care should be taken while handling and disposing radioactive materials to avoid the hazards of radioactivity. Exposure to radioactivity may cause harmful effects to the body.
4. Duration of the assay is very long.

ENZYME-LINKED IMMUNOSORBENT ASSAY OR ENZYME IMMUNOASSAY

In enzyme-linked immunosorbent assay (ELISA) technique, enzymes are used to label the antigens or antibodies.

There are two types of ELISA.

1. Single antibody method (competitive binding method).
2. Double antibody method.

Single Antibody Method (Competitive Method) (Fig. 7.2)

Known amount of enzyme-labeled antigen and an unknown amount of unlabeled antigen (in the patient sample) mixed is allowed to react with a specific antibody attached to a solid phase.

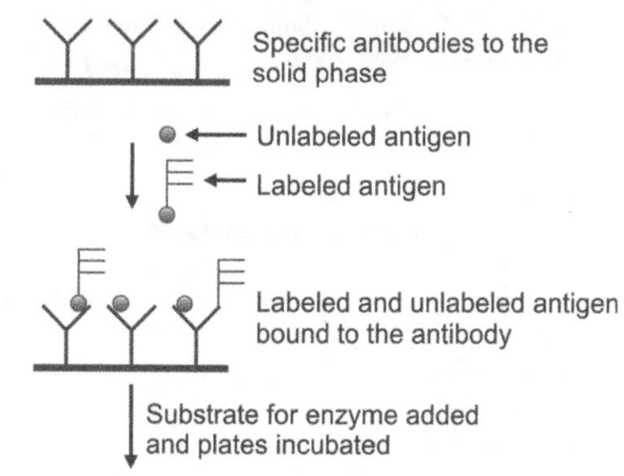

Fig. 7.2: Single antibody method for ELISA.

There is a competition between the labeled and unlabeled antigen for the binding with limited number of antibodies. After specific time of incubation, wells are washed. During washing the unbound antigens are washed off with buffer. After the complex has been washed with buffer, the enzyme substrate is added and the enzyme activity is measured by measuring product formed colorimetrically. The enzyme activity measured is proportional to the labeled antigen and inversely proportional to the amount of unlabeled antigen in the test sample.

Double Antibody Type of Elisa (Sandwich Method)

The unknown antigen (in the test sample) is allowed to bind with the specific antibody attached to a solid phase. Now a second antibody, which is labeled with the enzyme, is added. This antibody binds with the already bound antigen forming an antibody-antigen-antibody complex. The antigen is now sandwiched between two antibodies. After washing off the excess of antibodies, the enzyme substrate is added. The enzyme activity is measured by measuring the product formed colorimetrically. The enzyme activity is directly proportional to the amount of antigen present in the test sample **(Fig. 7.3)**.

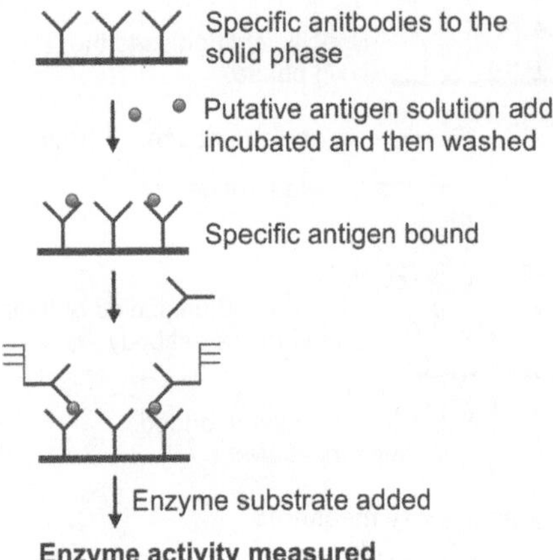

Fig. 7.3: The double antibody method for ELISA.

Indirect Elisa Method

The antibody molecules of the antiserum bind to the antigen and the remaining material is washed away. When this is exposed to enzyme labeled anti-immunoglobulin antibody results in binding to any specific antibody molecules absorbed from the original serum, resulting in degradation proportional to the amount of specific antibody in the original serum.

Applications of ELISA

ELISA is used in the clinical biochemistry laboratories to measure hormones, such as thyroid hormones, insulin, reproductive hormones, pituitary hormones, such as follicle stimulating hormone (FSH), luteinizing hormone (LH) thyroid stimulating hormone (TSH).

Used to measure the level of tumor markers in serum, such as AFP, PSA, HCG, CEA, CA 125, etc.

ELISA is used in the study of infectious diseases, such as detection of bacterial toxins, viruses, hepatitis B surface antigens, etc.

For the assay of antibodies in serum in infectious diseases including antiviral antibodies, e.g., to Epstein-Barr virus, rubella virus and antibacterial antibodies, e.g., to *Brucella, Salmonella.*

For the assay of autoantibodies, e.g., anti-DNA, ANA (antinuclear antibody).

Differences between RIA and ELISA

1. ELISA is cheaper than RIA.
2. Suitable for the use even in small laboratories.
3. Lacks radiological hazards of RIA
4. Reagents have more shelf-lives compared to RIA.
5. ELISA is equally sensitive and specific as RIA.

Materials Used in ELISA

1. Solid phase—plastic tubes or microtiter plates
2. Enzymes—horseradish peroxidase for which substrate is hydrogen peroxide (H_2O_2).
3. Alkaline phosphatase for which substrate is p-nitrophenyl phosphate (PNPP).

Equipment Required

Essential

1. Micropipettes—to dispense volumes of 10 μL, 50 μL , 100 μL and 200 μL as required in the particular ELISA procedure with disposable tips.
2. An incubator capable of maintaining the temperature at 37°C (± 1°C).
3. ELISA reader with the required filter (405 nm, 450 nm, 495 nm, etc.) to measure the color intensity of the solution (a sensitive spectrophotometer which can measure a volume less than 0.5 mL can also be used to read the color intensity or optical density of the solution) **(Figs. 7.4 and 7.5).**

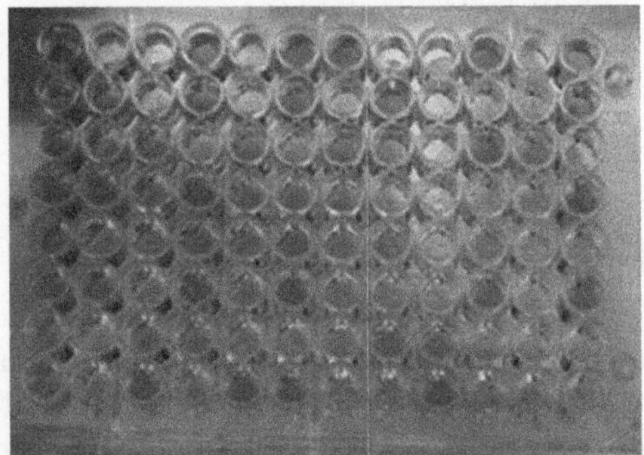

Fig. 7.4: Enzyme-linked immunosorbent assay strip.

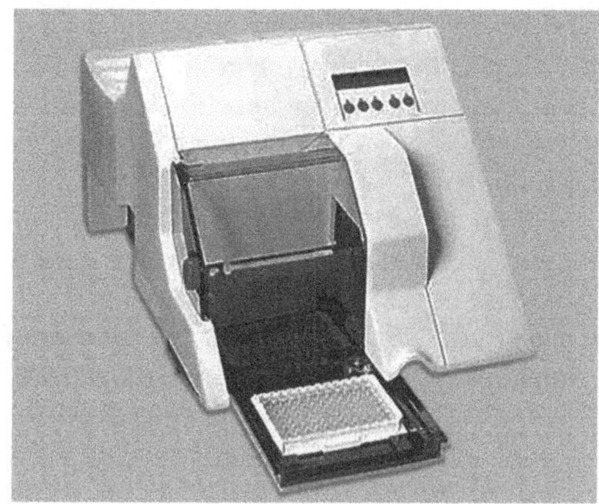

Fig. 7.5: Plate reader.

ELECTROCHEMILUMINESCENT ASSAY

Electrochemiluminescent Assay Principles

Electrochemiluminescent (ECL) processes are known to occur with numerous molecules including compound of ruthenium, osmium, rhenium or other elements.

Electrochemiluminescent is a process in which highly reactive species are generated from stable precursors at the surface of an electrode. These highly reactive species react with one another, producing light.

The development of ECL/origen immunoassays is based on the use of a ruthenium (II) tris [(bipyridyl Ru $(bpy)_3^{2+}$] complex and tripropylamine (TPA). The final chemiluminescent product is formed during the detection step.

The chemiluminescent reactions that lead to the emission of light from the ruthenium complex are initiated electrically, rather than chemically. This is achieved by applying a voltage to the immunological complexes (including the ruthenium complex) that are attached to streptavidin coated microparticles. The advantage of electrically initiating the chemiluminescent reaction is that the entire reaction can be precisely controlled.

Use of the Ruthenium Complex

The ECL technology uses a ruthenium chelate as the complex for the development of the light. Salts of ruthenium-tris (bipyridyl) are stable, water-soluble compounds. The bipyridyl ligands can be readily modified with reactive groups to form activated chemiluminescent compounds.

For the development of ECL immunoassays, [Ru $(bpy)_3^{2+}$] N hydroxysuccinimide (NHS) ester is used because it can be easily coupled with amino groups of proteins, haptens and nucleic acids. This allows the detection technology to be applied to a wide variety of analytes.

The ECL Reaction at the Electrode Surface

Two electrochemically active substances, the ruthenium complex and tripropylamine (TPA), are involved in the reaction that leads to the emission of light. Both substances remain stable, as long as a voltage is not applied **(Fig. 7.6A)**.

The ECL reaction of ruthenium tris (bipyridyl)$^{2+}$ and tripropylamine occurs at the surface of a platinum electrode. The applied voltage creates an electrical field, which causes all the materials in this field to react. Tripropylamine is oxidized at the electrode, releases an electron and forms an intermediate. Tripropylamine radical-cation, which further reacts by releasing a proton (H^+) to form a TPA radical (TPA).

In turn, the ruthenium complex also releases an electron at the surface of the electrode thus oxidizing to form the, Ru $(bpy)_3^{3+}$ cation. This ruthenium cation is the second reaction component for the following chemiluminescent with the TPA radical **(Fig. 7.6B)**.

The TPA and [Ru $(bpy)_3^{3+}$] react with one another, whereby, [Ru $(bpy)_3^{3+}$] is reduced to [Ru$(bpy)_3^{2+}$] and at the same time forms an excited state via energy transfer. This excited state is unstable and decays with the emission of a photon at 620 nm to its original state.

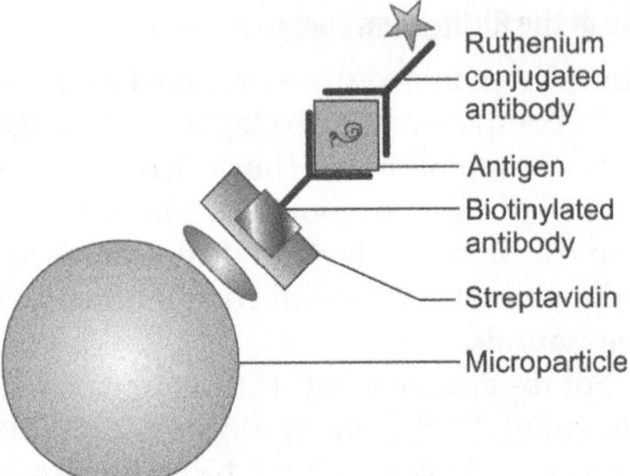

Fig. 7.6A: Electrochemiluminescent reaction.

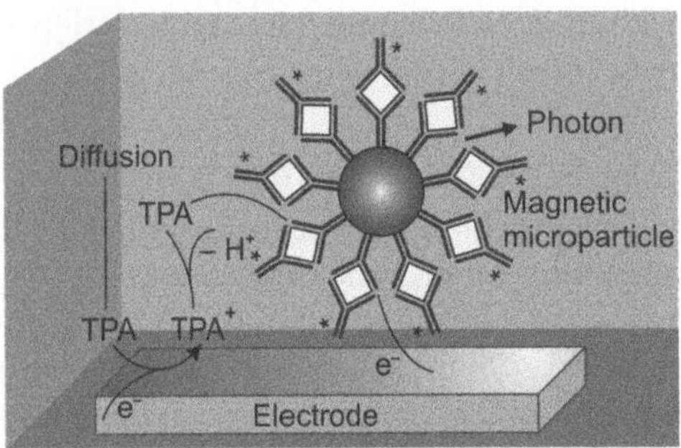

Fig. 7.6B: Electrochemiluminescent reaction.

The reaction cycle can now start again. Tripropylamine radical reduces to by-products, which do not affect the chemiluminescent process. TPA is used up and therefore must be present in excess. The reaction is controlled by diffusion of the TPA and the amount of ruthenium complex present. As TPA in the electrical field is depleted, the signal strength (light) is slowly reduced once the maximum is reached.

Although during measurement, TPA is used up, the ruthenium ground state complex is continuously regenerated. This means that the ruthenium complex can perform many lights generating cycle during the measurement process, therefore showing an inherent amplification effect, which contributes to the technology sensitivity. Many photons can be created form one antigen-antibody complex.

Advantages of ECL Technology

It is a highly innovative technology that offers distinct advantages over detection techniques. Stable non-isotopic label allows liquid reagent convenience.

- Enhanced sensitivity in combination with short incubation times means high quality assays and fast result turnaround.
- Large measuring range of five orders of magnitude minimizes dilutions and repeats, reducing handling time and reagents costs.
- Applicable for the detection of all analytes providing a solid platform for menu expansion.

Competitive Principle (Fig. 7.7)

This principal is applied to analytes of low molecular weight, such as FT3.

- In the first step, sample and a specific anti-T3 antibody labeled with a ruthenium complex are combined in an assay cup.
- After addition of biotinylated T3 and streptavidin-coated paramagnetic micro-particles, the still free binding sites of the labeled antibody become occupied, with formation of an antibody-hapten complex. The entire complex is bound to the microparticle via interaction of biotin and streptavidin.
- After the second incubation, the reaction mixture containing the immune complexes is transported into the measuring cell. The immune complexes are magnetically entrapped on the working electrode. However, unbound reagent and sample are washed away by ProCell.
- In the ECL reaction, the conjugate is a ruthenium-based derivative and the chemiluminescent reaction is electrically stimulated to produce light. The amount of light produced is indirectly proportional to the amount of antigen in the patient sample. Evaluation and calculation of concentration of the antigen are carried out by means of a calibration curve that was established using standards of known antigen concentration.

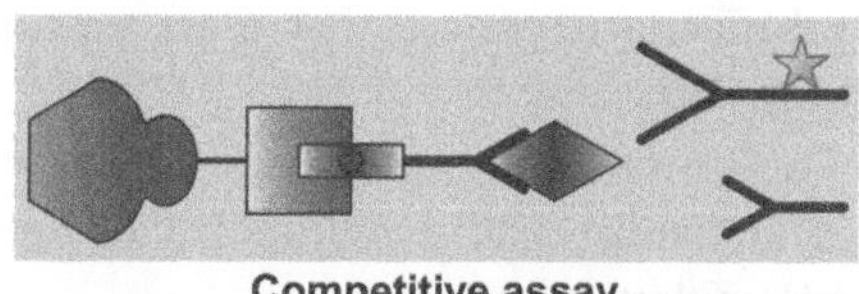

Competitive assay

First reaction
Second reaction
Light reaction
+ TPA ECL
Antigen
Ruthenium labeled antibody
Antigen → Tripropylamine
Biotinylated antigen
Streptavidin-coated microparticle

Competitive principle

Fig. 7.7: Competitive reaction.

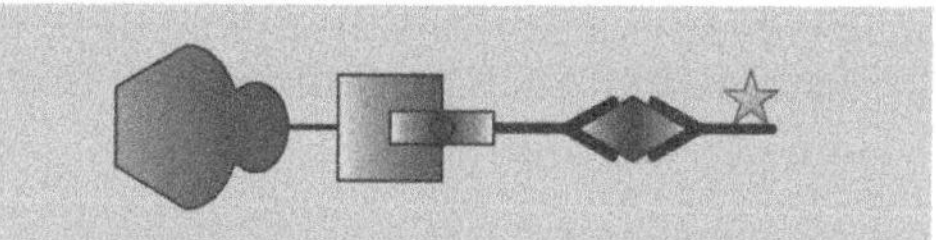

Sandwich matrix for high molecular weight

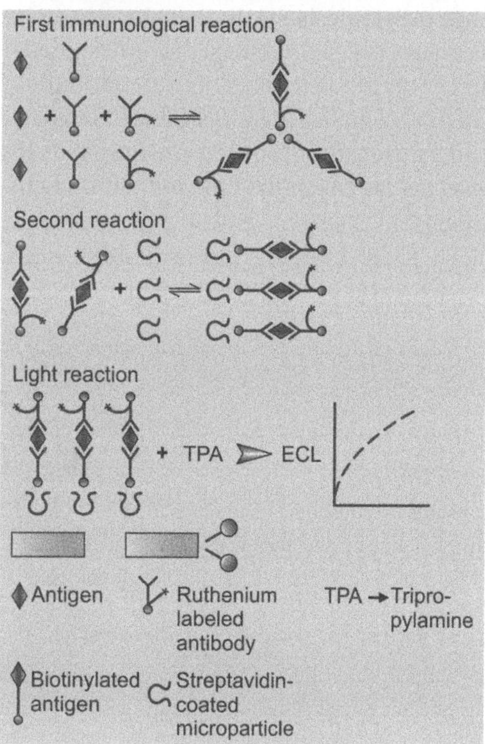

Sandwich principle

Fig. 7.8: Sandwich reaction.

Sandwich Principle (Fig. 7.8)

This principle is applied to higher molecular weight analytes like TSH.

1. Serum is combined with a reagent containing biotinylated TSH antibody and a ruthenium-labeled TSH-specific antibody. During the incubation time, antibodies capture the TSH present in the serum sample.
2. In the second step, streptavidin coated paramagnetic microparticles are added. During the second nine-minute time of incubation, the biotinylated antibody attaches to the streptavidin coated surface of the microparticles.
3. In the third step, the reaction mixture containing the immune complexes is transported into the measuring cell, the immune complexes are magnetically entrapped on the working electrode, but unbound reagent and serum sample are washed away by ProCell.
4. In the ECL reaction, the conjugate is a ruthenium-based derivative and the chemiluminescent reaction is electrically stimulated to produce light. The amount of light produced is directly proportional to the amount of antigen (TSH) in the patient sample.

Evaluation and calculation of concentration of the antigen are carried out by means of a calibration curve that was established using standards of known antigen concentration.

Bridging Principle (Fig. 7.9)

This principle is similar to the sandwich principle, except that the assay is designed to detect antibodies only (Immunoglobulins). This is accomplished by including biotinylated and ruthenium-labeled antigens in the reagents for which the targeted antibody has affinity.

1. In the first step, the serum antibodies bind with the biotinylated and ruthenium-labeled antigens to form an immune complex.
2. The immune complex then reacts with streptavidin coated microparticles via the biotinylated antigen.
3. In the third step, the reaction mixture containing the immune complexes is transported into the measuring cell, the immune complexes are magnetically entrapped on the working electrode, but unbound reagent and serum sample are washed away by ProCell.
4. In the ECL reaction, the conjugate is a ruthenium-based derivative and the

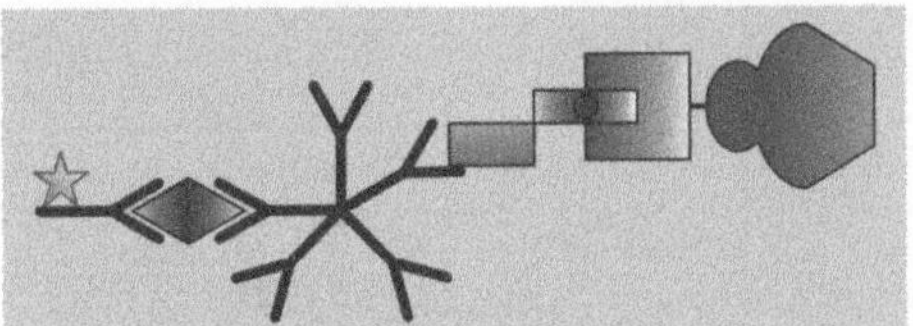

Bridge assay to determine IgA and IgM

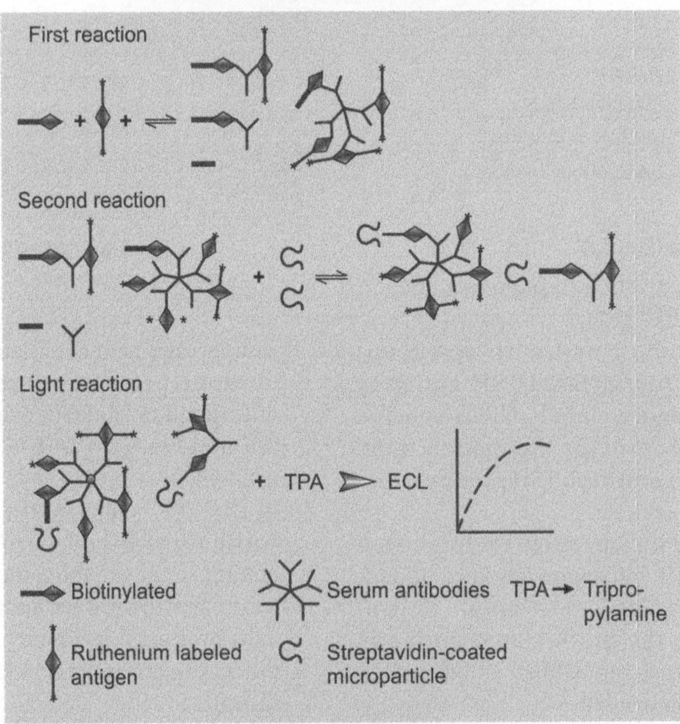

Bridging principle

Fig. 7.9: Bridging reaction.

chemiluminescent reaction is electrically stimulated to produce light. The amount of light produced is directly proportional to the amount of analyte in the sample.

Evaluation and calculation of concentration of the antibody are carried out by means of a calibration curve that was established using standards of known antibody concentration.

SELF TEST

1. What is an isotope? Give two examples.
2. What is the name of the instrument in which radioactivity is measured?
3. What is an antibody?
4. Expand the term ELISA.
5. Name any two enzymes used in ELISA.
6. Write the advantages of ELISA technique over RIA.
7. Name a few investigations, which can be done by ELISA.

MULTIPLE CHOICE QUESTIONS

1. **In RIA, labeled antigen and unlabeled antigen compete for the limited number of:**
   a. Antibodies
   b. Antigens
   c. Complex mixture
   d. Compliments
2. **The radioactivity is measured at the end of radioimmunoassay procedure:**
   a. Bound labeled antigen
   b. Unbound labeled antigen
   c. Labeled antibody
   d. Unlabeled antibody
3. **The radioactivity count is proportional to the test sample:**
   a. Inversely
   b. Directly
   c. Both directly and indirectly
   d. Completely
4. **Half-life of ^{125}I is:**
   a. 129
   b. 125
   c. 140
   d. 130
5. **In ELISA are used as labels:**
   a. Enzymes
   b. Antigens
   c. Antibodies
   d. Antibodies
6. **Labeled antigen and unlabeled antigen compete for the limited number of antibodies in type of ELISA:**
   a. Competitive
   b. Uncompetitive
   c. Non-competitive
   d. Double antibody
7. **The enzyme activity measured is directly proportional to the antigen concentration in the test sample in:**
   a. Double antibody type of ELISA
   b. Single antibody type of ELISA
   c. Double antibody type of RIA
   d. Single antibody type of RIA

8 UNIT Carbohydrates

LEARNING OBJECTIVES

At the end of this unit, the learner should be able to understand:

- Chemistry of carbohydrates.
- Digestion and absorption of carbohydrates.
- The brief explanation about metabolism of carbohydrates.
- Blood glucose determination using different methods.
- The types of diabetes and their symptoms and treatments.
- The regulation of blood glucose.

INTRODUCTION

Glucose is the most important carbohydrate available to the body for various purposes. The carbohydrates, which are taken through the diet, are acted upon by several enzymes and ultimately converted to glucose. Glucose is the primary energy source for the human body. RBCs and brain tissue mainly depend on glucose for their energy requirement.

There are two sources of glucose:

1. *Exogenous source*: The carbohydrate from the diet (Starch of vegetables, grains, liver and muscle).
2. *Endogenous source:* The stored liver glycogen, proteins and other non-carbohydrates, such as glycerol and lactic acid which are available in the body.

Chemistry

Definition: Carbohydrates are defined as polyhydroxy alcohols with free aldehyde or keto groups.

CLASSIFICATION

Monosaccharides

These are the simplest sugars. Monosaccharides are further subdivided into triose, tetrose, pentose, and hexose depending on the number of carbon atoms present. They contain an aldehyde or keto group. Those containing an aldehyde group are aldo sugar and those with keto group are keto sugars.

Number of carbon atoms	*Examples*	*Functional groups present*
Trioses (3 carbons)	Glyceraldehyde	Aldehyde (aldotriose)
	Dihydroxy-acetone	Ketone (Ketotriose)
Tetroses (4 carbons)	Erythrose	Aldehyde (aldotetrose)
Pentoses (5 carbons)	Ribose	Aldehyde (Aldopentose)
	Xylose	Aldehyde (Aldopentose)
	Xylulose	Ketone (Ketopentose)
Hexoses (6 carbons)	Glucose	Aldehyde (Aldohexose)
	Galactose	Aldehyde (Aldohexose)
	Fructose	Ketone (Ketohexose)

Disaccharides

These are molecules containing two same or different monosaccharide units. On hydrolysis, they yield two monosaccharide units. Two monosaccharide units are joined by a glycosidic bond.

Examples	Product formed upon hydrolysis	Glycosidic linkage	Sources
Maltose	Glucose +Glucose	α 1–4	Malt
Lactose	Galactose +Glucose	β 1–4	Milk
Sucrose	Glucose + Fructose	β 1–2	Sugar cane
Isomaltose	Glucose +Glucose	α 1–6	Digestion of amylopectin

Polysaccharides

These are polymer of same monosaccharide units.

These are classified into homo- and hetero-polysaccharides

Homopolysaccharides

Examples of homopolysaccharides are:

Examples	Monosaccharide unit	Sources
Starch	Glucose	Plant, rice
Dextrin	Glucose	From starch hydrolysis
Glycogen	Glucose	Liver, muscle
Cellulose	Glucose	Plant fibers
Inulin	Fructose	Dahlia roots

Starch

Starch is a mixture of two polysaccharides: amylose and amylopectin.

The major difference between amylose and amylopectin is:

Amylose

Unbranched and linear.

Blue color forms because the iodine molecules are trapped inside the helical structure. Color disappears upon heating and reappears upon cooling.

Amylopectin

Highly branched. The branch point appears after every 24–30 glucose units in straight chain form. Gives reddish violet color with iodine.

Heteropolysaccharides

These are made up of more than one type of monosaccharide derivatives. Examples

Include hyaluronic acid, chondroitin sulfate, heparin, keratan sulfate, heparan sulfate and dermatan sulfate.

Digestion of Carbohydrates (Fig. 8.1)

- The diet of human beings contains carbohydrates, fat and proteins, which are complex compounds of high molecular weight.
- They are absorbed only when they are hydrolyzed to simpler forms.
- The major carbohydrates of our diet, such as starch and glycogen, are the polysaccharides. These polysaccharides are hydrolyzed to maltose and glucose by the action of several enzymes.
- The digestion of carbohydrates starts in the mouth.
- Salivary amylase hydrolyzes α-1, 4-glycosidic linkages randomly within the polysaccharide chain and produce disaccharides and monosaccharides.
- After the food reaches duodenum, pancreatic amylase also helps in the digestion of polysaccharides.
- Further digestion takes place in the small intestine by the intestinal enzymes, which hydrolyze terminal α-1,4-glycosidic linkages.
- At the same time, disaccharides, such as maltase, lactase and sucrase digest disaccharides, such as maltose, lactose and sucrose respectively into their respective monosaccharide units.

Digestion of Important Food Products

- Although cellulose is not digested further it helps in easy peristalsis and provides bulk to the feces.
- Lactase deficiency leads to lactose intolerance.

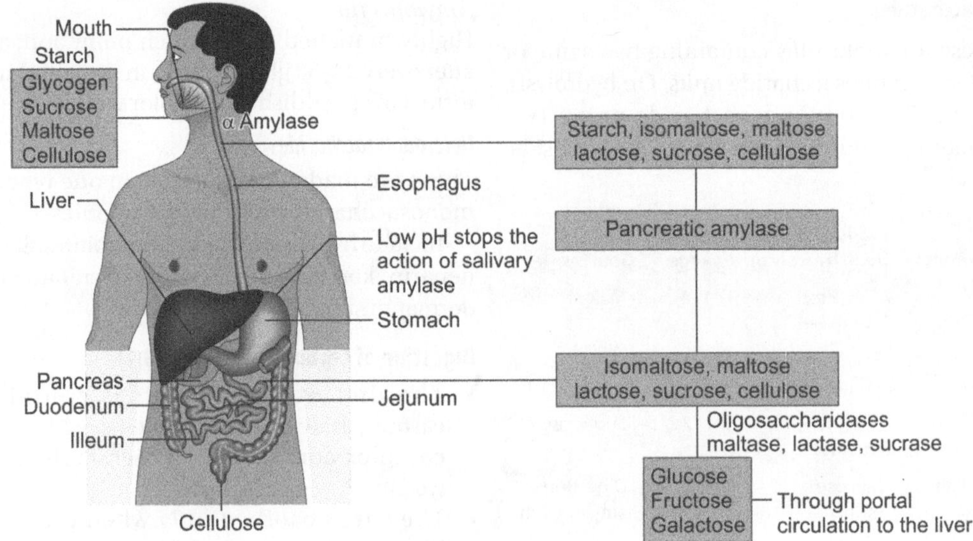

Fig. 8.1: Digestion of carbohydrates.

Absorption of Monosaccharides

- After digestion, all monosaccharides are almost completely absorbed from the small intestine.
- **Galactose and glucose** are absorbed very rapidly by the **active process**, which is linked to the transport of sodium and requires energy in the form of hydrolysis of the high-energy phosphate bond in ATP.
- Glucose cannot diffuse through the lipid bilayer of the cell membrane because of its polar nature.
- Absorption from intestinal lumen into intestinal cell is by a co-transport mechanism called **sodium dependent glucose transporter.**
- It occurs against the concentration gradient and requires a carrier protein.

Utilization of Glucose

The glucose molecule undergoes several metabolic pathways, such as storage, oxidation, synthesis of fat, conversion to other carbohydrates and conversion to amino acids.

1. *Storage:* Carbohydrates when taken in excess through the diet is deposited as glycogen in various tissues especially in the liver and muscle. Remaining glucose is converted to fatty acid and stored as triglycerides.
2. *Oxidation of glucose:* Carbohydrates undergo three types of oxidation depending upon the nature of the tissue and the availability of oxygen.
   a. *Complete oxidation:* If there is more demand for energy glucose may be completely oxidized to CO_2 and water by glycolysis and the TCA cycle.
   b. *Hexose monophosphate shunt (pentose phosphate pathway):* In certain tissues, such as adipose and liver tissues, glucose may be degraded to CO_2 in various reactions involving pentose.
   c. *Glycolysis:* At certain times in muscles especially during exercise, glucose is partially oxidized to lactic acid by glycolysis. This is also called anaerobic glycolysis. The lactic acid so produced is disposed of by the tissues especially the liver. The oxidation of glucose to pyruvate in the presence of oxygen is called aerobic glycolysis.

3. *Conversion to fat:* The amount of glycogen that is stored in the body is limited. Thus, the remaining glucose will be converted into fat. The fatty acid then form fats and are stored in adipose tissue.
4. *Conversion to amino acids:* From glucose or its metabolites, the carbon skeleton of some of the non-essential amino acids is derived.
5. *Conversion to other carbohydrates:* Small amount of glucose is also converted to other useful carbohydrates. They are:
   a. Ribose and deoxyribose: Required for the synthesis of nucleic acids.
   b. Mannose, fucose, glucosamine, galactosamine, neuraminic acid: Form parts of mucopolysaccharides and glycoproteins.
   c. Glucuronic acid: Involved in the formation of mucopolysaccharides and detoxification reactions.
   d. Galactose: A component of lactose.

Metabolic Pathways

A metabolic pathway consists of series of enzymatic reactions to produce particular products. The process of metabolism is divided into the anabolic pathway and the catabolic pathway.

- The anabolic pathway refers to the biosynthesis of a particular compound.
- The catabolic pathway refers to the breakdown of a particular compound.

In carbohydrate metabolism, glucose is the central molecule since most of the metabolic pathways of carbohydrates are linked with it.

Major Pathways

The major metabolic pathways of carbohydrates are:

Glycolysis: Oxidation of glucose into pyruvate (aerobic) or lactate (anaerobic).

Krebs cycle: Oxidation of acetyl-CoA into carbon dioxide (CO_2).

This is the final common oxidative pathway for carbohydrates, proteins and lipids through acetyl coenzyme A.

Gluconeogenesis: Synthesis of glucose from noncarbohydrate source.

Glycogenesis: Synthesis of glycogen from glucose.

Glycogenolysis: Breakdown of glycogen into glucose.

Hexose monophosphate shunt pathway (HMP Shunt Pathway): Glucose is oxidized to carbon dioxide and water.

Minor Pathways

Uronic acid pathway: Glucose is converted into glucuronic acids and pentoses.

Galactose metabolism: Here there is conversion of galactose into glucose and synthesis of lactose.

Fructose metabolism: Here the oxidation of fructose into pyruvate takes place.

Aminosugars and mucopolysaccharide metabolism.

Here, the synthesis of amino sugars and other sugars for the formation of mucopolysaccharides takes place.

Glycolysis

This is also called as Embden-Meyerhof-Paranas (EMP) pathway. The term glycolysis is derived from the Greek word *Glykys* meaning sweet and *Lysis* meaning splitting. Glycolysis is defined as the conversion of glucose into pyruvate in the aerobic condition or lactate in the anaerobic condition, along with the production of small quantities of energy (in the form of ATP). All the reactions of the glycolysis take place in the cytoplasm of the cell.

Significance of Glycolysis

- It is the only pathway occurring in all the cells of the body.
- Glycolysis is very essential for the brain, which is dependent on glucose for energy.

- Glycolysis is the only source of energy for the erythrocytes.
- During heavy exercise, when there is insufficient oxygen for muscle tissue, oxygen is obtained mainly through anaerobic glycolysis.
- Glycolytic pathway also provides carbon skeletons required for the synthesis of nonessential amino acids and glycerol.

Gluconeogenesis

- The synthesis of glucose from noncarbohydrate source is called as gluconeogenesis.
- The main noncarbohydrate sources are:
  - Lactate
  - Pyruvate and
  - Glucogenic amino acids
- The minor sources are:
  - Propionate and
  - Glycerol.
- Gluconeogenesis occurs mainly in the cytoplasm of liver cells.
- A small amount of gluconeogenesis occurs in the renal cortex.

Significance of Gluconeogenesis

1. A continuous supply of glucose is required for the brain and central nervous system, erythrocytes, testes and renal medulla. The human brain alone requires about 120 g of glucose/day. The major metabolic significance of gluconeogenesis is the maintenance of blood glucose level under conditions of the starvation. On prolonged starvation, gluconeogenesis is speeded up. At the same time, there is increased lipolysis and protein catabolism, which provides substrates for the gluconeogenesis.
2. Under anaerobic conditions, glucose is the only source of energy for skeletal muscles.
3. When certain metabolites, such as lactate, glycerol, etc., accumulate in the tissues, glucose synthesis is the effective way to reduce their levels.

Glycogenesis

- The synthesis of glycogen from glucose is called glycogenesis.
- Glycogen is the storage form of carbohydrates in the human body.
- Glycogen is mainly stored in the liver and muscles.
- After meals, excess glucose is converted into glycogen for the purpose of storage.
- The glycogen is present in the form of granules in the cytoplasm of liver and muscle cells.
- The main enzyme in the synthesis of glycogen is glycogen synthase.

Glycogenolysis

- The breakdown of glycogen into glucose is called glycogenolysis.
- It takes place in the cytoplasm of the liver and muscle cells.
- The main enzyme in glycogenolysis is glycogen phosphorylase.
- The branches of glycogen are removed by debranching enzymes.

Determination of Glucose in Body Fluids (Blood, Urine and CSF)

There are many methods available to measure the blood glucose level. They are:

1. *Enzymatic method*
   a. Hexokinase method
   b. Glucose oxidase-peroxidase method (GOD-POD)
   c. Glucose dehydrogenase method.
2. *Polarographic method:* PO_2 electrode method.
3. *Chemical methods*
   a. O-toluidine method
   b. Folin-Wu's method
   c. Nelson-Somogyi's method.

Sample Collection and Processing

- The blood sample is collected and processed. The selection of serum or plasma depends on the methods used.
- The serum is free of fibrinogen.
- Plasma contains fibrinogen.
- The fasting whole blood glucose concentration is 12% lower than plasma glucose.
- Usually, venous blood samples are used for the glucose estimation.
- If the serum is used then the assay should be done within 30 minutes of sample collection, since it does not contain any preservatives to stop the process of glycolysis.
- Glycolysis decreases serum glucose by 5 to 7%/hr in normal uncentrifuged blood kept at room temperature.
- Glycolysis can be inhibited by adding the sodium iodoacetate or sodium fluoride which stabilizes the glucose level.
- Fluoride ions prevent glycolysis by inhibiting the enzyme enolase. Fluoride is also a weak anticoagulant because it binds Ca^{2+} ions.
- Potassium oxalate 2 mg and sodium fluoride 2 mg/mL of blood are added to prevent clotting.
- The vacutainer available contains the fluoride.

  The blood glucose done at three intervals are:

Fasting

Fasting blood sugar is estimated 8 to 12 hours after the last meal. This is usually done in the early morning. The person should not consume anything other than water.

Postprandial

Postprandial blood glucose is estimated usually 2 hours after a normal meal or breakfast.

Random

The random blood glucose can be measured at any time of the day irrespective of the food taken.

Enzymatic Method

Hexokinase Method

Principle: Glucose is phosphorylated to glucose-6 phosphate by ATP in the presence of hexokinase and activator magnesium (Mg^{2+}). The glucose 6-phosphate formed is oxidized by glucose 6-phosphate dehydrogenase to give 6-phosphogluconolactone in the presence of NAD (nicotinamide adenine dinucleotide). During the reaction NAD^+ is converted to $NADH + H^+$. The amount of NADH produced is directly proportional to the amount of glucose present in the sample.

Glucose 6-phosphate dehydrogenase derived from yeast is usually used in the assay, which uses $NADP^+$ as a coenzyme.

NAD^+ is the coenzyme of the bacterial glucose 6-phosphate dehydrogenase.

NADH produced, is measured at 340 nm.

$$\text{Glucose} + \text{ATP} \xrightarrow[Mg^{2+}]{\text{Hexokinase}} \text{glucose 6-phosphate} + \text{ADP}$$

$$\text{Glu 6-p} + NAD^+ \xrightarrow{\text{Glu 6-P DH}} \text{6-p Gluconolactone} + \text{NADH} + H^+$$

Note: $NADP^+$ can be used instead of NAD^+.

Plasma is deproteinized by adding solutions of barium hydroxide ($Ba(OH)_2$) and zinc sulfate ($ZnSO_4$). The clear supernatant is mixed with reagent containing ATP, NAD^+, hexokinase, glu-6-phosphate dehydrogenase. The mixture is incubated at room temperature or 25°C until the reaction is complete and NADH produced is measured. Standards and reagent blank run simultaneously with the sample. The NADH formed is measured spectrophotometrically at 340 nm. The formation of NADH is proportional to the glucose concentration.

1. Bilirubin, lipids and some drugs may interfere with the assay.
2. The procedure is linear up to 500 mg% of glucose concentration. If the concentration exceeds 500 mg% the sample must be diluted with normal saline in the beginning of the assay.

Glucose Oxidase-Peroxidase Method

Principle

The enzyme, glucose oxidase (GOD) catalyzes the oxidation of the glucose to gluconic acid and H_2O_2. Addition of the enzyme peroxidase (POD) splits H_2O_2 to H_2O and nascent oxygen. The oxygen oxidizes the added colorless chromogen ortho-dianisidine to a colored compound, which can be read colorimetrically. The intensity of color formed is directly proportional to the glucose concentration. This method is highly specific and gives an accurate glucose value. The glucose oxidase will act only on beta D-glucose.

$$\text{Glucose} + H_2O + O_2 \xrightarrow{\text{Glucose oxidase}} \text{Gluconic acid} + H_2O_2$$

$$H_2O_2 \xrightarrow{\text{Peroxidase}} H_2O + O$$

$$\text{O-Dianisidine} \xrightarrow{\text{Nascent oxygen}} \text{Oxidized colored product}$$

Many of the laboratories use this method to analyze glucose using autoanalyzers. The commercially available GOD/POD kit can also be used to analyze the blood glucose using a colorimeter. The kit contains working and standard solutions.

The procedure for manual estimation using the kit is as follows:

Reagents	*Blank*	*Standard*	*Test*
Working solution	1.0 mL	1.0 mL	1.0 mL
Standard	—	10 μL	—
Sample	—	—	10 μL
Distilled water	10 μL	—	—

Mix and incubate at 37°C for 15 minutes or at room temperature for 30 minutes and read the absorbance of the Test (A_T), standard (A_S) and reagent blank (A_B) at 505 nm or with Green filter against distilled water.

Calculations

$$(\text{mg/dL}) = \frac{A_T - A_B}{A_S - A_B} \times 100$$

To convert mg/dL to mmol/L

mmol/L = mg/dL × 0.056

Linearity = 500 mg/dL

Standard graph: The glucose oxidase and peroxidase method can be used in the laboratory. Standard calibration graph plotted with various concentration of standard and the concentration of blood glucose in the test sample is determined.

The reagent preparation and procedure is as follows:

Reagents

1. *Buffer solution:* 0.2 M phosphate buffer, pH 7.4.

   Solution A: 0.2 M monobasic sodium dihydrogen phosphate ($NaH_2PO_4 \cdot 2H_2O$) is prepared by dissolving 7.8 g in 250 mL water.

   Solution B: 0.2M dibasic disodium hydrogen phosphate ($Na_2HPO_4 \cdot 2H_2O$) is prepared by dissolving 8.9 g in 250 mL water.

   The two solutions are mixed as follows and the pH is adjusted to 7.4.

   36.4 mL of solution A + 213.6 mL of solution B.
2. *Phenol:* 0.05% 100 mg of phenol taken directly.
3. *Color reagents:*
   a. 4-Aminoantipyrine: 0.01%—20 mg.
   b. Horseradish peroxidase: 0.73 IU/mL—1 mg/100 mL of buffer.
   c. Glucose oxidase: 30 IU/mL—22 mg/100 mL of buffer.

   Mix a + b + c. Refrigerate (do not freeze). To this add 100 mg of phenol.

4. *Glucose standard (stock):* 1 g of glucose is dissolved in 100 mL water. For storage 100 mg of benzoic acid (0.1% benzoic acid) + 100 mL water + 1 g of glucose.
   Working standard preparation:
   a. 50 mg/dL—0.5 stock + 9.5 mL of water.
   b. 100 mg/dL—1 mL stock + 9 mL of distilled water.
   c. 150 mg/dL—1.5 mL stock + 8.5 of distilled water.
   d. 200 mg/dL—2 mL stock 8 mL of distilled water.
   e. 250 mg/dL—2.5 mL stock 7.5 mL of distilled water.
   f. 300 mg/dL—3 mL stock + 7 mL of distilled water.
   g. 350 mg/dL—3.5 mL stock + 6.5 mL of distilled water.
   h. 400 mg/dL—4 mL stock + 6 mL of distilled water.

Procedure

Standard glucose (0.02 mL of each) are pipetted out into S_1-S_8 series of test tubes. Simultaneously run the blank with 0.02 mL of water. Serum of 0.02 mL pipetted into a test tube labeled test. Then 1 mL of water is added to all the tubes, mixed well and 2 mL of color reagent are added. Contents are mixed and incubated at 37°C for 15 minutes. The absorbance of the red color developed is read at 505 nm. Color is stable for 1 hour at room temperature.

Advantages

1. True glucose values are obtained by this method, since it specifically oxidizes glucose to give gluconic acid and has very little effect on any other sugar.
2. This method is unaffected by other blood constituents.
3. This method is sensitive and is applied to various automated analyzes.
4. This method is useful in measuring CSF glucose.

Disadvantages

1. Glucose oxidase methods are not applicable directly to urine samples, owing to the high concentration of peroxidase inhibitor and other interfering substances.
2. Uric acid, ascorbic acid, bilirubin, glutathione and tetracyclines will interfere with the assay.

Glucose Dehydrogenase Method

Principle: The enzyme glucose dehydrogenase catalyzes the oxidation of glucose to glucono-lactone. Since the enzyme, GDH is specific for β-D glucose and the enzyme mutarotase is added to shorten the time required to reach the equilibrium. The amount of NADH produced is directly proportional to the glucose concentration, which is measured at 340 nm.

1. The reaction is highly specific for glucose.

Glucose oxidase: standard graph

Contents	*B*	S_1	S_2	S_3	S_4	S_5	S_6	S_7	S_8	*T*
Standard (mL)	-	0.02	0.02	0.02	0.02	0.02	0.02	0.02	0.02	-
Concentration of standard (mg/dL)	-	50	100	150	200	250	300	350	400	-
Serum (mL)	-	-	-	-	-	-	-	-	-	0.02
Water (mL)	1.02	1	1	1	1	1	1	1	1	1
Color reagent (mL)	2	2	2	2	2	2	2	2	2	2
Mix and incubate at 37°C for 15 minutes or at room temperature for 30 minutes and read at 505 nm										

2. The reaction is not interfered by anticoagulants and other substances, which are normally present in the plasma.
3. The absorbance is usually linear with glucose concentrations up to 1000 mg%.
4. Lipemic samples cause interference. Blank set up with normal for lipemic samples.
5. The procedure is not widely used.

Chemical Methods

Ortho-Toluidine Method

Principle: The ortho-toluidine in glacial acetic acid when heated with glucose produces a colored complex, with an absorption maximum at 630 nm. The aldehyde group of glucose apparently condenses with amino group of the O-toluidine to form N-glycosylamine and a Schiff's base, which gives the blue green colored product.

The reaction is not specific for glucose and other aldohexoses, such as mannose and galactose will also react. But these aldohexoses are usually present in very small amounts. The reagent thiourea is added for stabilization of the color.

Specimen: Venous blood is collected in an oxalate-fluoride coated tube.

Reagents

1. *Ortho-toluidine reagent:* To 1.5 g thiourea (AR grade) mix 40.0 mL O-toluidine and dilute to 1 liter with glacial acetic acid. Store in a brown bottle and this will be stable for 6 months.
2. *Trichloroacetic acid, 10%:* Dissolve 10 g TCA (Trichloroacetic acid) in water and make up the volume to 100 mL.
3. *Glucose standard:* 100 mg of glucose in 100 mL saturated benzoic acid solution, or water.

Procedure

Reagents	*Blank (B)*	*Standard (S)*	*Test (T)*
Distilled water	1.4 mL	1.2 mL	1.2 mL
Standard glucose solution	—	0.2 mL	—
Sample	—	—	0.2 mL
TCA, 10%	0.6	0.6 mL	0.6 mL
Mix and after 5 minutes centrifuge for 10 minutes			
Supernatant in 3 tubes	1.0 mL	1.0 mL	1.0 mL
O-Toluidine	5.0 mL	5.0 mL	5.0 mL
Keep in boiling water for 10 minutes			
Read the absorbance at 630 nm or red filter			

Calculation

$$\frac{\text{OD of T} - \text{OD of B}}{\text{OD of S} - \text{OD of B}} \times 100 = \text{mg of glucose/100 mL}$$

Note: O-toluidine is highly corrosive. Use dispenser for O-toluidine reagent.

Thiourea used to stabilize the color.

Anhydrous acetic acid is preferred.

Special Features

Advantages

1. The method can be directly applied to serum or plasma, CSF and urine.
2. For whole blood of hemolyzed samples, deproteinization with TCA is required.
3. The color of the reaction mixture is stable up to 45 minutes and then the color slowly decreases.
4. Among the non-enzymatic methods, this is the most widely used because of high specificity and simplicity.

Disadvantages

1. Bilirubin may interfere, because of partial conversion of bilirubin which is green in color.

2. If the patient is uremic, higher values are obtained with this method.

Standard Graph

The glucose can be estimated even by plotting a standard graph. This method is helpful for the students to learn more about pipetting and plotting a graph with different concentration of glucose ranging from 50 mg to 400 mg.

The reagents are same as explained in the above method except the standards.

1. *Standard glucose (stock):* 500 mg of glucose is dissolved in 100 mL of water. It contains 5.0 mg of glucose/mL.
2. *Working standards*: Series of working standards of various concentrations are prepared which ranges from 50 to 400 mg/dL (**Fig. 8.2**).
   a. 50 mg/dL—1.0 mL stock + 9.0 mL water
   b. 100 mg/dL—2.0 mL stock + 8.0 mL water
   c. 150 mg/dL—3.0 mL stock + 7.0 mL water
   d. 200 mg/dL—4.0 mL stock + 6.0 mL water
   e. 250 mg/dL—5.0 mL stock + 5.0 mL water
   f. 300 mg/dL—6.0 mL stock + 4.0 mL water
   g. 350 mg/dL—7.0 mL stock + 3.0 mL water
   h. 400 mg/dL—8.0 mL stock + 2.0 mL water

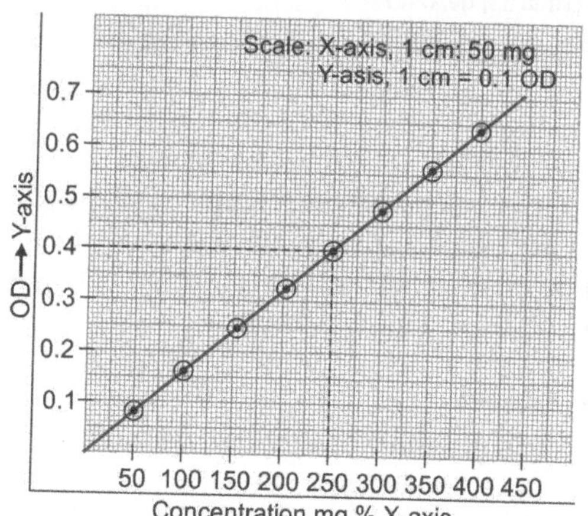

0.4 OD corresponds to 250 mg% of glucose from the graph

Fig. 8.2: Standard graph.

Folin-Wu's Method

Principle: The protein is removed by using the tungstic acid. The protein free filtrate containing glucose reduces alkaline copper reagent. Phosphomolybdic acid added develops blue color. The optical density of blue color is measured with colorimeter using the blue filter (490 nm). Other reducing substances present in the blood will give a positive result. This includes glutathione, uric acid, glucuronic acid and ascorbic acid.

Reagents

1. *Sodium tungstate:* 10%: Dissolve 10 g of sodium tungstate in about 70 mL water. Then make up to 100 mL with water.
2. Sulfuric acid 0.667 N.
3. *Alkaline copper reagent:* Dissolve 40 g anhydrous sodium carbonate in 400 mL water. Add 7.5 g tartaric acid and 4.5 g copper sulfate. Make up to one liter with water.
4. *Phosphomolybdic acid:* Add 35 g molybdic acid and 5 g sodium tungstate to 200 mL of 10% sodium hydroxide solution. Add 200 mL water. Boil until the ammonia scent is no longer deleted, cool and transfer to a 500 mL flask. Carefully add 125 mL syrupy phosphoric acid, keeping the flask cooled under a tap. Make up to 500 mL with water.
5. *Stock standard glucose solution:* 100 mg/100 mL. Add 2 to 4 spatulas benzoic acid to 120 mL of boiled water, mix, cool and filter. Transfer exactly 100 mg

Contents	*B*	S_1	S_2	S_3	S_4	S_5	S_6	S_7	S_8	*T*
Working standard (mL)	-	0.1	0.1	0.1	0.1	0.1	0.1	0.1	0.1	-
Concentration (mg/dL)	-	50	100	150	200	250	300	350	400	-
Serum (mL)	-	-	-	-	-	-	-	-	-	0.1
Water (mL)	1	0.9	0.9	0.9	0.9	0.9	0.9	0.9	0.9	0.9
O-toluidine (mL)	7	7	7	7	7	7	7	7	7	7
Keep in boiling water bath for 10 mins, cool and read the absorbance at 620 nm										
	0.07->0	0.08	0.16	0.24	0.32	0.42	0.48	0.56	0.64	0.40

glucose to a 100 mL flask. Add benzoic acid solution up to 100 mL mark and mix thoroughly.

6. *Standard glucose solution for use:* 10 mg per 100 mL. Dilute 1 mL stock to 10 mL solution with water. This gives 1 mL = 0.1 mg solution (prepare fresh everyday).

Calculation

$$\frac{T-B}{S-B} \times 100$$

Note: Place the tubes after water starts boiling. The period of boiling is exactly 8 minutes.
Procedure for Folin-Wu's method:

Reagents	*B*	*S*	*T*
Distilled water	-	-	7
Blood	-	-	1
Sodium tungstate 10%	-	-	1
Sulfuric acid 0.667N	-	-	1
Wait 10 minutes. Filter.			
Filtrate	-	-	2
Distilled water	2	-	-
Standard glucose for use	-	2	-
Alkaline copper reagent	2	2	2
Keep in boiling water for 8 minutes. Cool.			
Phosphomolybdic acid	2	2	2
Water up to	25 mL	25 mL	25 mL
Read the absorbance at 490 nm			

Nelson-Somogyi's Method

In this method, the proteins are precipitated by using equal volumes of barium hydroxide and zinc sulfate. The interfering substances are removed along with the precipitate. The results obtained may be more accurate better than the results obtained with Folin-Wu's method.

The modified alkaline copper tartrate reagent is stable.

The method gives results near to the true glucose values. The disadvantage is that a little excess of either $Ba(OH)_2$, or $ZnSO_4$ causes lot of error in the estimation.

Normal Range: (Plasma)

Fasting glucose	80–100 mg%
Post-prandial	90–140 mg%
Random	90–150 mg%
Newborn	40–90 mg%

The CSF glucose concentration is about 60% of the blood glucose value and simultaneous measurement of the blood glucose estimation is required along with the CSF.

Glycosurias

- The presence of reducing substances in urine is called glycosuria.
- The presence of glucose in urine is called glucosuria.
- The presence of fructose in urine is called fructosuria.
- The presence of lactose in urine is called lactosuria.

- The reducing substances, which are excreted in the urine, are glucose, fructose, lactose, galactose and pentoses. The non-carbohydrates, which are known to have reducing activity, are homogentisic acid, salicylic acid and ascorbic acid. In normal conditions, glucose does not appear in urine.

The different types of glycosurias seen are:

Hyperglycemic Glycosuria

Hyperglycemia is the most common cause for the excretion of glucose in urine.

When the blood glucose level exceeds the renal threshold value of 180 mg/dL, glucose may appear in urine.

Hyperglycemic glycosuria is commonly seen in diabetes mellitus patients.

Renal Glycosuria

The excretion of glucose in urine due to the decrease of renal threshold is called renal glycosuria. In these cases, the glucose tolerance is normal. The blood sugar levels are within normal limits. The renal threshold is decreased in pregnancy.

This can also occur due to renal tubular defects.

Alimentary Glycosuria

This is seen in persons with sudden absorption of glucose from the gastrointestinal tract. As a result, it may appear in urine.

This is called alimentary glucosuria since the alimentary canal (gastrointestinal tract) is involved.

Transient Glycosuria

In some persons, glucose may appear in urine due to certain emotional stress conditions, such as anger, anxiety, etc.

In these conditions, excessive secretion of catecholamine may lead to hyperglycemia and glycosuria.

Fructosuria

This is linked to fructokinase deficiency or hereditary fructose intolerance

Fructose ⟶ fructose-1-phosphate

Galactosuria

- This is seen in galactose 1-phosphate uridyltransferase deficiency **(Fig. 8.3)**.
- It is a rare congenital disease in infants.
- Galactose accumulated in blood lead to galactosemia.

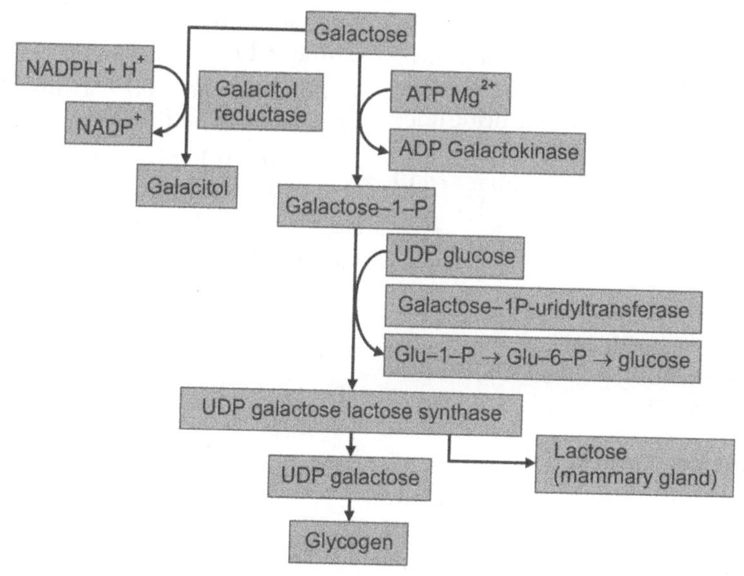

Fig. 8.3: Galactose metabolism.

The galactose excreted in the urine (galactosuria).

Lactosuria

Lactose is found in the urine of normal pregnant women during third trimester of pregnancy and lactation.

It is the second most common type of glycosuria.

In pregnancy with suspected gestational diabetes mellitus, it is very important to differentiate lactosuria from glycosuria.

Qualitative Tests for Glycosurias

Benedict's qualitative reagent is used for the test. The reagent contains Cu^{2+} ions complexed to citrate in alkaline solution. Reducing substances convert Cu^{2+} ions to Cu^{+} ions forming yellow $Cu(OH)_2$ or red Cu_2O.

Preparation of Benedict's reagent: Dissolve 173 g of sodium citrate and 100 g of anhydrous sodium carbonate in about 500 mL in slightly hot deionized water. Into this slowly added 17.3 g copper sulfate with constant stirring, cool, transfer to a liter volumetric flask and make up to 1 liter with water.

Technique: Add 8 drops of urine to 5 mL of Benedict's reagent in test tube and boil for 5 minutes. A precipitate forms, varying from greenish to yellowish brown to reddish brown if the urine contains reducing sugars. The original color remains as such if the urine does not contain any reducing sugars.

- The blue color indicates the absence of sugar in urine
- The yellow color means 1% sugar in the urine
- Orange indicates 1.5%
- Brick red means 2% or more.
- The presence of any reducing sugar will give a positive Benedict's test.

Semiquantitative Measurement of Glucose

Enzyme coated paper strips are commercially available. The strip is dipped in the urine and the color is examined after 20 to 30 seconds and compared with the standard.

The glucose oxidase, peroxidase method is the principle lying behind this method.

Qualitative tests for reducing sugars.

Seliwanoff's test for fructose in urine: Seliwanoff's reagent (resorcinol in HCl) 3 mL and 0.5 mL urine are boiled for 30 seconds. A red color appears if fructose presents.

Methylamine test for lactose: To 5 mL urine is added 1 mL methylamine hydrochloride and 1 mL sodium hydroxide are added and kept at 56°C for 30 minutes. An appearance of red color indicates the presence of lactose.

Mucic acid test for galactose: When urine is boiled with mucic acid, crystals are formed indicating the presence of lactose or galactose.

Bial's test for pentoses: When 5 mL Bial's reagent (orcinol in HCl) is boiled with 0.5 mL urine a green color is produced if the urine contains pentoses.

Fructose Determination in Serum

Reagents

Resorcinol: 100 mg of resorcinol is dissolved in 250 mg of thiourea in 100 mL of acetic acid.

HCl: 20 mL concentrated HCl made up to 100 mL with water.

Stock standard: Fructose 10 mg in 10 mL of saturated benzoic acid.

Working standard: 0.1 mg/mL. Dilute 1 mL of stock to 10 mL with water.

Procedure: 0.1 mL serum + 2.9 mL water + 0.5 mL 0.3 N barium hydroxide + 0.5 mL zinc sulfate mix and centrifuge. The supernatant is used for the assay.

	Blank	*Standard*	*Test*
Water (mL)	1.0	1.0	0.5
Standard	—	0.05	—
Supernatant	—	—	0.5
Resorcinol	0.5	0.5	0.5
HCl	3.5	3.5	3.5
Mix and incubate at 80°C for 10 minutes, cool and read at 540 nm			

Calculation

$$\frac{T-B}{S-B} \times \frac{0.05}{0.0125} \times 100$$

$$\frac{T-B}{S-B} \times 400 = mg/dL$$

Normal range: 90 to 520 mg/dL

The method can be used for the estimation of semen fructose.

Glucose Tolerance Tests (GTT)

- A normal person should be able to reduce a glucose load from his/her blood within a specified time. This is known as normal tolerance.
- If the person has an elevated blood glucose concentration for longer than the normal time, the condition is called as reduced tolerance.
- If the glucose concentration becomes very low or normal very early than the normal time then the condition is called as increased tolerance.
- The tests that are used to measure these changes in blood glucose after a glucose load are called glucose tolerance tests.

There are 2 types: (i) oral, (ii) intravenous GTT. They are mainly used in the detection of diabetes. Oral GTT is more commonly used in all the laboratories. It is convenient to give glucose through oral route.

Indications for Performing GTT

1. Family history of diabetes mellitus.
2. Signs and symptoms comparable with diabetics without any complications.
3. Glucosuric patients with normal fasting blood sugar.
4. Border line postprandial blood sugar.
5. Reactive hypoglycemia for 3 hours or longer period after food intake.
6. Pregnancy with history of abortions, stillbirths or a large baby.

Preparation of the Patients

1. Patient should not be under fear or anxiety about the possibility of being a diabetic. If so, it can lead to false positive results. So it is the duty of the technician to prepare the patient emotionally or mentally and calm.
2. Adequate carbohydrate intake. Before the test, the patient should have been on a diet containing at least 150 g of carbohydrate per day with low fat for at least 3 days. An adequate deposit of glycogen in the liver and other tissues is essential for the production of a normal response. If the subject is in a state of relatively low carbohydrate diet for some time before the test, the rise in blood sugar levels following the ingestion of glucose will more pronounced and its fall to the normal level is delayed.
3. It is desirable for the subject to fast for 10 to 12 hours before the test.
4. The test patient must not have ingested tea or coffee on the day of test.
5. The patient should not have excessively exercise or be physically strained.
6. If the patient is not well, the test should be postponed.
7. The patient should not receive any drugs for at least 3 days before the test.

Factors affecting GTT

1. *Factors associated with hyperglycemia:* Aldosterone, catecholamines, diphenylhydantoin (DPH), nicotine, oral contraceptives, thiazides, glucagon and growth hormone.
2. *Factors associated with hypoglycemia:* Ethanol, INH, and sulfonamide drugs.
3. The age factor is also important. The glucose tolerance tends to become lower in old age.

Method

The test is usually carried out in the early morning after fasting overnight.

Fasting blood sample and urine is then collected. 75 g (or 100 g) of glucose dissolved in about 150 to 200 mL of water is given to drink.

Venous blood for the estimation of blood glucose is collected at ½ hour intervals for 2 to 2½ hours or hourly intervals for 3 hours after the ingestion of glucose. Urine specimens are also collected at the same time.

Blood glucose is estimated in each sample and the urine is tested for the presence of the sugar.

Comments

1. Some prefer the administration of 1.75 g/kg body weight of glucose. However, the amount of glucose makes very little difference to the response of the test.
2. It is preferable to give 100 mL of water after the ingestion of glucose, which takes away the sweet taste and decreases the risk of vomiting.
3. Plasma specimens are more satisfactory than whole blood for glucose analysis, because plasma gives more reliable results and it is independent of hematocrit values.
4. Variation in hematocrit values can be accounted for differences in whole blood glucose values.

Interpretation

Normal Glucose Tolerance Curve (Fig. 8.4)

The normal curve has the following features:

1. The fasting blood glucose in this category is usually within the range of 60 to 100 mg/dL.
2. The blood glucose does not rise above 160 mg/dL.
3. The blood glucose at 2 hour after the load is 110 mg/dL.
4. The urine remains free of glucose throughout the test.
5. The timing of the peak value is not defined as a part of the normal pattern of response, but it is usually seen either in the 30 minutes or in 60 minutes blood sample.

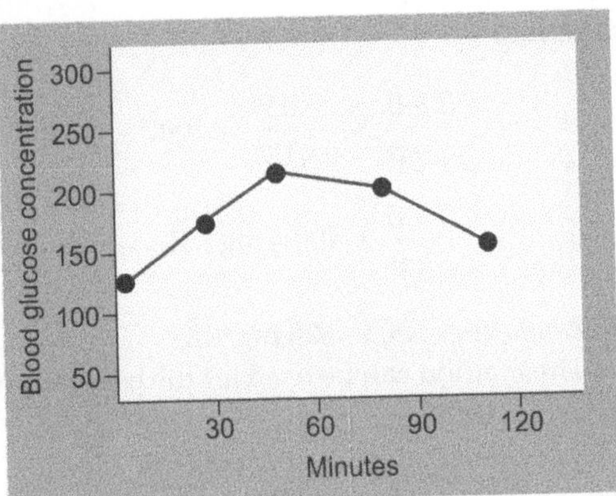

Fig. 8.4: Normal glucose tolerance test.

Sample no.	*mg glucose/ 100 mL blood*	*Urine glucose*
Fasting	90	Negative
30 minutes	120	Negative
60 minutes	150	Negative
90 minutes	140	Negative
120 minutes	90	Negative

Abnormal Glucose Tolerance Response (Fig. 8.5)

Reduced glucose tolerance:

The main features are:

1. The fasting level is above 120 mg.
2. The glucose level crosses 200 mg/100 mL in 30 to 60 minutes.
3. The blood glucose level is more than 110 mg/dL even after 2 hour.

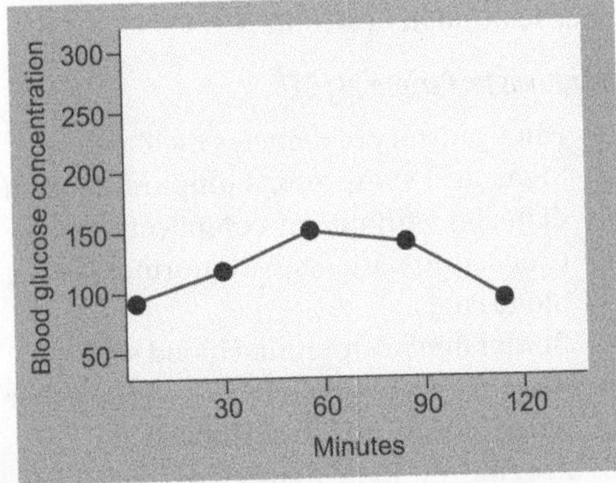

Fig. 8.5: Abnormal glucose tolerance test.

4. There may be glucose in at least two of the urine specimens.

Sample no.	mg glucose/100 mL blood	Urine glucose
Fasting	120	Negative
30 minutes	160	Positive
60 minutes	200	Positive
90 minutes	180	Positive
120 minutes	150	Negative

Conditions associated with diminished glucose tolerance:

1. Due to lack of insulin, there will be decreased tissue utilization of glucose, which is seen in diabetes mellitus.
2. Increased glycogenolysis and gluconeogenesis seen in glucocorticoid excess and hyperthyroidism.
3. Increased rate of absorption, which is seen in thyrotoxicosis.
4. Decreased glycogen storage, which is seen in severe hepatic diseases and glycogen storage diseases.

Increased Glucose Tolerance

Increased glucose tolerance curve is characterized by a flat response.

Conditions associated with increased tolerance.

1. Hypothyroidism
2. Hypoadrenalism
3. Hypopituitarism
4. Malabsorption from the GIT
5. Renal glycosuria
6. Hyperinsulinism

   This is also characterized by

   i. Fasting hypoglycemia

   ii. Slight increase in blood glucose following glucose ingestion.

Intravenous Glucose Tolerance Test

Preparation of Patient

Poor absorption of orally given glucose may result in a flat tolerance curve. Some patients are unable to tolerate a large amount of carbohydrate load. In these patients, an intravenous glucose tolerance test may be performed to eliminate the factors related to the rate of the glucose absorption. This test is also used to monitor the first phase of insulin response in clinical studies.

The preparation of patient is the same as that of oral GTT. The dose of glucose is 0.5 g/kg body weight (25 g/dL solution). The dose is administered intravenously over 3 minutes through one hand and blood is collected at every 10 minutes from the opposite arm after the mid injection time for 1 hour and rate of glucose clearance is calculated.

Spot Test

Single blood sample is collected for glucose estimation after the 50 g (with 150 mL of water) of glucose loaded orally.

Exactly one hour after the glucose load, the blood sample is collected for glucose estimation.

The blood glucose must not cross the upper limit of the random glucose that is 150 mg/dL.

If the glucose level crosses 150 mg/dL, then perform the oral GTT for confirmation.

DIABETES MELLITUS

It is a group of metabolic diseases in which a person has high blood sugar (>126 mg/dL), either because the body does not produce enough insulin, or because cells do not respond to the insulin that is produced.

Some patients may develop life-threatening conditions like ketoacidosis and coma.

The diabetic patients are at increased risk of developing specific complications, such as retinopathy, which leads to blindness, renal failure, nephropathy, neuropathy and atherosclerosis. The last complication may result in stroke, gangrene and coronary diseases.

There are mainly two types of diabetes:

a. Insulin dependent diabetes mellitus (IDDM), Type I or Juvenile onset diabetes.
b. Non-insulin dependent diabetes mellitus (NIDDM), Type II or adult onset diabetes mellitus.

Insulin Dependent Diabetes Mellitus or Type I (Fig. 8.6)

Mode of inheritance: Not a transmitted disease, genetic predisposition.

This comprises around 5 to 10% cases of diabetes mellitus. Patients usually develop the following symptoms:

a. Polyuria
b. Polydipsia
c. Polyphagia
d. Weight loss.

Polyuria

A large amount of glucose may be excreted in the urine.

Along with glucose water is also excreted due to osmotic diseases.

Therefore, a large amount of urine is excreted and this condition is called polyuria.

Polydipsia

Loss of fluid stimulates thirst center. Hence, the person drinks more water than normal and this condition is polydipsia.

Polyphagia

Since lipid and protein breakdown is increased, weight loss is common.

Person eats more frequently and this condition is called polyphagia.

The patient may show boils, abscesses, cellulites, etc.

1. Patients have a deficiency of insulin and are dependent on insulin to sustain life and prevent ketosis.
2. Onset usually occurs in children and youth less than 20 years old.
3. Evidence suggests that most patients with type I diabetes have acute immune destruction of β-cells of pancreas.
4. The complication of this type is cataract, neuropathy (nerve diseases) and nephropathy (kidney diseases).

Non-insulin Dependent Diabetes Mellitus or Type II

Mode of inheritance: Weight gain or obesity, excess sugar in the bloodstream.

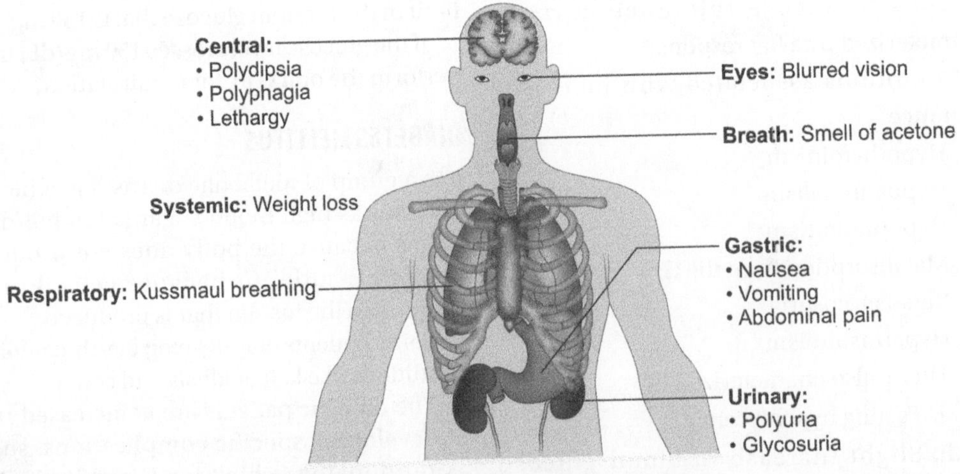

Fig. 8.6: Diagram showing symptoms of diabetes.

1. This group comprises approximately 90% of the diabetic population. The patients have minimum symptoms and usually not prone to ketosis.
2. Patients are not dependent on insulin to prevent ketosis. Serum insulin levels may be normal or may fluctuate. Most of the persons with NIDDM have impaired insulin action.
3. Obesity is common with NIDDM and weight reduction usually improves the hyperglycemia. Many people with NIDDM may require diet change and oral hypoglycemic agent or insulin to control hyperglycemia.
4. Usually occurs after the age of 40 years, sometimes occurs in young persons also.

Symptoms of Diabetes (Figs. 8.7A and B)

- Frequent urination
- Excessive thirst
- Extreme hunger or constant eating
- Unexplained weight loss
- Presence of glucose in the urine.

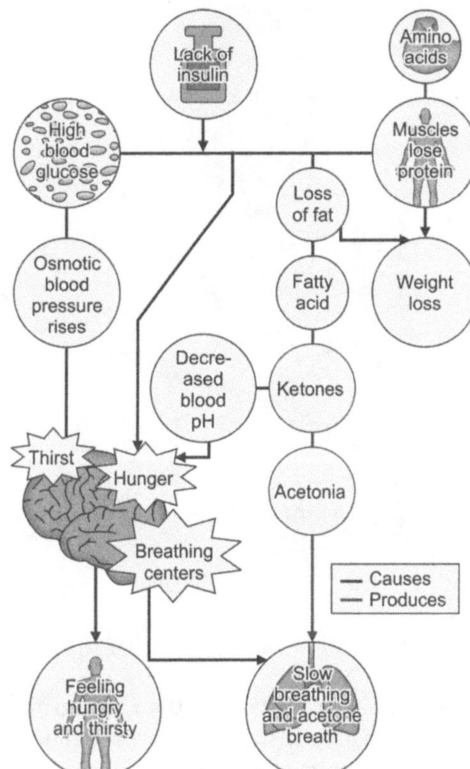

Fig. 8.7A: Causes and symptoms of diabetes.

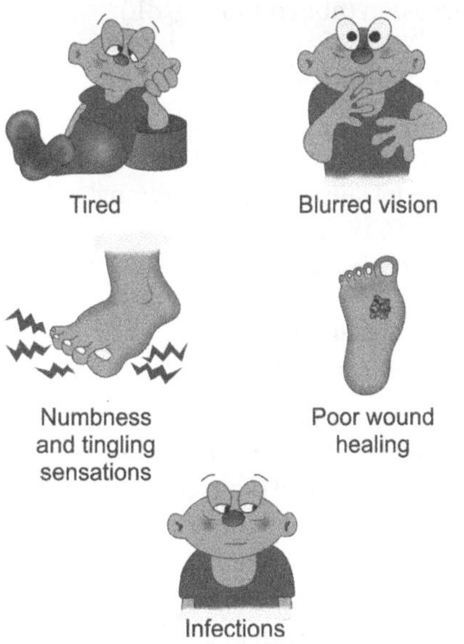

Fig. 8.7B: Symptoms of diabetes.

Diagnosis

The diagnosis of diabetes mellitus depends on the demonstration of hyperglycemia.

For the type I, the diagnosis is easy because hyperglycemia is more severe and is accompanied by serious metabolic disturbances.

Checking for Diabetes

The presence of diabetes should be checked in the persons with the following characteristics:

- All adults older than 40 years of age should have a measurement of fasting blood glucose every 3 months
- Persons with body mass index (BMI) of 25 kg/m^2 and above
- Persons with family history of diabetes
- Individual with history of gestational diabetes mellitus

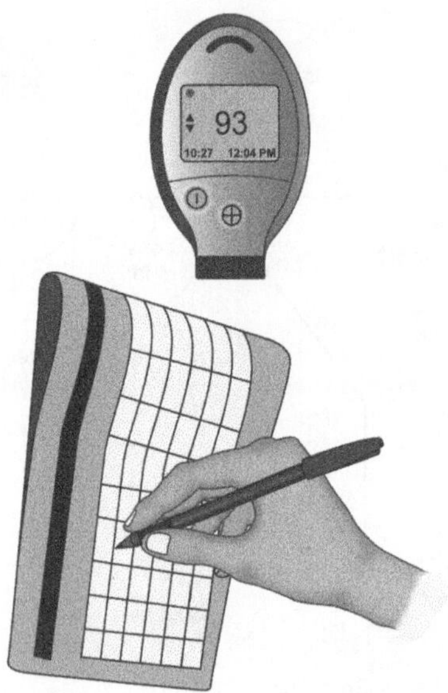

Fig. 8.8: Glucose monitoring.

- Delivery of a baby with high serum triglyceride levels
- Individual with HDL less than 35 mg/dL
- Person with a history of impaired glucose tolerance or impaired fasting glucose
- Elevated fasting glucose on more than one occasion (above 140 mg/dL).

Treatment (Fig. 8.8)

- Monitor blood glucose levels
- Diet, exercise, medication
- *Type I:* Daily insulin injections
- *Type II:* Weight loss
- Alternative medicine.

Diabetes due to Secondary Causes or Syndromes

In some patients, the hyperglycemia is due to specific disorders. This includes:

1. Pancreatic disease with endocrine insufficiency, where insulin secretions are markedly decreased.
2. Cushing's syndrome in which there is excess secretion of glucocorticoids.
3. Acromegaly where there is excessive secretion of growth hormone.
4. Excessive secretion of glucagon due to a tumor of the pancreas.
5. Hyperaldosteronism (excessive production of aldosterone).

Metabolic Changes in Diabetes Mellitus

Hyperglycemia

Causes

- Decreased or impaired transport and uptake of glucose in muscles and adipose tissues.
- Decreased activity of the key glycolytic enzymes.
- Increased gluconeogenesis due to lack of insulin.
- Increased amino acids of blood acts as source for gluconeogenesis.

Protein Metabolism

Protein synthesis is decreased in all the tissues due to decreased production of ATP and absolute or relative insulin deficiency.

Fat Metabolism

- Fatty acid synthesis is decreased.
- Lipid breakdown (lipolysis) is increased.
- The fatty acids are broken down to give large number of acetyl-CoA.
- In the deficiency of insulin, acetyl-CoA will enter the pathway of cholesterol synthesis or ketone formation. Therefore, cholesterol is increased in those with diabetes mellitus.

Glycogen Metabolism

Glycogen synthesis is decreased. This is because of decreased activity of glycogen synthase due to insulin deficiency.

Glycosylated Hemoglobin

HbA1c level increases 3–4 times in untreated diabetes mellitus.

Sorbitol Pathway

Hyperglycemia leads to conversion of glucose to sorbitol.

Clinical Complications of Diabetes Mellitus

If the diabetes is not controlled, one has to face the major complications of diabetes mellitus:

- Retinopathy
- Neuropathy
- Angiopathy
- Nephropathy
- Increased susceptibility to infections
- Hyperlipidemia
- Ketoacidosis
- Hyperglycemic hyperosmolar nonketotic coma (HHNC)

  Except HHNC all are seen frequently in type I DM.

  Most of the following complications are seen in uncontrolled diabetes mellitus:

Retinopathy

- Hyperglycemia leads to sorbitol formation
- This may leads to retinal microvascular abnormalities.
- It in turn may lead to retinopathy and blindness (glycosylation of retinal proteins also causes cataract formation).

Neuropathy

- It is the most common complication of diabetes mellitus.
- It is identified by a variety of symptoms, such as pain, numbness tingling or burning sensation in extremities, dizziness and double vision.
- Secondary manifestations of neuropathy include cardiac failure, excessive sweating and impotence (male).

Angiopathy

- It means damage to basement membrane of blood vessels.
- Angiopathy increases the risk of stroke and coronary artery disease.
- It may cause atherosclerosis in medium sized arteries, such as cerebral arteries (leading to paralysis) coronary arteries (leading to myocardial infarction), or peripheral vessels. (leads to gangrene of limbs).
- If small vessels are affected, it is called microangiopathy.
- Microangiopathy may lead to diabetic retinopathy and nephropathy.

Nephropathy

- Damage to the glomerulus of nephron of the kidney and associated capillaries.
- This damage leads to decreased filtering capacity of the kidneys.
- Capillary damage is caused by angiopathy, which is a common feature in diabetic nephropathy.

Urinary Protein

- Examination of urinary protein is useful for the diagnosis of nephropathy in diabetic patients.
- Normal urinary albumin excretion is less than 150 mg/day. If it is more, it indicates nephropathy.

Hyperlipidemia and Atherosclerosis

- Serum cholesterol, triglyceride and VLDL levels are increased in type II diabetes mellitus.
- HDL decreased in diabetics.
- All these factors increase the risk of atherosclerosis in diabetics.

Diabetic Ketoacidosis

- Deficiency of insulin activity in diabetes increases lipid breakdown.
- The lipid breakdown increases the concentration of acetyl-CoA.
- In normal condition, acetyl-CoA combines with oxaloacetate and enters the Krebs cycle for energy production.
- In diabetes, insulin deficiency causes depletion of oxaloacetate. Therefore, the acetyl-CoA cannot enter the Krebs cycle. So, it enters the alternate pathways such as cholesterol formation or ketone body

formation. Therefore, the cholesterol and ketone body increase in blood.

- Increased ketone body level in blood is called **Ketonemia**. Ketonemia leads to excretion of ketone bodies in urine. The condition is called **ketonuria**. The person's breath smells of acetone. The conditions of ketonemia, ketonuria and acetone smell of breath together constitute the condition called **ketosis**.
- The accumulation of acidic ketone bodies in blood decreases its pH resulting in metabolic acidosis. Since it is seen due to diabetes, it is called diabetic ketoacidosis.
- Ketone bodies are excreted as their sodium or potassium salts. This leads to loss of bases from the body. To compensate for this hyperventilation occurs. This is called **acidotic breathing or Kussmaul respiration**.
- If the patient is not treated properly, he or she may enter unconscious state, coma and death.

Hyperglycemic Hyperosmolar Nonketotic Coma (HHNC)

- It is characterized by glucose level above 600 mg/dL.
- Blood pH is normal or slightly decreased. Keto acids are normal, serum osmolality is above 350 mosm/kg.
- Osmotic diuresis due to glycosuria causes severe water and electrolyte depletion.
- Coma results from dehydration of cerebral cells.
- Even though diabetic ketoacidosis is common in type I, HHNC is primarily seen in type II. So, the condition is common in older patients.
- Giving hypotonic intravenous drugs with insulin treats this.

Lactic Acidosis

- It is caused by the accumulation of lactic acid.
- Accumulation of lactic acid occurs due to overproduction or underutilization of lactic acid.
- Lactic acidosis may be seen in diabetic patients treated with hypoglycemic drugs such as biguanides and phenformin. These drugs inhibit gluconeogenesis and TCA cycle.

Infection

- Diabetics are highly susceptible to infection, ulceration and gangrene in the extremities.
- Skin disorders are more commonly seen in diabetics than in non-diabetics.

Pregnancy

In an uncontrolled diabetic mother, fetal abnormalities, premature birth, big babies (macrosomia), chances of abortion, intrauterine death of fetus and hypocalcemia may occur (cesarean section and hypertensive disorders may also be seen).

Gestational Diabetes Mellitus (GDM)

- If the carbohydrate intolerance is noticed for the first time during pregnancy in non-diabetic women, it is referred to as gestational diabetes mellitus.
- A known diabetic patient, who becomes pregnant, is not included under this category.
- If the FBS value is more than 130 mg% during pregnancy, it is considered as gestational diabetes.
- The frequency of abnormal glucose tolerance during pregnancy range from 1 to 15%. But the incidence of gestational diabetes mellitus is 1 to 5%.
- The glucose tolerance may come to normal after delivery or during pregnancy itself.
- Strong family history of diabetes mellitus, a history of stillbirth or neonatal death, a history of bearing a infant with congenital anomaly are the clues suggesting gestational

diabetes mellitus. Delivery of large babies is one of the results of gestational diabetes.

- Symptoms of gestational diabetes are mild and it is not expressed in the mother. But it is associated with increased incidence of congenital malformations, increased risk of recurrence of diabetes after 10 years of parturition and prenatal mortality.
- Early diagnosis and control during the 8th to 12th weeks of pregnancy can significantly decrease the risk of congenital malformations.

Spot test: The spot test is the preferred test in the beginning to screen the GDM.

- The spot test is performed between 24th to 28th weeks of gestation on all pregnant women.
- Glucose load of 50 g given orally irrespective of time or meal.
- Determine the plasma glucose after 1 hour of glucose load.
- Oral GTT is preferred when estimated spot test blood glucose level rises above 150 mg/dl.

Diagnosis of GDM with GTT

- Perform oral glucose tolerance test in the morning after 10 to 12 hours of fasting.
- Measure fasting plasma glucose.
- Give 75 or 100 g glucose orally.
- Collect blood and urine samples simultaneously at the interval of 1 hour.
- Measure plasma glucose in all the blood samples and also check the urine for the presence of glucose.
- The positive GDM presents the values as shown below:
  - Fasting - 110 mg/dL
  - 1 hour - above 190 mg/dL
  - 2 hours - above 165 mg/dL
  - 3 hours - above 145 mg/dL
- Any one of the urine sample must be positive for Benedict's test.
- If the results are normal in a clinically suspected case, repeat the test during the 3rd trimester.

Glycosylated Hemoglobin

- Hemoglobin to which glucose is bound.
- Glycation is one of the nonenzymatic processes where the addition of sugar residue to amino groups of proteins takes place.
- Glycosylated hemoglobin is tested to monitor the long-term control of diabetes mellitus. The level of glycosylated hemoglobin is increased in the red blood cells of persons with poorly controlled diabetes mellitus.
- The formation of glycated hemoglobin is an irreversible process, and the blood level depends on both the lifespan of the red blood cell and the blood glucose concentration.
- Since the glucose stays attached to hemoglobin for the life of the red blood cell (normally about 120 days), the level of glycosylated hemoglobin reflects the average blood glucose level over the past 3 months.
- The human adult usually consists of HbA1: 97%, HbA2: 2.5% and HbF : 0.5%.
- The values of glycated hemoglobin are free of day-to-day glucose fluctuations and unaffected by exercise or food ingestion.
- Glycated hemoglobin testing is recommended for both, (a) checking blood sugar control in people who might be pre-diabetic and (b) monitoring blood sugar control in patients with more elevated levels, termed diabetes mellitus.
- Glycosylated hemoglobin is also known as glycohemoglobin or as hemoglobin A1C.

Determination of Glycated Hemoglobin by Affinity Chromatography Technique

Principle

Affinity gel columns are used to separate bound, glycosylated hemoglobin from the nonglycosylated fraction. The gel contains immobilized m-aminophenylboronic acid on cross-linked, beaded agarose. The boronic acid reacts with the cis-diol groups of glucose bound to hemoglobin to form a reversible 5-membered ring complex, thus selectively holding the glycosylated hemoglobin on the column. The nonglycosylated hemoglobin is eluted. The complex is next dissociated by sorbitol, which permits elution of the glycosylated hemoglobin. Absorbance of the bound and nonbound fractions, measured at 415 nm, is used to calculate the percent of glycosylated hemoglobin.

The major advantages of affinity chromatography are:

- No interference from nonglycosylated hemoglobin
- Negligible interference from the labile intermediate form of HbA1C and
- The method has been evaluated in some detail.

Specimen: Venous blood in tubes containing EDTA, heparin or fluoride and mixed well. Whole blood may be stored at 4°C for 1 week.

Reagents

1. *Wash buffer*: Ammonium acetate: 250 mmol—(19.27 g/1 L).
   Magnesium chloride: 50 mmol—(10.16 g/1 L)
   Sodium azide: 0.2 g.
   Dissolve 19.27 g ammonium acetate, 10.16 g magnesium chloride and 0.2 g of sodium azide in about 800 mL water. Adjust the pH to 8.0 with ammonia and dilute to one liter with water. Store at room temperature.
2. *Elution buffer*: Sorbitol: 200 mmol,
   Tris: 100 mmol
   Sodium azide: 0.2 g.
   Dissolve 36.4 g D (-) sorbitol, 12.1 g, Tris and 0.2 g sodium azide in about 800 mL water. Adjust the pH to 8.5 with 1 N HCl and dilute to one liter. Store at room temperature.
3. HCl, 0.1 mol/L.
4. HCl, 0.001 mol/L.

Preparation of Hemolysate

1. Centrifuge the blood specimen and remove the plasma and Buffy coat by aspiration.
2. Pipette 100 µL of packed cells to a small test tube.
3. Add 2.0 µL of water and mix well.
4. Let stand for about 5 minutes mix, and centrifuge. The supernatant should be clear.

Preparation of Columns

The gel columns contain 0.5 mL of immobilized gel (Glyco-Gel B) and should be stored at 4°C and protected from direct sunlight. If the gel becomes darkly colored (red-purple), that should be discharged.

1. Bring columns to room temperature.
2. Remove top stopper only, then pour off and discard the liquid in the column.
3. Remove bottom cap and place column in a suitable rack or test tube.
4. Add 2.0 mL of equilibration wash buffer (WB), let drain, and discard eluate. Column flow stops when the liquid level reaches a disk on the surface of the gel.

Procedure

1. Place the washed column in a clean 16 × 125 mm tube marked NB (for non-bound fraction).
2. Add 50 µL of clear hemolysate on top of disk. Allow it for draining.
3. Add 0.5 µL of wash buffer and let drain. This serves to ensure complete transfer of the sample through the disk and onto the gel.
4. Add 5.0 mL of WB and let drain. Total volume of eluate is 5.55 mL.
5. Transfer column to a clean tube marked B (for bound, or glycosylated fraction).
6. Add 3.0 mL of elution buffer (EB) and let drain.
7. Mix the contents of the NB and B tubes respectively and transfer to corresponding cuvettes.

8. Measure the absorbance of NB and B against water at 415 nm.

$$\frac{3.0 \times A_B}{5.55 \times A_{NB} + 3.0 \times A_B} \times 100 = \%\ \text{glycosylated Hb}$$

Regeneration of Columns

This procedure should be done immediately.

1. To the used column add 5 mL of 0.1 mol/L HCl, let drain and discard eluate.
2. Add 3 mL of HCl, 0.001 mol/L, let drain, and discard eluate.
3. Add 3 mL of HCl, 0.001 mol/L, pick up the column and insert the top stopper. Then place bottom cap over the column tip.
4. Label the column "1" to show it has been used once, "2" if it has been used twice, etc. Columns may be used 5 times and are then discarded.
5. Store all columns in the dark at 4°C when not in use.

Reference Ranges

Values for glycosylated hemoglobin are usually expressed as a percentage of total blood hemoglobin. Based on several studies of normal subjects, suggests the following reference ranges:

Hb A_1 (A_1a + b + c) = 5.0–8.0%

HbA1c only = 3.0–6.0%

Reference range may increase with age, in agreement with similar observations of fasting blood glucose levels. In poorly controlled patients with diabetes mellitus, values may extend to twice the upper limit or more but rarely exceed 20%. Values over 20% should prompt further studies to determine the possible presence of Hb F, if this is known to interfere in the method.

Hypoglycemia

- This is a condition where blood glucose concentration is below the fasting range. But it is difficult to define specific limits.
- A decline in the glucose may be seen 2 hours after a meal and often plasma glucose level is as low as 50 mg/dL. This may be observed even after oral glucose load.
- There are no symptoms, which are specific for hypoglycemia.
- The classical signs and symptoms of hypoglycemia are weakness, sweating, nausea, rapid pulse and epigastric discomfort.
- These symptoms may also be noted in other conditions, such as hyperthyroidism, pheochromocytoma and in anxiety.
- The gradual onset of hypoglycemia may not produce any symptoms.
- The brain mainly depends on blood glucose and very low levels of plasma glucose (40 mg/dL) cause severe central nervous system dysfunction.
- During prolonged hypoglycemia, the ketone bodies are the source of energy.

The signs and symptoms with prolonged hypoglycemia are:

- Headache, confusion, giddiness, lethargy to seizures and may lead to loss of consciousness and even death. These symptoms are also known as neuroglycopenia
- The most common hypoglycemia is **reactive hypoglycemia**, due to symptoms that occur 2–3 hours of food intake. The symptoms are usually mild and gradually caused by serious disease.
- The glucose concentration in neonates is much lower than the adult and it declines shortly after birth when liver glycogen is depleted.
- Reactive hypoglycemia is a clinical disorder in which the patient has postprandial symptoms, after normal food accompanied by a blood glucose level 45 to 50 mg/dL. It is important to rule out fasting hypoglycemia, before diagnosing reactive hypoglycemia. Reactive hypoglycemia is a

benign condition that may be considered as a variant of normal physiology.
- The best diagnostic test for reactive hypoglycemia is to obtain a blood sample when a patient has symptoms. Blood glucose in the normal range demonstrates that the symptoms are not due to hypoglycemia.

Blood Glucose Regulation

- The blood glucose is regulated by several metabolic pathways which are mainly modulated through many hormones.
- The major pathways are glycogenesis (the conversion of glucose to glycogen).
- Glycogenolysis (the breakdown of glycogen to glucose and other intermediate products), gluconeogenesis (the formation of glucose from non-carbohydrate sources, such as amino acids, glycerol or lactate).
- Glycolysis (the conversion of glucose to pyruvate) and oxidation to CO_2 and H_2O occurs through the TCA cycle, oxidation to $CO_2 + H_2O$ also occurs by monophosphate shunt pathways.
- During a brief fast, a decrease in the level of blood glucose is prevented by the breakdown of glycogen stored in the liver. A small amount of glucose may also be derived from the kidneys.
- The liver glycogen contributes glucose through glycogenolysis.
- The liver and kidney contain glucose 6-phosphatase, which convert glucose-6 phosphate to glucose, which is through gluconeogenesis.
- The glucose 6-phosphatase enzyme is absent in skeletal muscle so muscle glycogen cannot contribute directly to the blood glucose.
- If the fasting condition prolongs, the gluconeogenesis plays a role in maintaining the blood glucose level.
- In contrast after a meal, the absorbed glucose is converted to glycogen for storage in the liver and muscle or fat for storage in the adipose tissue.
- During the fluctuations in the supply and demand of carbohydrates, the glucose concentration is normally maintained within a narrow range by hormones which modulate the movement of glucose into and out of the circulation.
- Insulin is the main hormone which decreases the blood sugar.
- Hormones like glucagon and growth hormone increase blood sugar levels.

Postprandial Blood Sugar Regulation

After the meal or breakfast, absorption of glucose from the intestine increases the blood glucose. Increased glucose level in the blood stimulates β-cells of pancreas to secrete insulin. The insulin promotes the uptake of glucose by the tissues, and promotes glycogenesis and lipogenesis. Therefore, the glucose level is regulated at the normal range.

Fasting Blood Sugar Regulation

In normal conditions, 4–5 hours after a meal, blood glucose level decreases near to fasting levels. Further decrease in blood glucose is prevented by the hyperglycemic hormones, which stimulate liver glycogenolysis. If fasting is prolonged, glucose is synthesized by gluconeogenesis pathway.

The liver is the central organ, which maintains blood glucose level.

Normal Blood Glucose Levels

- If glucose is estimated in the post-absorptive state, i.e., an overnight fast of 12 hours, it is called fasting blood sugar (FBS). In normal persons, the fasting blood sugar level is 70 to 100 mg/dL. The plasma values are slightly higher than the whole blood glucose, since RBCs contains only 73% of water compared to the 93% of water of plasma.
- If blood glucose is estimated 2 hours after the meal, it is called postprandial blood sugar (PPBS). In normal persons, the PPBS level is 90–140 mg/dL.

- If blood glucose is estimated randomly, it is called random blood glucose (RBS). The normal random blood glucose level is 90 to 150 mg/dL.
- When the blood glucose level is in the normal range, it is called normoglycemia.
- Increase in blood glucose level above the normal level is called hyperglycemia. It is a harmful condition.
- Decrease in blood glucose level below 50 mg/dL is called as hypoglycemia. Prolonged hypoglycemia is fatal.
- In normal condition, glucose is not be excreted in the urine.
- Excretion of glucose in urine is called as glucosuria.

Blood Glucose Regulation by Hormones

Insulin

- Insulin is the peptide hormone produced by the β-cells of islets of Langerhans of the pancreas.
- Human insulin consists of 51 amino acids in two chains namely alpha and beta joined by two disulfide bridges with a molecular weight of 6000. Carboxyterminal region of the β-chain appears to be crucial for the biological actions of insulin.
- Insulin from most animals is immunologically and biologically similar to human insulin and all insulin-dependent patients were treated with pure insulin obtained from beef or pig pancreas.
- It is an anabolic hormone, which stimulates the uptake of glucose into muscle and other tissues.
- Insulin promotes the conversion of glucose to glycogen or fat for storage.
- Inhibits the glucose production by the liver through gluconeogenesis and glycogenolysis.
- It also stimulates protein synthesis and inhibits protein breakdown.

Glucagon

- The polypeptide hormone secreted by the α-cells of pancreas.
- It stimulates the production of glucose in the liver by glycogenolysis and gluconeogenesis.
- Inhibits glycolysis.
- Depresses glycogen synthesis.
  Insulin antagonizes the effect of glucagon and also inhibits the glucagon release from the pancreas.

Epinephrine

- This is a catecholamine hormone secreted by adrenal medulla.
- Stimulates glycogenolysis and decreases glucose utilization.
- Stimulates glucagon secretion and inhibit insulin secretion by the pancreas.

Growth Hormone

- A polypeptide hormone secreted by anterior pituitary gland.
- It stimulates gluconeogenesis and lipolysis.
- It antagonizes insulin stimulated glucose uptake.

Cortisol

- Secreted by the adrenal cortex
- Stimulates gluconeogenesis
- Increases the breakdown of protein and fat.

Thyroxin

- Secreted by the thyroid gland
- Increases the rate of intestinal glucose absorption.

Somatostatin

A polypeptide hormone found in the several areas of the body but is concentrated in the hypothalamus and the cells of pancreas.

- Inhibits the release of growth hormone.
- It also decreases the secretion of glucagon and insulin by the pancreas.
  Motivating the reciprocal relationship of two hormones.

SELF TEST

1. What are the major metabolic pathways of glucose?
2. Define glycolysis.
3. Write about the clinical significance of glycolysis.
4. What are the disorders associated with glycolysis?
5. Name the regulatory enzymes of glycolysis.
6. What is TCA cycle?
7. Define gluconeogenesis.
8. Why gluconeogenesis is important?
9. What is glycogenesis?
10. Define glycogenolysis.
11. Explain galactosemia.
12. Name the enzyme deficient in galactosemia.
13. Write the important features of galactosemia.
14. How can you diagnose galactosemia?
15. Explain essential fructosuria.
16. Name the enzyme deficient in essential fructosuria.
17. What will happen with high fructose intake?
18. Why must blood sugar be maintained in the normal range?
19. How is postprandial blood sugar regulated?
20. How is fasting blood sugar regulated?
21. Name the hypoglycemic hormone.
22. What does "hyperglycemic hormone" mean?
23. Name the hyperglycemic hormones.
24. Explain the actions of hyperglycemic hormones.
25. Name the different methods of estimations of glucose.
26. Write the principle of the O-toluidine method.
27. What is the principle of Folin-Wu's method?
28. State the principle of glucose the oxidase method.
29. What is insulin?
30. How insulin is synthesized?
31. Describe the structure of insulin.
32. What are the physiological actions of insulin?
33. Explain the action of insulin on carbohydrate metabolism.
34. Explain the action of insulin on lipid metabolism.
35. Name the products of proinsulin.
36. What is the importance of insulin estimation?
37. What is the importance of proinsulin estimation?
38. What is the importance of C-peptide estimation?
39. State the actions of glucagon.
40. What is diabetes mellitus?
41. What are the types of diabetes mellitus?
42. Explain type 1 diabetes mellitus.
43. Compare types of diabetes mellitus.
44. Write a note on gestational diabetes mellitus.
45. Explain impaired glucose tolerance.
46. What does "secondary diabetes mellitus" mean?
47. What are the criteria for the diagnosis of diabetes?
48. Explain the metabolic changes in diabetes mellitus.
49. Enumerate the clinical features of diabetes mellitus.
50. Mention the clinical complications of diabetes mellitus.
51. Briefly explain the following clinical complications of diabetes mellitus.
    - Retinopathy
    - Neuropathy
    - Angiopathy
    - Nephropathy
52. Explain diabetic ketoacidosis.
53. Add a note on glycated hemoglobin.
54. What is glucose tolerance test?
55. How can you prepare patient for GTT?
56. Write the procedure for GTT.
57. What are the factors affecting GTT?
58. Write a note on hypoglycemia.

MULTIPLE CHOICE QUESTIONS

1. **The preservative used during the collection of blood for glucose estimation is:**
   a. Potassium oxalate
   b. Heparin
   c. Sodium fluoride
   d. Sodium oxalate
2. **The specific method used for glucose estimation is:**
   a. Ortho-toluidine method
   b. Folin-Wu's method
   c. PO_2 electrode method
   d. Glucose-oxidase peroxidase method
3. **If 500 mg glucose is dissolved in 100 mL water then the concentration of glucose in the 2 mL solution is:**
   a. 5 mg
   b. 200 mg
   c. 10 mg
   d. 20 mg
4. **The normal range for fasting blood sugar is:**
   a. 90–140 mg%
   b. 60–90 mg%
   c. 90–150 mg%
   d. None
5. **The amount of glucose given during a spot test is:**
   a. 50 g
   b. 100 mg
   c. 100 g
   d. 75 g
6. **The reference range for glycated hemoglobin is:**
   a. 5–8 g% Hb
   b. 20–12 g% Hb
   c. 40–50 g% Hb
   d. 2–4 %g Hb

9

UNIT

Hormones

Learning Objectives

At the end of this unit, the learner should be able to understand:

- The hormones secreted from anterior and posterior pituitary hormones.
- The various gland and their hormones.
- The functions of different hormones in the humans.
- Signs and symptoms of decreased and increased hormones.

INTRODUCTION

Hormones are substances secreted by highly specialized cells and carried by extracellular fluid (mainly blood) and act on the target organ where they alter the activity of the cells quantitatively, which influence:

1. Metabolism
2. Growth
3. Reproduction
4. Adaptation to the environment.

- Hormones carry messages from glands to cells to maintain chemical levels in the bloodstream that achieve homeostasis.
- Glands manufacture hormones.
- Hormones circulate freely in the bloodstream, waiting to be recognized by a target cell, their intended destination.
- The target cell has a receptor that can only be activated by a specific type of hormone. Once activated, the cell knows to start certain function within its walls.
- There are two types of hormones—steroids and peptides.
- In general, steroids are sex hormones related to sexual maturation and fertility. Steroids are made from cholesterol.
- Cortisol is an example of a steroid hormone.
- Peptides regulate other functions, such as sleep and sugar level. They are made from long strings of amino acids, so sometimes they are referred to as "protein" hormones.
- Growth hormone helps us to burn fat and build up muscles.
- Insulin starts the process of converting sugar into cellular energy.
- As special categories, autocrine hormones act on the cells of the secreting gland, while paracrine hormones act on nearby, but unrelated cells.

CHEMICAL CLASSES OF HORMONES

Vertebrate hormones fall into three chemical classes.

1. Amine-derived hormones are derivatives of the amino acids tyrosine and tryptophan. Examples are catecholamines and thyroxin.
2. Peptide hormones consist of chains of amino acids. Examples of small peptide hormones are TRH and vasopressin. Peptides composed of scores or hundreds of amino acids are referred to as proteins.

Examples of protein hormones include insulin and growth hormone. More complex protein hormones bear carbohydrate side chains and are called glycoprotein hormones. Luteinizing hormone, follicle-stimulating hormone and thyroid-stimulating hormone are glycoprotein hormones.

3. Lipid and phospholipid-derived hormones derive from lipids, such as linoleic acid and arachidonic acid and phospholipids. The main classes are the steroid hormones that derive from cholesterol and the eicosanoids. Examples of steroid hormones are testosterone and cortisol. Sterol hormones, such as calcitriol are a homologous system. The adrenal cortex and the gonads are primary sources of steroid hormones. Examples of eicosanoids are the widely studied prostaglandins.

GENERAL ENDOCRINOLOGY (FIG. 9.1)

In classical endocrinology, the hormones are grouped into:

1. Pituitary hormones
2. Thyroid hormones
3. Parathyroid hormones
4. Pancreatic hormones
5. Suprarenal cortical hormones
6. Suprarenal medullary hormones
7. Ovarian hormones
8. Testicular hormones
9. Hypophyseal hormones.

MECHANISM OF HORMONAL ACTION (FIG. 9.2)

- The hormone binds to a site on the extracellular portion of the receptor.
- The receptors are transmembrane proteins that pass through the plasma membrane 7 times, with their N-terminal exposed at the exterior of the cell and their C-terminal projecting into the cytoplasm.
- Binding of the hormone to the receptor activates a **G protein**.
- This initiates the production of a **second messengers,** such as **cyclic AMP**, (**cAMP**) which is produced by **adenylyl cyclase** from **ATP, inositol 1,4,5-trisphosphate** (**IP_3**).
- The second messenger, in turn, initiates a series of intracellular events, such as

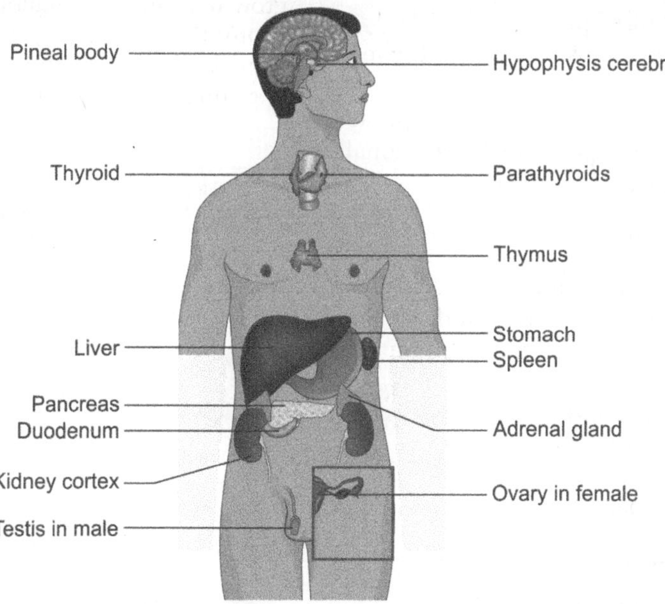

Fig. 9.1: Diagram showing the situation of major endocrine glands.

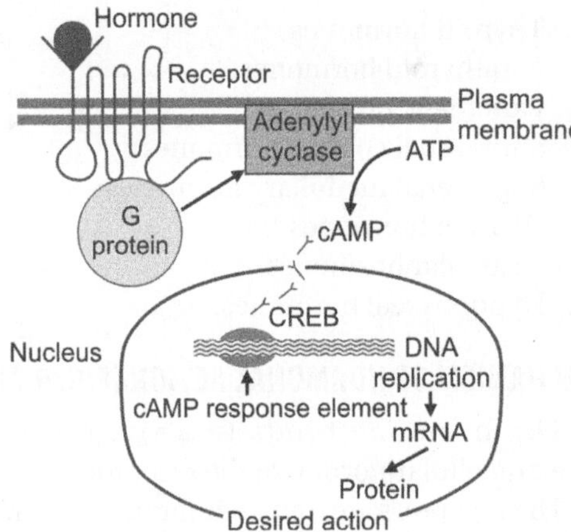

Fig. 9.2: Mechanism of hormonal action.

phosphorylation and activation of enzymes; release of Ca^{2+} into the cytosol from stores within the endoplasmic reticulum.

- In the case of cAMP, these enzymatic changes activate the **transcription factor CREB** (c**A**MP **r**esponse **e**lement **b**inding protein).
- Bound to its **response element** in the promoters of genes that are able to respond to the hormone, activated CREB turns on gene transcription, then to translation to produce the desired protein.
- The biochemical response is achieved finally.
- The cell begins to produce the appropriate gene products in response to the hormonal signal, it had received at its surface.

PITUITARY HORMONES

The endocrine is a gland, which secretes hormones also called ductless glands, as the hormone is carried not by the duct, but by blood.

Pituitary gland comprises:

- Anterior pituitary lobe
- Posterior pituitary lobe
- Intermediate lobe.

Anterior Pituitary Hormones

a. Growth hormone (GH)
b. Thyroid-stimulating hormone (TSH)
c. Follicular-stimulating hormone (FSH)
d. Luteinizing hormone (LH)
e. Adrenocorticotropic hormone (ACTH)
f. Prolactin (PRL)
g. Alpha-melanocyte stimulating hormone (α–MSH).

Growth Hormone

Human growth hormone (GH) (also called somatotropin) is a protein of 191 amino acids. The GH-secreting cells are stimulated to synthesize and release GH by the intermittent arrival of growth hormone releasing hormone (GHRH) from the hypothalamus.

- **Direct effects** are the result of growth hormone binding its receptor on target cells. Fat cells (adipocytes), for example, have growth hormone receptors, and growth hormone stimulates them to break down triglyceride and suppresses their ability to take up and accumulate circulating lipids **(Fig. 9.3)**.
- **Indirect effects** are mediated primarily by an insulin-like growth factor-I (IGF-I), a hormone that is secreted from the liver and other tissues in response to growth hormone. A majority of the growth promoting effects of growth hormone is actually due to IGF-I acting on its target cells (e.g., on long bones) **(Fig. 9.3)**.

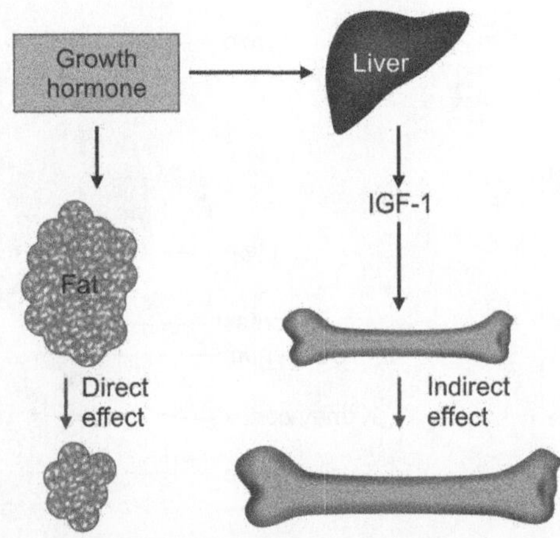

Fig. 9.3: Direct and indirect effects of GH.

Pathophysiology

In childhood: Hyposecretion of GH produces the stunted growth of a dwarf.

Dwarfism can also result from an inability to respond to GH.

This can result from inheriting two mutant genes encoding the receptors for
- GHRH
- GH

Growth hormone deficiency symptoms.
Symptoms of GH deficiency in children include the following:
- Short stature
- Low growth velocity (speed) for age and pubertal stage
- Increased amount of fat around the waist
- The child may look younger than other children his/her age
- Delayed tooth development
- Delayed onset of puberty.

Symptoms of GH deficiency in adults include the following:
- Low energy
- Decreased strength and exercise tolerance
- Decreased muscle mass
- Weight gain, especially around the waist
- Feelings of anxiety, depression, or sadness causing a change in social behavior.

The effect of excessive secretion of growth hormone is also very dependent on the age of onset and is seen as two distinctive disorders:

Hypersecretion leads to gigantism in children.

Gigantism is the result of excessive growth hormone secretion that begins in young children or adolescents. It is a very rare disorder, usually resulting from a tumor of somatotropes

In adults, a hypersecretion of GH leads to acromegaly.

Acromegaly results from excessive secretion of growth hormone in adults, usually the result of benign pituitary tumors. The onset of this disorder is typically insidious, occurring over several years. Clinical signs of acromegaly include overgrowth of extremities, soft-tissue swelling, abnormalities in jaw structure and cardiac disease. The excessive growth hormone and IGF-I also lead to a number of metabolic derangements, including hyperglycemia.

Thyroid-stimulating Hormone

The TSH (also known as thyrotropin) is a glycoprotein consisting of:
- A beta chain of 112 amino acids and an alpha chain of 89 amino acids. The alpha chain is identical to that found in two other pituitary hormones, FSH and LH. Thus, its beta chain that gives TSH its unique properties.
- The secretion of TSH is stimulated by the arrival of thyrotropin releasing hormone (TRH) from the hypothalamus.
- Inhibited by the arrival of somatostatin from the hypothalamus.
- As its name suggests, TSH stimulates the thyroid gland to secrete its hormone **thyroxin (T_4) (Fig. 9.4).**
  Normal value 0.3–5 mIU/mL

Follicular-stimulating Hormone

In female, it acts on the ovary to stimulate the development of ovarian follicle.
- In male, FSH acts on the testes for the maturation of sperm.
- It is a glycoprotein hormone, such as LH, hCG and TSH consists of two noncovalently associated subunits alpha and beta.
- The beta subunit confers its immunological and functional specificity.

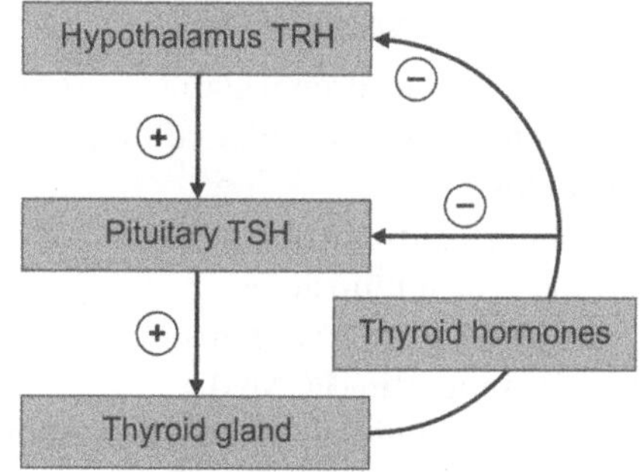

Fig. 9.4: Release of thyroid hormones.

- The gonadotropic cells of the anterior pituitary secrete both FSH and LH in response to gonadotropin releasing hormone (GnRH).
- It controls growth and reproductive activities of gonadal tissues.

Normal value

In adult woman:

Follicular cycle	—	3–20 mIU/mL
Mid cycle	—	9–26 mIU/mL
Luteal cycle	—	1–12 mIU/mL
Menopausal	—	18–153 mIU/mL
In males:	—	1–12 mIU/mL

Luteinizing Hormone

- In females, it stimulates the ovarian follicle to mature and also to secrete the estrogen. Therefore, estrogens modulate the secretion of LH and FSH, which in turn regulate menstrual cycles in females.
- In males, it stimulate the secretion of testosterone.
- The determination of the concentration of the LH is essential for the prediction of ovulation, in the evaluation of infertility and the diagnosis of pituitary and gonadal disorders.

Normal value

In female:

Follicular cycle	2–15 mIU/mL
Mid cycle	12–105 mIU/mL
Luteal cycle	0.6–19 mIU/mL
Menopausal	16–64 mIU/mL
In males:	2–12.5 mIU/mL

Adrenocorticotropic Hormone (ACTH)

- It stimulates the adrenal gland to secrete the adrenal, cortical, and medullary hormones.
- Adrenocorticotropic hormone (ACTH) is a peptide of 39 amino acids.
- It is cut from a larger precursor pro-opiomelanocortin (POMC).
- ACTH acts on the cells of the adrenal cortex stimulating them to produce their hormone.

Pathophysiology

- If ACTH secretion is increased by the pituitary or by ectopic production from a tumor, it results in Cushing's syndrome.
- The decreased ACTH production leads to Addison's disease.

Prolactin (Somatomammotropin)

- Prolactin is a protein of 198 amino acids.
- During pregnancy, it helps in the preparation of the breasts for future milk production. After birth, prolactin promotes the synthesis of milk.
- Prolactin secretion is stimulated by TRH and repressed by estrogens and dopamine.

Pathophysiology

- Hyperprolactinemia is a cause of infertility in females.
- Secretion of prolactin is stimulated by TRH and inhibited by PIF.

  Normal range:

  Females: 5.4–22.5 ng/mL (mid cycle) 4.5–15 ng/mL (menopausal women).

  Male: 4.2–15 ng/mL.

Posterior Pituitary Hormone

Vasopressin

- It was originally named because of its ability to control blood pressure when administered in pharmacological amounts.
- But more appropriately, it is called antidiuretic hormone (ADH), because of its important function to promote reabsorption of water from the distal convoluted tubules.
- If there is defect in the ADH secretion or the decreased action, it may lead to diabetes insipidus.
- Diabetes insipidus is characterized by excretion of large volumes of diluted urine.
- *Primary diabetes insipidus:* An insufficient secretion of hormone, which is due to the destruction of the hypothalamic–hypophyseal tract.
- Arises due to basal skull fractures.

- Tumor or infection.
- It may be hereditary also.

Biochemical Findings

- Decreased specific gravity
- Decreased ADH
- Diluted urine
- Polyurea.

Oxytocin

- Produced in hypothalamus and transported to posterior pituitary gland.
- Appropriate stimulation releases the hormones into the blood.
- The neural impulses that result from stimulation of the nipples are the primary stimuli for oxytocin release.
- Vaginal and uterine distention is the secondary stimuli.
- Estrogen also stimulates the production of oxytocin.
- Oxytocin causes contraction of uterine smooth muscles and thus is used in pharmacological amount to induce labor in humans.
- The most likely physiologic function of oxytocin is stimulation for the contraction of cells surrounding mammary alveoli. This promotes the movement of milk into the system and allows milk ejection.

Thyroid Gland (Fig. 9.5)

Secretes thyroid hormones **T_4 and T_3**

Thyroid Hormones

The thyroid gland synthesizes and secretes: **T_4 and T_3**

- The thyroid gland releases its hormone upon stimulation by TSH.
- Thyroxin (T_4) is a derivative of the amino acid tyrosine with four atoms of iodine.
- In the liver, one atom of iodine is removed from T_4 converting it into triiodothyronine (T_3).
- T_3 is the active hormone.

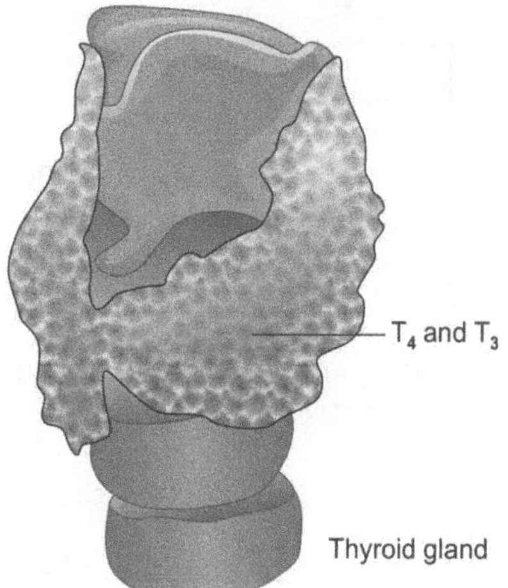

Fig. 9.5: Thyroid gland and hormones.

- It has many effects on the body. Among the most prominent of these are:
  - An increase in metabolic rate (seen by a rise in the uptake of oxygen).
  - An increase in the rate and strength of the heartbeat.
- The thyroid cells responsible for the synthesis of T_4 take up circulating iodine from the blood.
- Thyroid hormones stimulate:
  - The gluconeogenesis
  - RNA synthesis
  - Protein synthesis.
- Increased T_3 concentration causes protein catabolism and negative nitrogen metabolism.
- This is one of the reasons for weight loss in hyperthyroidism.

Synthesis of T_3 and T_4:

Tyrosine + I^+ = Monoiodotyrosine (MIT)

Monoiodotyrosine + monoiodotyrosine = Diiodotyrosine (DIT)

MIT + DIT = T_3 = Tri-iodotyrosine

DIT + DIT = T_4 = Tetraiodothyronine (Thyroxin)

Hypothalamic pituitary thyroid negative/positive feedback system **(Fig. 9.6)**.

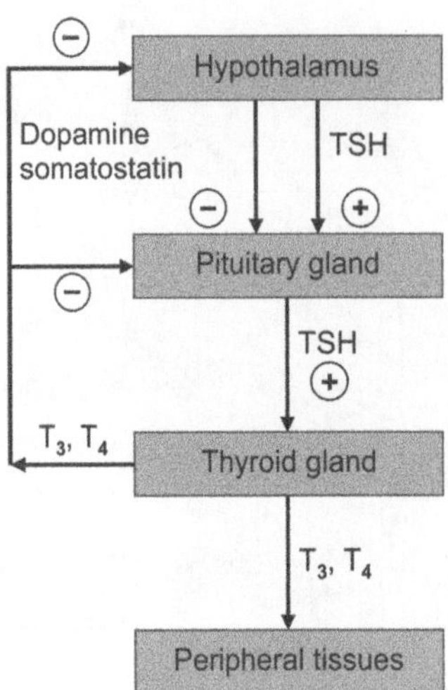

Fig. 9.6: Negative/positive feedback system.

Pathophysiology

Hypothyroidism

Hypothyroid diseases; caused by inadequate production of T_3.

Over 90% of cases of hypothyroidism occur because of autoimmune destruction of the thyroid gland (Hashimoto's disease).

Radioiodine or surgical treatment of hyperthyroidism.

Cretinism: Hypothyroidism in infancy and childhood leads to stunted growth and intelligence. It can be corrected by giving thyroxin if started early enough.

Myxedema: Hypothyroidism in adult's leads to lowered metabolic rate and vigor.

It can be reversed by giving thyroxin.

Goiter (Fig. 9.7): Enlargement of the thyroid gland. Can be caused by:

- Inadequate iodine in the diet with resulting low levels of T_4 and T_3.
- An autoimmune attack against components of the thyroid gland (called Hashimoto's thyroiditis).
- The region for hypothyroid disease produces an enlarged gland.
- The activity of the thyroid is under negative feedback control:

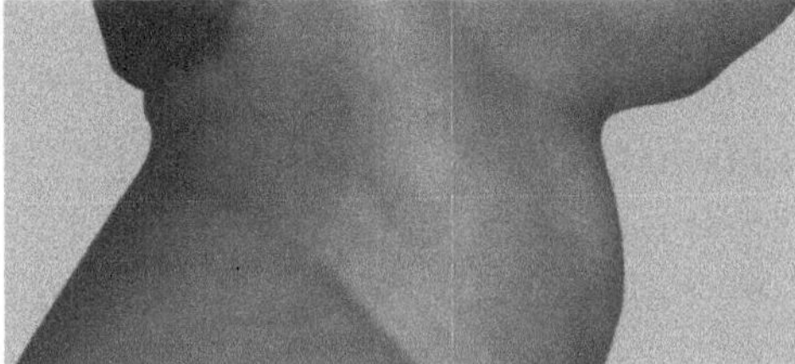

Fig. 9.7: Goiter.

  - The synthesis and release of TRH and TSH is normally inhibited as the levels of T_4 and T_3 rise in the blood.
  - When the iodine supply is inadequate, T_4 and T_3 levels fall.
  - This stimulates the hypothalamus and pituitary to increased TRH and TSH activity respectively. This stimulates the thyroid gland to enlarge (fruitlessly).

Symptoms

- Decrease basal metabolic rate (BMR)
- Slow heart rate
- Diastolic hypertension
- Sluggish behavior
- Sleepiness
- Constipation
- Sensitivity to cold
- Dry skin and hair.

A diagnosis of hypothyroidism can be suspected in patients with fatigue, cold intolerance, constipation, and dry, flaky skin. A blood test is needed to confirm the diagnosis.

When hypothyroidism is present, the blood levels of thyroid hormones can be measured directly and are usually decreased. However, in early hypothyroidism, the level of thyroid hormones (T_3 and T_4) may be normal. Therefore, the main tool for the detection of hypothyroidism is the measurement of the TSH, the thyroid stimulating hormone.

Biochemical Findings

- Decreased T_3, T_4 and increased TSH especially in primary hypothyroidism.
- Decreased T_3, T_4 and decreased TSH in secondary hypothyroidism.

Treatment

A pure, synthetic T_4 is widely used available. In majority of patients, synthetic T_4 is readily and steadily converted to T_3 naturally in the bloodstream, and this conversion is appropriately regulated by the body's tissues.

Hyperthyroidism

Hyperthyroid diseases; caused by excessive secretion of thyroid hormones.

Graves' Disease

It is caused by a generalized overactivity of the thyroid gland. In this condition, the thyroid gland usually loses its capacity to respond to the normal control by the pituitary gland via TSH. Graves' disease is hereditary and is more common in women than men. The triggers of Graves' disease include stress, smoking, radiation to the neck, medications, infectious organisms (viruses). The disease can be diagnosed by a nuclear medicine thyroid scan and blood test. This disease may be associated with eye disease (Graves' ophthalmopathy) **(Fig. 9.8)** and skin lesions.

Osteoporosis

High levels of thyroid hormones suppress the production of TSH through the negative-feedback mechanism mentioned above. The resulting low level of TSH causes an increase in the numbers of bone-reabsorbing osteoclasts resulting in osteoporosis.

Symptoms

- Rapid heart rate
- Nervousness

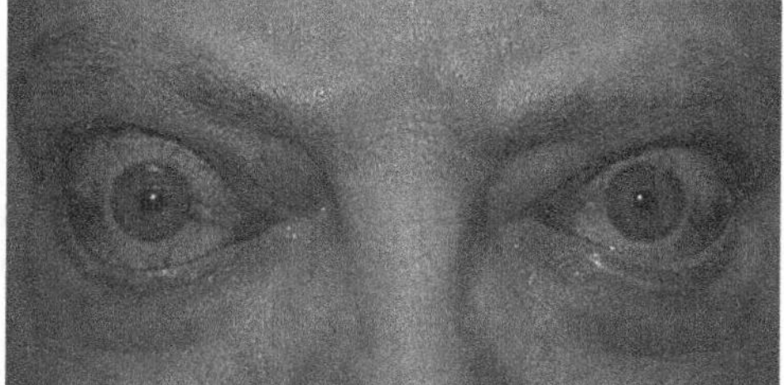

Fig. 9.8: Eve disease in Graves' disease.

- Inability to sleep
- Weight loss in spite of hyperthyroidism
- Weakness
- Excessive sweating
- Sensitivity to heat.

Diagnosis

Measuring the level of thyroid-stimulating hormone (TSH), produced by the pituitary gland (which in turn is also regulated by the hypothalamus's TSH releasing hormone) in the blood is typically the initial test for suspected hyperthyroidism. A low TSH level typically indicates that the pituitary gland is being inhibited or "instructed" by the brain to cut back on stimulating the thyroid gland, having sensed increased levels of T_4 and/or T_3 in the blood. In rare circumstances, a low TSH indicates primary failure of the pituitary, or temporary inhibition of the pituitary due to another illness (euthyroid sick syndrome) and so checking the T_4 and T_3 is still clinically useful.

Measuring specific antibodies, such as anti-TSH-receptor antibodies in Graves' disease, or anti-thyroid-peroxidase in Hashimoto's thyroiditis—a common cause of hypothyroidism—may also contribute to the diagnosis.

Treatment

The large and generally accepted modalities for treatment of hyperthyroidism in humans involve initial temporary use of suppressive thyrostatics medication (antithyroid drugs), and possibly later use of permanent surgical or radioisotope therapy. All approaches may cause under active thyroid function (hypothyroidism), which is easily managed with levothyroxine or triiodothyronine supplementation.

Biochemical Findings

Increased T_3 and T_4 and TSH decreased.

Normal levels:

$T_3 = 0.8\text{–}2.0\ \mu g/mL$

$T_4 = 4.5\text{–}12.0\ \mu g/dL$

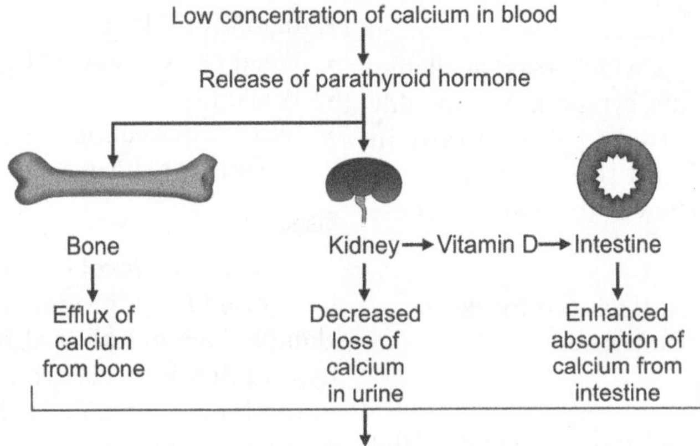

Fig. 9.9: Calcium homeostasis.

T3 and T4 exist in two forms—bounded and free. Bounded T3 and T4 attach to proteins in the blood, while free T3 and T4 flow through the bloodstream independently. Because free T3 and T4 can interact with the body's tissues, they are often considered a better indicator of thyroid function when used alongside other thyroid hormone tests.

- Normal free T3 levels range from 0.8–1.8 ng/dL
- Normal free T4 levels in adults typically range from 0.7–1.9 ng/dL

Parathyroid Hormones (PTH)

Functions

Calcium homeostasis (regulation) **(Fig. 9.9)**

The PTH restores normal calcium concentration by acting directly on bone and kidney and acting indirectly on intestinal mucosa.

Bone: It increases the resorption in both organic and inorganic phases, which lose Ca^{2+} into ECF.

Kidney: It reduces renal clearance or excretion of calcium and hence increases ECF concentration of calcium.

GIT: It increases efficiency of calcium absorption from the intestine by promoting the synthesis of calcitriol. It acts upon the intestine to increase Ca^{2+} absorption and plays a permissive role of PTH on bone and kidney.

The PTH increases renal phosphate clearance also. Thus the net effect of PTH on bone and kidney is to increase ECF Ca^{++} concentration and decrease ECF PO_4 concentration.

Excessive secretion of parathyroid hormone is seen in two forms.

Primary Hyperparathyroidism

- It is a disorder of the parathyroid glands.
- Most people with this disorder have one or more enlarged, overactive parathyroid glands that secrete too much parathyroid hormone.
- In secondary hyperparathyroidism, a problem, such as kidney failure makes the body resistant to the action of parathyroid hormone.
- This excess PTH triggers the release of too much calcium into the bloodstream.
- The bones may lose calcium, and too much calcium may be absorbed from food.
- The levels of calcium may increase in the urine, causing kidney stones.
- PTH also acts to lower blood phosphorous levels by increasing excretion of phosphorus in the urine.

Inadequate production of parathyroid hormone—**hypoparathyroidism** results in

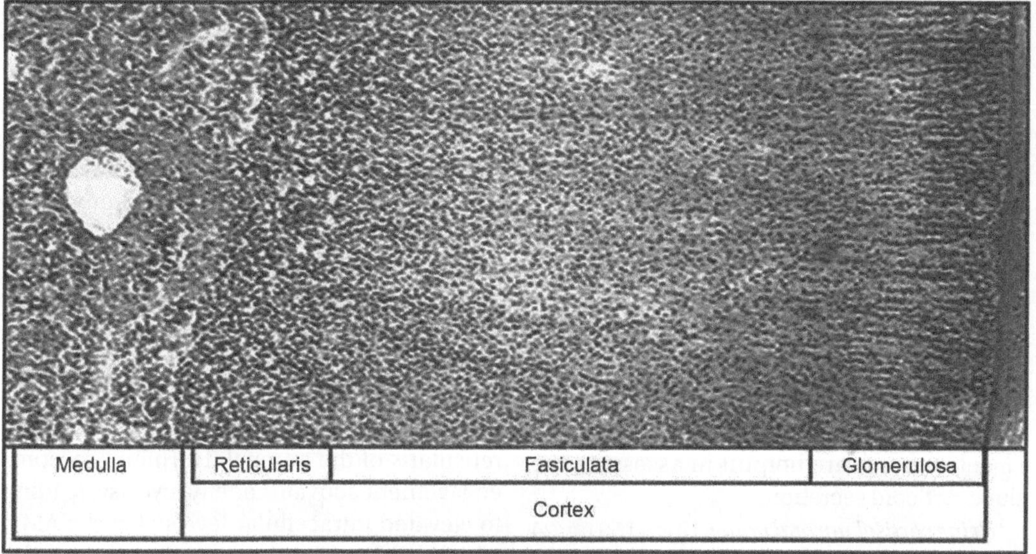

Fig. 9.10: Histology of adrenal gland.

decreased concentrations of calcium and increased concentrations of phosphorus in blood. Common causes of this disorder include surgical removal of the parathyroid glands and disease processes that lead to destruction of parathyroid glands. The resulting hypocalcemia often leads to tetany and convulsions, and can be acutely life threatening.

Adrenal Gland

The adrenal gland comprises cortex and medulla.

Cortex has again three zones **(Fig. 9.10)**:

Zona glomerulosa → produces mineralocorticoids.

Zona fasciculata → produces glucocorticoids.

Zona reticularis → secretes sex steroids, such as androgens and estrogens.

Glucocorticoids

It is a steroid hormone; it is mainly derived from cholesterol.

The functions of glucocorticoid in the human body are:

- The glucocorticoids get their name from their effect of raising the level of blood sugar. They do this is by stimulating gluconeogenesis in the liver.
- The conversion of fat and protein into intermediate metabolites that are ultimately converted into glucose.
- The most abundant glucocorticoid is **Cortisol** (also called hydrocortisone).
- Cortisol and the other glucocorticoids also have a potent anti-inflammatory effect on the body.
- They depress the immune response, especially cell mediated immune response
- They are widely used in therapy:
  - To reduce the inflammatory destruction of rheumatoid arthritis and other autoimmune diseases.
  - To prevent the rejection of transplanted organs.
  - To control asthma.

Assessment of Glucocorticoid Secretion

The plasma or serum cortisol level determination is one of the methods for assessing the secretion of glucocorticoids.

The cortisol level is determined by radioimmunoassay, enzyme-linked immunosorbent assay and fluoroimmunoassay.

Normal Value

8–26 μg/dL at AM (250–850 nmol/L)

5–18 μg/dL at PM (110–390 nmol/L)

Note: Prednisolone therapy cause spurious values. Bilirubin concentration of 200 mL/L will elevate cortisol results.

Estimation of urinary free cortisol and 17-ketosteroids are helpful in assessing the glucocorticoid secretion.

Urine cortisol normal value: Up to 150 μg/24 hour.

Urinary ketosteroids

Male	:	8–20 mg/24 hour
Female	:	6–15 mg/24 hour

Control of Cortisol Secretion

Cortisol and other glucocorticoids are secreted in response to a single stimulator—adrenocorticotropic hormone (ACTH) from the anterior pituitary. ACTH is itself secreted under control of the hypothalamic peptide corticotropin-releasing hormone (CRH). The central nervous system is thus the commander and chief of glucocorticoid responses, providing an excellent example of close integration between the nervous and endocrine systems.

Virtually any type of physical or mental stress results in elevation of cortisol concentrations in blood due to enhanced secretion of CRH in the hypothalamus. This fact sometimes makes it very difficult to assess glucocorticoid levels, particularly in animals. Observing the approach of a phlebotomist, and especially being restrained for blood sampling, is enough stress to artificially elevate cortisol levels several fold.

Cortisol secretion is suppressed by classical negative feedback loops. When blood concentrations rise above a certain threshold, cortisol inhibits CRH secretion from the hypothalamus, which turns off ACTH secretion, which leads to a turning off of cortisol secretion from the adrenal. The combination of positive and negative control on CRH secretion results in pulsatile secretion of cortisol. Typically, pulse amplitude and frequency are highest in the morning and lowest at night.

ACTH binds to receptors in the plasma membrane of cells in the zona fasciculata and reticularis of the adrenal. Hormone-receptor engagement activates adenyl cyclase, leading to elevated intracellular levels of cyclic AMP, which leads ultimately to activation of the enzyme systems involved in biosynthesis of cortisol **(Fig. 9.11)** from cholesterol.

Mode of Action

Glucocorticoids bind to the cytosolic glucocorticoid receptor. This type of receptor is activated by ligand binding. After a hormone binds to the corresponding receptor, the newly-formed receptor-ligand complex translocates itself into the cell nucleus, where it binds to many glucocorticoid response elements (GRE) in the promoter region of

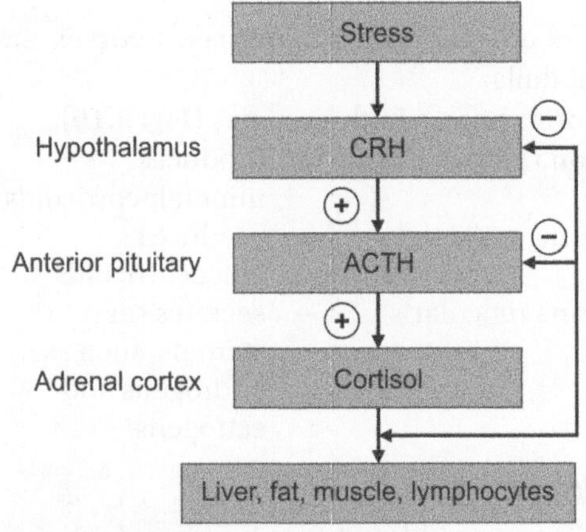

Fig. 9.11: Synthesis of cortisol.

the target genes (**Fig. 9.11**). The opposite mechanism is called transrepression. The activated hormone receptor interacts with specific transcription factors and prevents the transcription of targeted genes.

Pathophysiology

Addison's Disease (Adrenal Insufficiency)

Addison's disease is a rare endocrine or hormonal disorder that occurs in all age groups.

In this condition, the adrenal gland reduces insufficient amounts of steroid hormones (glucocorticoids and often mineralocorticoids).

The disease is also called adrenal insufficiency, or hypocortisolism.

Causes:

1. Failure to produce adequate levels of cortisol can occur for different reasons. The problem may be due to a disorder of the adrenal glands themselves (primary adrenal insufficiency)
   - Destruction of the adrenal glands by infection.
   - Their destruction by an autoimmune attack.
2. Inadequate secretion of ACTH by the pituitary gland (secondary adrenal insufficiency): An inherited mutation in the ACTH receptor on adrenal cells.

This form of adrenal insufficiency is much more common than primary adrenal insufficiency and can be traced to a lack of ACTH. Without ACTH to stimulate the adrenals, the adrenal glands' production of cortisol drops, but not aldosterone. A temporary form of secondary adrenal insufficiency may occur when a person who has been receiving a glucocorticoid hormone, such as prednisone for a long time abruptly stops or interrupts taking the medication. Glucocorticoid hormones, which are often used to treat inflammatory illnesses, such as rheumatoid arthritis, asthma, or ulcerative colitis, block the release of both corticotropin-releasing hormone (CRH) and ACTH. Normally, CRH instructs the pituitary gland to release ACTH. If CRH levels drop, the pituitary is not stimulated to release ACTH, and the adrenals then fail to secrete sufficient levels of cortisol.

Another cause of secondary adrenal insufficiency is the surgical removal of benign, or noncancerous, ACTH-producing tumors of the pituitary gland (Cushing's disease).

Other Causes

Less common causes of primary adrenal insufficiency are:

- Cancer cells spreading from other parts of the body to the adrenal glands
- Amyloidosis
- Surgical removal of the adrenal glands
- Symptoms
- Hypoglycemia
- Extreme sensitivity of insulin
- Intolerance to stress
- Weight loss
- Nausea
- Severe weakness
- Patients have low blood pressure.

The essential role of the adrenal hormones means that a deficiency can be life threatening. Fortunately, replacement therapy with glucocorticoid and mineralocorticoids can permit a normal life.

A diagnosis of Addison's disease is made by laboratory tests. The aim of these tests is first to determine whether levels of cortisol are insufficient and then to establish the cause.

ACTH Stimulation Test

This is the most specific test for diagnosing Addison's disease. In this test, blood cortisol, urine cortisol, or both are measured before and after a synthetic form of ACTH is given by injection. In the so-called short, or rapid, ACTH test, measurement of cortisol in blood is repeated 30 to 60 minutes after an intravenous ACTH injection. The normal response after an injection of ACTH is a rise in blood and urine cortisol levels. Patients with either form of adrenal insufficiency respond poorly or do not respond at all.

Routine Investigation may Show

- Hypoglycemia
- Hyponatremia
- Hypokalemia
- Eosinophilia and lymphocytosis.

Cushing's Syndrome

Cushing's syndrome is a hormonal disorder caused by prolonged exposure of the body's tissues to high levels of the hormone cortisol. In Cushing's syndrome, the level of adrenal hormones, especially of the glucocorticoids (cortisol) is too high.

Cause

- Excessive production of ACTH by the anterior lobe of the pituitary.
- Excessive production of adrenal hormones themselves (e.g., because of a tumor).
- **Ectopic ACTH syndrome:** Some benign or malignant (cancerous) tumors that arise outside the pituitary can produce ACTH. This condition is known as ectopic ACTH syndrome. Lung tumors cause over 50% of these cases.
- As a result of glucocorticoid therapy for some other disorder, such as rheumatoid arthritis or decreased glucocorticoid hormone synthesis.

Symptoms **(Fig. 9.12)**

- Hyperglycemia
- High blood pressure
- Severe protein catabolism results in thinning of skin, muscle wasting, osteoporosis and negative nitrogen balance
- There is a peculiar redistribution of fat in trunks
- Moon face
- Central obesity and typical buffalo hump

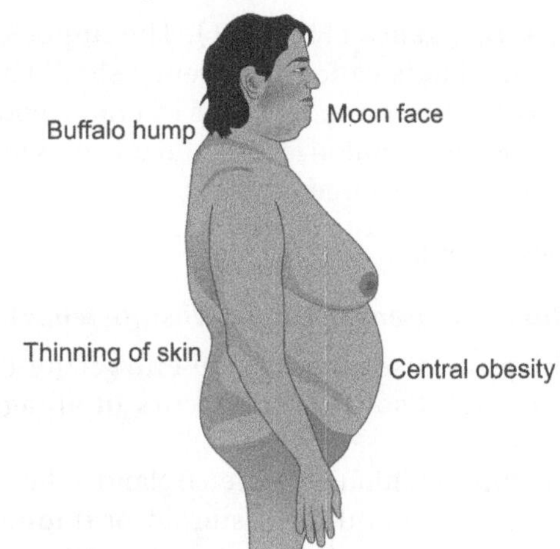

Fig. 9.12: Features of Cushing's syndrome.

- Resistant to infection and inflammatory response is impaired
- Facial hair growth.

Diagnosis is based on a review of the patient's medical history, physical examination and laboratory tests.

24-Hour Urinary Free Cortisol Level

This is the most specific diagnostic test. The patient's urine is collected over a 24-hour period and tested for cortisol. If the cortisol level is higher than 50–100 micrograms a day for an adult suggests Cushing's syndrome. The normal range may vary from laboratory-to-laboratory depending on the techniques they use.

Dexamethasone Suppression Test

This test is used to distinguish patients with excess production of ACTH due to pituitary adenomas from those with ectopic ACTH-producing tumors. Patients are given dexamethasone, a synthetic glucocorticoid, by mouth every 6 hours for 4 days. For the first 2 days, low doses of dexamethasone are given, and for the last 2 days, higher doses are given. The 24-hour-urine sample collections are made before dexamethasone is administered and on each day of the test. Since cortisol and other glucocorticoids signal the pituitary to lower secretion of ACTH, the normal response after taking dexamethasone is a drop in blood and urine cortisol levels. Different responses of cortisol to dexamethasone are obtained depending on whether the cause of Cushing's syndrome is a pituitary adenoma or an ectopic ACTH-producing tumor.

The dexamethasone suppression test can produce false-positive results in patients with depression, alcohol abuse, high estrogen levels, acute illness, and stress. Conversely, drugs such as phenytoin and phenobarbital may cause false-negative results in response to dexamethasone suppression. For this reason, patients are usually advised by their physicians to stop taking these drugs at least one week before the test.

CRH Stimulation Test

This test helps to distinguish between patients with pituitary adenomas and those with ectopic ACTH syndrome or cortisol-secreting adrenal tumors. Patients are given an injection of CRH, the corticotropin-releasing hormone that causes the pituitary to secrete ACTH. Patients with pituitary adenomas usually experience a rise in blood levels of ACTH and cortisol. This response is rarely seen in patients with ectopic ACTH syndrome and practically never in patients with cortisol-secreting adrenal tumors.

Mineralocorticoids

- It is a steroid hormone and mainly derived from the cholesterol.
- The mineralocorticoids get their name from their effect on mineral metabolism. The most important of them is the steroid **aldosterone**.
- Aldosterone acts on the kidney promoting the reabsorption of sodium ions (Na^+) into the blood.
- Water follows the salt and this helps maintain normal blood pressure.
- Aldosterone also acts on sweat glands to reduce the loss of sodium in perspiration.
- Acts on taste cells to increase the sensitivity of the taste buds to sources of sodium.
- The secretion of aldosterone is stimulated by:
  - A drop in the level of sodium ions in the blood.
  - A rise in the level of potassium ions in the blood.
  - Angiotensin II.
  - ACTH.

Primary Aldosteronism or Cohn's Syndrome

- Results from an aldosterone-secreting tumor which leads to elevated levels of plasma aldosterone.
- The plasma pH in this condition increases because of hypokalemic alkalosis and the plasma osmolality also increases.

Adrenal Medulla

Secretes

- Dopamine
- Adrenaline (epinephrine)
- Noradrenaline (norepinephrine).

Functions

- The adrenal medulla consists of masses of neurons that are part of the sympathetic branch of the autonomic nervous system.
- Instead of releasing their neurotransmitters at a synapse, these neurons release them into the blood. Thus, although part of the nervous system, the adrenal medulla functions as an endocrine gland.
- The adrenal medulla releases:
  - **Adrenaline** and **Noradrenaline**
  - Both are derived from the amino acid tyrosine
  - Release of adrenaline and noradrenaline is triggered by nervous stimulation in response to physical or mental stress.

Some of the Effects are

- Increase in the rate and strength of the heartbeat resulting in increased blood pressure

- Blood shunted from the skin and viscera to the skeletal muscles, coronary arteries, liver, and brain
- Rise in blood sugar
- Increased metabolic rate
- Bronchi dilate
- Pupils dilate
- Hair stands on end
- Reduced clotting time
- Increased ACTH secretion from the anterior lobe of the pituitary
- Promotes glycogenolysis
- Increases gluconeogenesis
- Stimulates lipolysis
- Helps in the uptake of amino acids.

Importance of Catecholamine and its Principle Metabolite Estimation

- Catecholamines are derived from tyrosine. They are named so because of the presence of the catechol nucleus.
- The major catecholamines are epinephrine, norepinephrine and dopamine produced by the adrenal medulla.
- Increased catecholamine production may result in permanent hypertension.
- *Pheochromocytoma:* Excess production of catecholamine.
- Catecholamine assays are helpful in the detection of cases of pheochromocytoma. Pheochromocytoma is relatively rare and usually benign tumors arise from chromaffin cells. This results in hypersecretion of the catecholamines.
- It is important to diagnose it because it is surgically curable and even more significantly, it can cause death from acute hypertensive attacks.
- Excessive production of catecholamines (epinephrine and norepinephrine) and their principal metabolites (metanephrine and vanillylmandelic acid-VMA) result in hypertension.
- Epinephrine is stored in chromaffin (staining strongly with chromium salts as cells of adrenal gland) granula and catabolized to vanillylmandelic acid (VMA).
- VMA excreted in urine is an indication of the production of catecholamine.
- VMA can be estimated in the 24 hour urine sample colorimetrically.

Specimen: 24 hour urine

- Normal value of excretion of VMA is 2–6 mg/24 hours.
- It is increased in pheochromocytoma.
- Generally, the total urine metanephrine test on a 24 hours sample is the preferred screening test.

Pathophysiology

The tumor of the adrenal medulla results in over secretion of its hormones and leads to a condition called pheochromocytoma.

Pancreas

Alpha cells of pancreas secrete glucagon and beta cells of islets of Langerhans of pancreas secrete insulin.

Insulin

Insulin is a polypeptide hormone synthesized from the beta cells of islets of Langerhans of pancreas.

It is synthesized as a larger precursor called pre-pro-insulin. Pre-pro-insulin has 109 amino acids. It is immediately converted into pro-insulin in the endoplasmic reticulum by the removal of 23 amino acids. So the pro-insulin formed contains 86 amino acids. The pro-insulin is transported to Golgi apparatus and is cleaved to from insulin and C-peptide.

The C-peptide contains 33 amino acids. Insulin formed from pro-insulin contains 53 amino acids from which 2 amino acids are cleaved to from insulin with 51amino acids.

Insulin mainly controls blood glucose by the following mechanisms:

1. Increases the uptake of glucose by the peripheral cells.
2. Increases the utilization of glucose by stimulating the glycolysis.
3. Stimulates glycogenesis and inhibit glycogenolysis.
4. Inhibits lipolysis.
5. Inhibits gluconeogenesis.

Structure of Human Insulin

- Human insulin contains 51 amino acids arranged in 2 polypeptide chains, namely α chain and β chain.
- The α chain contains 21 amino acids and the β chain contains 30 amino acids.
- The α and α chains are held together by a pair of interchain disulfide bonds and an intrachain disulfide bond. One interchain disulfide bond is between 7th cysteine of α chain and 7th cysteine of achain. Another disulfide bond is between 20th cys of α chain and 19th cys of α-chain. Intrachain disulfide bond is between 6th and 11th cysteine residues of α chain.
- The insulin formed is packed into granules in the Golgi apparatus with two zinc ions and one calcium ion.
- By exocytosis, these insulin granules are released into the circulation along with C-peptide.
- Both C-peptide and insulin are produced in equimolar concentrations.
- C-peptide has no biological activity.

Insulin mainly controls blood glucose by the following mechanisms:

1. Increases the uptake of glucose by the peripheral cells
2. Increases the utilization of glucose by stimulating glycolysis
3. Stimulates glycogenesis and inhibits glycogenolysis
4. Inhibits lipolysis
5. Inhibits gluconeogenesis.

Degradation of Insulin

- Insulin is rapidly degraded in the liver
- The half-life of insulin in the plasma is 4 to 5 minutes
- Insulin is mainly cleaved by insulinase and hepatic glutathione insulin transdehydrogenase.

Physiological Actions of Insulin

Insulin plays a major role in the regulation of carbohydrate, lipids and protein metabolism.

Effect on Carbohydrate Metabolism

- Insulin increases the uptake of glucose by tissues
- Insulin is necessary for the uptake of glucose by:
  - Skeletal, cardiac and smooth muscles
  - Adipose tissue
  - Leukocytes and
  - Mammary glands.
- Insulin is not required for the uptake of glucose by:
  - Brain
  - Liver
  - Kidney
  - Erythrocytes
  - Blood vessels
  - Nerves
  - Intestinal mucosa and
  - Retina.

About 80% of the glucose uptake in the body is not dependent on insulin. The remaining 20% of the glucose uptake is promoted by insulin.

Utilization of Glucose

- Insulin increases the utilization and storage of glucose.
- About 50% of glucose ingested is utilized to meet the energy needs of the body through glycolysis.
- About 40% glucose converted into fat.
- The remaining 10% is converted into glycogen.
- Insulin stimulates glycolysis and glycogenesis and inhibits gluconeogenesis and glycogenolysis.

Effect on Lipid Metabolism

Lipogenesis

Adipose tissue is most sensitive to the action of insulin.

- Insulin enhances the synthesis of triacylglycerol from glucose by providing more acetyl CoA and NADPH.

- Insulin increases the activity of acetyl-CoA carboxylase that is a key enzyme in fatty acid synthesis.
- Insulin provides NADPH required for fatty acid synthesis by increasing the activity of glucose-6-phosphate dehydrogenase.

Antilipolysis

In adipose tissue, insulin inhibits lipolysis. This is by inhibiting the activity of hormone sensitive lipase. So mobilization of fatty acids from the adipose tissue and liver are decreased.

Effect on Ketogenesis

- Insulin decreases ketone body formation (ketogenesis) by decreasing the activity of HMG-CoA synthase.
- Insulin also favors the utilization of acetyl-CoA for oxidation in Krebs cycle and lipogenesis. So, acetyl-CoA is not available for keto genesis.

Effect on Protein Metabolism

- Insulin increases protein synthesis by increasing the uptake of amino acids into the cells. So, insulin is an anabolic hormone.
- Insulin promotes cell growth and replication. Thus, insulin is an essential growth factor for all the mammalian cells.

Regulation of Insulin Secretion

The main regulator of insulin is glucose. There are some stimulators of insulin secretion and some inhibitors of insulin release.

Stimulation of Insulin Secretion

Insulin secretion is stimulated by:

- Glucose
- Amino acids
- Pancreatic and gastrointestinal hormones, such as:
  - Glucagon
  - Gastrin
  - Secretin
  - Pancreozymin, etc.
- Some medications, such as sulfonylureas, etc.

Inhibitors of Insulin Release

- Hypoglycemia
- Somatostatin (somatostatin is produced from delta cells of pancreas)
- Many drugs, such as:
  - β adrenergic blockers
  - Diazoxide
  - Phenytoin
  - Phenothiazine
  - Nicotinic acid, etc.

Note

- Proinsulin has relatively low biological activity (about 10% of insulin activity).
- C-peptide is devoid of biological activity.
- Both C-peptide and insulin are secreted into circulation in equimolar amounts but fasting levels of C-peptide are 5 to 10 times higher than fasting level of insulin. This is because the half-life of C-peptide in circulation is more than that of insulin and is about 35 minutes.
- The degradation of C-peptide occurs in the kidney. About 50% of the degradation of insulin occurs in the liver and remaining is in the kidney.
- Patients who are treated with beef or pig insulin develop antibodies against insulin in the blood.
- Insulin brings about its action by binding with insulin receptors in the cells.

Insulin Estimation

Importance of Insulin Estimation

- The main importance is the evaluation of patients with fasting hypoglycemia
- To predict diabetes mellitus
- To assess β cell activity
- To classify the type of diabetes mellitus
- To check insulin resistance.

Importance of Pro-insulin Estimation

- For the diagnosis of β cell tumor
- To find familial hyperproinsulinemia
- To cross check insulin estimation.

Importance of C-peptide Estimation

- For the evaluation of fasting hypoglycemia
- For the diagnosis of β cell tumor
- To assess β cell activity
- To monitor the therapy of pancreatectomy and pancreas or islet cell transplant.

Estimation of Insulin by Radioimmunoassay Technique

Radioimmunoassay is the technique of choice for the measurement of insulin in the biological fluids. The ELISA method is used less frequently.

Specimen

- Serum or plasma in the fasting condition can be used as specimen. Urine and CSF can also be used.
- Heparin should be used for the collection of plasma and not EDTA. This is because EDTA samples give falsely elevated levels of insulin.
- Hemolysis should be avoided since it results in false high-levels of insulin.
- In whole blood, insulin is stable for 4 to 5 hours at room temperature. Serum or plasma can be stored for 7 days at 4°C and 2–3 months at—20°C.
- 0.2 to 0.5 g of albumin is added to 100 μL of urine sample to avoid denaturation.

Principle

Iodine 125 (^{125}I) labeled insulin competes with insulin in the patient's sample for binding to an insulin specific antibody, which is immobilized on the walls of a polypropylene tube. Then the supernatant is decanted and using a gamma counter, bound Iodine 125 is estimated. The calibration curve is obtained by plotting percent of total radioactivity bound against the concentration of calibrators.

By comparing with the calibration curve, the insulin in the sample can be measured.

Reagents

1. Insulin antibody coated tubes, which are stable for one year at 4°C.
2. Iodine-125-labeled buffered insulin. It is reconstituted with 100 mL distilled water. Keep for 10 minutes and mix by inversion. The reagent is stable for one month at 4 °C
3. Calibrators—0, 5, 15, 50, 100, 200, and 400 μIU/mL insulin in lyophilized processed human serum. The zero calibrator (B_0 or maximum binding) is reconstituted with 6 mL of distilled water while other calibrators are reconstituted with 3 mL-distilled water. After reconstitution, these calibrators are stable for one month at -20°C.

Procedure

1. Bring all the reagents and specimens to room temperature.
2. Label two insulin antibody coated polypropylene tubes as (T total counts) and two tubes as NSB (nonspecific binding).
3. Label two tubes each for B_0, calibrators and patients specimens.
4. Add 200 μL of calibrator and specimen to the labeled tubes.
5. Add ^{125}I insulin to each tube immediately and mix gently. Keep aside the tubes for total count.
6. Incubate all the tubes at 37°C in a water bath for 3 hours or at room temperature for 18 to 24 hours.
7. Remove the supernatant completely and keep it to drain for 2 to 3 minutes.
8. After the complete removal of moisture, count for one minute in a gamma counter.

Calculations

Estimate the corrected counts per minute (cpm) for each pair of tubes.

Corrected cpm = average cpm-average NSB

Maximum binding (B_0) = average cpm B_0 - NSB

$$\text{Percent bound} = \frac{\text{Sample cpm}}{B_0} \times 100$$

Plot the graphs for the calibrators on a graph (logit-log graph) by taking percent bound on the vertical axis against concentration on the horizontal axis. By interpolating the calibration curve, insulin concentration of the unknown can be estimated.

Insulin—Reference Values

- The fasting insulin level in a normal nonobese person ranges from 2–25 μIU/mL.
- Higher insulin levels are seen in
  - Obese non-diabetic persons
  - Some type II diabetic patients.
- Decreased insulin level is seen in
  - Type 1 diabetes mellitus and
  - In trained athletes.

Proinsulin Estimation

- It is a difficult procedure since proinsulin estimation requires the removal of insulin and C-Peptide from the fasting plasma samples.
- C-Peptide and insulin are removed by chromatographic techniques and then proinsulin can be estimated.
- Normal plasma proinsulin level ranges from 2 to 2.6 pmol/L.

C-Peptide Estimation

- It can be estimated by RIA method.
- Several kits are commercially available for C-peptide estimation.
- Normal fasting serum concentration of C-peptide ranges from 0.78 to 1.89 ng/mL (0.25–0.6 nmol/L).
- Glucose or glucagon stimulated values range from 2.73 to 5.64 ng/mL (0.9–1.8 nmol/L). C-peptide in the urine ranges from 48 to 100 μg/L.

Glucagon

- It is a polypeptide secreted by the α-cells of islets of Langerhans of pancreas.
- It is called as anti-insulin hormone since its actions are entirely opposite to that of insulin. Glucagon stimulates the production of glucose in the liver by promoting glycogenolysis and gluconeogenesis.

Estimation of Glucagon

Method: Competitive RIA method.

Principle

^{125}I labeled glucagon competes with glucagon in the patient serum for binding to polyclonal glucagon antibodies. Using polyethylene glycol and second antibody bound glucagon can be separated from free glucagon. Bound radioactivity for the patient's specimen is compared with that of glucagon calibrators.

Specimen

- Fasting blood samples collected in chilled EDTA tubes.
- Since glucagon is very unstable in blood. A proteolytic inhibitor should be added. Proteolytic inhibitor may be trasylol, (100 μL is added to 2 mL of blood).
- Plasma is separated in a refrigerated centrifuge at 4°C. Do not expose to light and keep -20°C.

Procedure

1. Label 12 × 75 mm glass tubes in duplicate for nonspecific binding (NSB), maximum binding (B_0), total counts, controls, specimens and calibrators. Five calibrators must be taken in duplicate; labeled as 25, 50,100,250,500 and 1000 ng/L.
2. 200 μL each of calibrator, control and specimen are added to respectively labeled tubes.
3. 100 μL of glucagon rabbit antiserum is added to each tube except NSB and total counts.
4. Mix properly, cover the tubes with parafilm and incubate at 4°C for 24 hours.
5. 100 μL of ^{125}I, labeled glucagon is added to all tubes and mix properly. Total count tube should be kept aside. Remaining tubes are covered with parafilm and incubated at 4 °C for 24 hours.
6. Add 1 mL of precipitating solution, which contains goat anti-rabbit gamma globulin

and dilute each with polyethylene glycol at 4°C.

7. Mix well and centrifuge at 1500 rpm for 15 minutes in a refrigerated centrifuge.
8. Discard the supernatant completely.
9. In a gamma counter, count each tube for 1 minute.
10. Average NSB counts are subtracted from each of the other count overages for maximum binding (B_0), divide all corrected counts by the average corrected counts. Plot the graph of percent bound versus calibrator concentration.

Normal Values

- Normal fasting plasma concentration of glucagon ranges from 70 to 180 ng/L (20-52 pmol/L).
- Highly elevated (500 times) values are seen in cell tumors.

Female Sex Hormones

It is very important to know how hormones can affect the female body, mind and emotions the better able we will be to minimize their negative effects and enhance their positive ones.

Infancy

Newborn babies (boys and girls) may have slightly enlarged breasts, sometimes accompanied by a little milk production, due to the female hormone, estrogen, in the mother's body passing through the placenta during pregnancy and stimulating breast development in the baby. Finally disappearing during childhood.

Puberty

At puberty, hormones will begin to make major, lasting changes to a girl's body:

Breasts will get bigger and take on the shape of an adult woman's breasts.

She will develop underarm and pubic hair and will get noticeably taller as a significant growth spurt occurs.

Her periods will start, usually as the growth spurt is beginning to slow down.

From beginning to end, the process of puberty usually takes at least 4 years.

The hypothalamus starts to release hormone, which stimulates the pituitary gland to produce luteinizing hormone (LH) and follicle-stimulating hormone (FSH), which in turn cause a girl's ovaries to start producing other hormones.

Female Sex Hormones at Different Stages

The most important hormones made by the ovaries are known as female sex hormones, such as estrogen and progesterone. The ovaries also produce some of the male hormone, testosterone. During puberty, estrogen stimulates breast development and causes the vagina, uterus (womb) and Fallopian tubes to mature. It also plays a role in the growth spurt and alters the distribution of fat on a girl's body, typically resulting in more being deposited around the hips, buttocks and thighs. Testosterone helps to promote muscle and bone growth.

From puberty onwards, LH, FSH, estrogen and progesterone all play a vital part in regulating a woman's menstrual cycle, which results in her periods. Each individual hormone follows its own pattern, rising and falling at different points in the cycle but together they produce a predictable chain of events. One egg (out of several hundred thousand in each ovary) becomes 'ripe' (mature) and is released from the ovary and run towards fallopian tube and into the womb. If that egg is not fertilized, the levels of estrogen and progesterone produced by the ovary begin to fall. Without the supporting action of these hormones, the lining of the womb, which is full of blood, is shed, resulting in a period.

Pregnancy

If the egg released from the ovary is fertilized and a pregnancy results, a woman's hormones change dramatically. The usual fall in estrogen and progesterone at the end of the menstrual cycle does not occur, so no period is seen. A new hormone, hCG (human chorionic gonadotropin), produced by the developing placenta, stimulates the ovaries to produce the higher levels of estrogen and progesterone that are needed to sustain a pregnancy. By the fourth month of pregnancy, the placenta takes over from the ovaries as the main producer of estrogen and progesterone. These hormones cause the lining of the womb to thicken, increase the volume of blood circulating, and relax the muscles of the womb sufficiently to make room for the growing baby. Around the time of childbirth, other hormones come into play that help the womb to contract during and after labor, as well as stimulate the production and release of breast milk.

After Childbirth

The levels of estrogen, progesterone and other hormones fall sharply, causing a number of physical changes. The womb shrinks back to its non-pregnant size, pelvic floor muscle tone improves and the volume of blood circulating round the body returns to normal.

The Menopause

The next significant hormonal change for most women occurs around the time of the last period—the menopause. Over 3 to 5 years leading up to a woman's last period, the normal functioning of her ovaries begins to deteriorate. This can cause her menstrual cycle to become shorter or longer, and sometimes it becomes quite erratic. Eventually, the ovaries produce so little estrogen and finally periods stop altogether.

Ovary

Ovarian follicles secrete the following hormones:

a. Estrogen is secreted from the follicular tissue.
b. Progesterone is secreted from the corpus luteum.
c. Androgens.

Estrogen

- Estradiol is secreted by the ovary and placenta.
- It is synthesized in the granulose cells of the ovary by the aromatization of the androgens synthesized in the thecal cells and in the placenta.
- The aromatization is stimulated by follicle stimulating hormone (FSH, follitropin) which in turn stimulates the production of human luteinizing hormone (LH, lutropin) receptors necessary for the synthesis of androgen precursors.
- It is responsible for the development of female sexual differentiating characters, such as uterus, vagina, pelvis and pubic and axillary hairs.
- It regulates the menstrual cycle and is essential for breast development.
- Influences the secretion of LH from anterior pituitary.
- The measurement of estradiol is important for the evaluation of normal sexual development (menarche), causes of infertility (anovulation, amenorrhea, dysmenorrhea), and menopause. Normal estradiol levels are lowest at menses and in the early follicular phase and then rise in the late follicular phase just before the LH surge, initiating ovulation.
- As LH peaks, estradiol begins to decrease before rising again during luteal phase.
- If conception does not take place, estradiol falls further to its lowest levels, thus initiating menses.
- If conception occurs, estradiol levels continue to raise reaching levels of 100 to 500 pg/mL during the first trimester, 5000 to 15,000 pg/mL during the second trimester and 10,000 to 40,000 pg/mL during the third trimester.
- At menopause, estradiol levels remain low.

Normal Values

Women: 23–145 pg/mL—follicular
112–443 pg/mL—mid cycle
48–241 pg/mL—luteal cycle.
Men: 2–50 pg/mL

Progesterone

- It is a steroid hormone synthesized from parent compound cholesterol.
- Causes the development of the endometrium and prepares it for the implantation of a fertilized ovum for conception.
- Stimulates the mammary gland.

Normal Value

0.175–0.7 ng/mL—follicular and mid cycle
4.7–20 ng/mL—luteal cycle.

Testes

Secretes testosterone.

Testosterone

- Promotes the growth and function of the epididymis, vas deference, prostate and seminal vesicles.
- It enhances and maintains the mobility and fertilizing power of sperm.
- Promotes protein synthesis in the body.

Normal value

Men: 2.8–8.2 ng/mL.
Adult women: 0.1–1 ng/mL (mid cycle only)

The method of estimation: Immunoassay techniques, such as RIA, ELISA and FIA are most frequently used to estimate the above hormones in the laboratory.

SELF TEST

1. What are hormones?
2. What are the hormones secreted from anterior pituitary gland?
3. Write the functions of growth hormone.
4. Explain the following with reasons:
   a. Gigantism
   b. Dwarfism
   c. Pheochromocytoma
5. Name the hormones secreted from the posterior pituitary gland.
6. Name the hormones secreted from the adrenal cortex.
7. State the hormones secreted from the adrenal medulla.
8. Give the functions of glucocorticoids.
9. What is the normal serum value of cortisol?
10. Write short notes on:
    a. Cushing's syndrome
    b. Addison's disease
11. Briefly discuss the functional mechanism of ADH.
12. Name the hormones secreted from the testes and mention their functions.
13. State the ovarian hormones.
14. Give the normal value for testosterone in male.
15. Which cells of the pancreas secrete insulin?
16. How does insulin help to regulate the blood glucose level?
17. What is Cohn's syndrome?
18. State the hormone, which stimulates the thyroid gland to secrete its hormone.
19. Write a note on:
    a. Hypothyroidism
    b. Goiter
    c. Hyperthyroidism
    d. Normal value of T_3 and T_4.
20. Name the techniques used to estimate the T_3 and T_4.

MULTIPLE CHOICE QUESTIONS

1. **Binding of hormones to receptor activates:**
   a. Glycoprotein
   b. G protein
   c. M protein
   d. Lipoproteins

2. **The hormonal action on the target organs depends on all the following factors, *Except:***
   a. Cyclic AMP
   b. Adenylate cyclase
   c. Receptor
   d. ADP
3. **Which of the following is NOT an anterior pituitary hormone?**
   a. Prolactin
   b. Follicular-stimulating hormone
   c. Antidiuretic hormone
   d. Alpha-melanocyte stimulating hormone
4. **Human growth hormone is also called as:**
   a. Cortisol
   b. Somatomammotropin
   c. Alpha-melanocyte stimulating hormone
   d. Somatotropin
5. **Concerning prolactin, all of the following statements are true, *Except:***
   a. HypoprolactInemia is a cause of infertility in females
   b. It is a protein of 198 amino acids
   c. Its secretion is stimulated by TRH
   d. Its secretion is repressed by dopamine
6. **Vasopressin:**
   a. Is secreted from anterior pituitary gland
   b. Deficiency results in diabetes mellitus
   c. Deficiency occurs due to basal skull fractures
   d. Deficiency leads to oliguria
7. **Which one of the following is NOT a hypothyroid disease?**
   a. Cretinism
   b. Myxedema
   c. Graves' disease
   d. Goiter
8. **Concerning the hypothyroidism, one of the following is INCORRECT:**
   a. Sensitivity to heat
   b. Rapid heart rate
   c. Increased BMR
   d. Reduced TSH
9. **Concerning calcium homeostasis by PTH, all of the following statements are true, *Except:***
   a. Increases the resorption bone
   b. Reduces renal clearance or excretion of calcium during hypocalcemia
   c. Inacts upon the intestine to increase Ca^{2+} absorption
   d. Increases renal phosphate clearance
10. **Concerning the glucocorticoids all of the following statements are true *Except:***
    a. Stimulates glycolysis
    b. Has anti-inflammatory effect
    c. Prevents the rejection of transplanted organs
    d. Is used to control asthma
11. **Cushing's syndrome:**
    a. Results from deficiency of glucocorticoids
    b. Present with low blood glucose
    c. Sensitive to infection
    d. Patients have obesity
12. **Cohn's syndrome results from the deficiency of:**
    a. Elevated aldosterone
    b. Elevated cortisol
    c. Reduced mineralocorticoids
    d. Reduced dopamine
13. **Concerning the adrenal gland hormones, one of the following statements is INCORRECT:**
    a. They are derived from tyrosine
    b. They rise the blood pressure
    c. Elevated BMR
    d. Reduced ACTH secretion from the anterior pituitary
14. **Insulin:**
    a. Stimulates gluconeogenesis
    b. Is synthesized directly
    c. Inhibits lipolysis
    d. Increases the uptake of glucose from the peripheral cells.

15. Concerning the estrogen, all of the following are true, *Except:*
a. Stimulates the mammary gland
b. Increases the adipose tissue fat
c. Participate in pregnancy if it occurs
d. Broadening the pelvis

16. All of the following are the adrenal gland hormones, *Except:*
a. Epinephrine
b. Antidiuretic hormone
c. Mineralocorticoids
d. Glucocorticoids

17. Which one of the following does not secret steroid hormones?
a. Ovary
b. Testes
c. Adrenal medulla
d. Placenta

18. Receptors within cell cytoplasm are specific to:
a. Peptide hormones
b. Protein hormones
c. Catecholamine
d. Cortisol

19. The maximum number of hormone secreting cells of anterior pituitary are:
a. Thyrotropes
b. Corticotropes
c. Lactotropes
d. Somatotropes

20. Which of the following is rapid acting?
a. T_4
b. TBG
c. T_3
d. Thyroglobulin

21. In myxedema, serum findings are all, *Except:*
a. Low T_3, T_4
b. High TSH
c. Low cholesterol
d. Normal creatinine

22. Conversion of vitamin D_3 to 1-25 dihydroxycholecalciferol occurs in:
a. Kidney
b. Adrenal cortex
c. Bone
d. Intestine

23. Thyroid hormone:
a. Decrease the absorption of carbohydrate from the intestine
b. Exerts a positive feedback action on TSH production
c. Indirectly increases the nitrogen excretion
d. Does not have any action on the cardiac muscle

24. Concerning aldosterone, one of the following statements is incorrect:
a. Deficiency results in hypotension
b. Increases sodium reabsorption from urine
c. Release is stimulated by an increase in angiotensin II
d. Is secreted by the zona fasciculata

25. Concerning insulin, all the following are true, *Except:*
a. Stimulates glycolysis in liver
b. Stimulates lipogenesis in liver and fat tissues
c. Is synthesized in the endoplasmic reticulum of the beta cells
d. Receptors are increased in the presence of uremia

26. Calcitonin:
a. Is produced by the parafollicular cells outside the thyroid glands
b. Is a steroid hormone
c. Is decreased in the presence of hypercalcemia
d. Increases incorporation of calcium into bone matrix

27. Parathyroid hormone:
a. Is not a peptide hormone
b. Is released in response to hypocalcemia
c. Increases phosphate reabsorption in the kidneys
d. Increases calcium excretion in the kidneys

28. **Amyloidosis:**
    a. The protein stained with eosin
    b. The deposition is intracellular
    c. Has a polymorphous structure
    d. AL type is seen in 15% of patients with multiple myeloma
29. **All the following are the anterior pituitary hormones, *Except:***
    a. Growth hormone
    b. Oxytocin
    c. ACTH
    d. FSH
30. **Biochemical findings of hypothyroidism are:**
    a. Normal TSH, decreased T_3 and T_4
    b. Increased T_3 and T_4 and decreased TSH
    c. Decreased T_3 and increased TSH
    d. Decreased TSH and decreased T_3 and T_4
31. **The hormone which helps in maintaining calcium homeostasis is:**
    a. Adrenocorticotropic hormone
    b. Luteinizing hormone
    c. Parathyroid hormone
    d. TSH
32. **The hormone which increases in Cushing's syndrome is:**
    a. Glucocorticoids
    b. Mineralocorticoids
    c. TSH
    d. Dopamine

CASE STUDIES

1. A patient presents with a blood pressure of 175/90 mm Hg, and complaints of tiredness and muscle weakness. The laboratory a result reveals that plasma sodium is slightly increased and plasma potassium is significantly decreased compared to normal. Hematocrit is also low. Plasma renin activity is markedly decreased, and serum aldosterone is increased. Which of the following is the most likely diagnosis?
   a. Addison's disease
   b. Conn's syndrome
   c. Cushing's syndrome
   d. Pheochromocytoma

   Answer is B: Conn's syndrome, or primary hyperaldosteronism, results from an adrenal tumor that secretes excessive aldosterone. The increased mineralocorticoid effects of aldosterone lead to renal sodium and water retention and increased renal potassium excretion (hypokalemia). The volume expansion also explains the decrease in hematocrit. The increased blood volume, increased blood pressure, and hypernatremia will all tend to suppress renin secretion in an attempt to compensate for the increased aldosterone.
2. A 60-year-old woman presents to her physician prior to beginning chemotherapy for newly diagnosed small cell lung carcinoma. Her examination is notable for obesity, blood pressure of 170/100, facial hair, abdominal striae, and an acneiform rash on her chest and back. Laboratory values are normal except for serum glucose of 300 mg/dL. Her chest X-ray shows a right perihilar mass and severe diffuse osteoporosis. Which of the following accounts for her physical examination, laboratory and X-ray findings?
   a. Adrenal gland destruction by metastases
   b. Anterior pituitary gland disruption by metastases
   c. Ectopic production of PTH
   d. Ectopic production of ACTH.

   The answer is D. This woman has all the classic findings of Cushing's syndrome: obesity, hypertension, hirsutism, acne, striae, glucose intolerance, and osteoporosis. Cushing's syndrome may be caused by an excess production of cortisol by bilateral adrenal hyperplasia or an adrenal neoplasm; by excess production of ACTH by a pituitary adenoma; or by ectopic production of ACTH by a tumor, most commonly a small cell lung.

3. A 35-year-old woman with disseminated histoplasmosis complains of profound weakness, easy fatigability, anorexia, weight loss, and diarrhea. Laboratory investigation reveals serum sodium of 131 mEq/L, serum potassium of 5.8 mEq/L and pH of 7.58. Skin hyperpigmentation is seen on physical examination. Which of the following is the most likely diagnosis?
   a. Primary adrenocortical insufficiency
   b. Conn's syndrome
   c. Cushing's syndrome
   d. Secondary adrenocortical insufficiency.

   Answer is C. The evidences shown indicate that this patient has adrenal insufficiency due to diminished aldosterone production. The primary form of adrenocortical insufficiency results from any condition that destroys the adrenal cortex. Clinical manifestations of hypoaldosteronemia appear when 90% of the adrenal cortex is destroyed. The most frequent form is due to an autoimmune process. The remaining cases are secondary to infections (such as tuberculosis or fungal infections) or metastatic disease involving both adrenals. Secondary adrenocortical insufficiency differs from the primary form—(1) It is caused by disorders affecting the pituitary gland or hypothalamus and leading to reduced ACTH production, and (2) It is not associated with skin hyperpigmentation. Skin hyperpigmentation results from increased production of ACTH precursor (which stimulates melanocytes), present in Addison's disease but obviously lacking in secondary adrenocortical insufficiency.

4. A 50-year-old man is evaluated for congestive heart failure. In addition to a dilated cardiomyopathy, he displays multiple signs and symptoms including intellectual function, fatigue, lethargy, cold intolerance, listlessness, thickened facial features, periorbital edema, dry and coarse skin, and peripheral edema. Serum studies demonstrate a T_4 of 1.4 μg/dL and a TSH of 22 μU/mL. Which of the following diagnoses is supported by these data?
   a. Cretinism
   b. Graves' disease
   c. Hashimoto's thyroiditis
   d. Myxedema.

   Answer is D. The diagnosis of myxedema, due to long-standing hypothyroidism in adults, is warranted. The clinical manifestations are those listed in above with the question. Myxedema can result from the many causes of hypothyroidism: Hashimoto's thyroiditis, idiopathic primary hypothyroidism, iodine deficiency, drugs, pituitary lesions, hypothalamic lesions, and damage to the thyroid by surgery or radiation.

5. A 50-year-old female develops swelling in her neck and diarrhea. X-ray shows dense calcification in her thyroid. Doctor asked her to have a nuclear scan and it showed a cold nodule that does not concentrate radioiodine. Her doctor does serum assays for several hormones. After the hormone is assayed, he tells her general practitioner that the patient probably has medullary carcinoma of the thyroid since one of the hormones is markedly raised. What hormone did the physician ordered?
   a. Calcitonin
   b. Thyroid stimulating hormone
   c. Thyroid hormone
   d. Parathyroid hormone

   Answer is A. Medullary thyroid cancer is a malignancy of the thyroid parafollicular cells. Thyroid cells normally produce the hormone calcitonin. A malignancy of these cells, therefore, can also produce calcitonin. Assay of calcitonin is a very good diagnostic test for medullary carcinoma of the thyroid. Thyroid stimulating hormone is an anterior pituitary hormone and is not produced by the thyroid gland at all.

6. A patient with small-cell carcinoma of the lung complains of muscle weakness, fatigue, confusion, and weight gain. Serum sodium is found to be 115 mEq/L. Which of the following abnormal laboratory results would also be expected in this patient?
   a. Decreased plasma atrial natriuretic peptide concentration
   b. Decreased serum osmolarity
   c. Decreased urinary sodium concentration
   d. Increased plasma aldosterone concentration.

   Answer is B. Bronchogenic carcinomas can secrete ectopic vasopressin antidiuretic hormone (ADH), leading to the syndrome of inappropriate ADH (SIADH). As long as water intake is not decreased, the increased plasma vasopressin causes excessive water reabsorption by the renal distal tubule and collecting duct. The increased total body water can explain the weight gain. Edema is usually absent because the extra free water is distributed to both intracellular and extracellular volumes. The extra-plasma water produces a dilutional hyponatremia, which can explain the weakness, fatigue, and confusion. There will also be a dilutional decrease in serum osmolarity. With SIADH, the urine sodium is usually increased compared to normal. This leads to inappropriately concentrated urine. The volume expansion resulting from the excessive water retention may be responsible for the increased urinary sodium. Volume expansion would increase plasma ANP and increase renal sodium excretion. The volume expansion would also inhibit renin secretion from the kidney with subsequent decrease in plasma aldosterone. Decreased plasma aldosterone would then allow for increased renal excretion of sodium.

7. A 48-year-old women presents with complaints of moderate weight loss over the past 4 months, intolerance, palpitations, and fine tremors in the hands. Physical examination reveals the presence of a diffuse goiter and exophthalmos. Which of the following laboratory findings would be expected in this individual?
   a. Decreased serum T_4
   b. Decreased resin T_3 uptake
   c. Increased plasma concentration of thyroid stimulating hormone
   d. Increased plasma concentration of thyroglobulin.

   Answer is D. The above case is of an individual with Graves' disease. Hypersecretion of thyroid hormone because of stimulation of the TSH receptor by thyroid-stimulating immunoglobulins results in excessive movement of thyroglobulin from the colloid to the plasma. The presence of exophthalmos is thought to be part of the autoimmune disorder in Graves' disease. It is postulated that the thyroid and orbital muscles may share a common antigen. Lymphocytic infiltration and inflammation of orbital muscle then produces the ophthalmopathy.

8. A 45-year-old male presents with complaints of recurrent headaches. He also admits to impotence and loss of libido that has gradually worsened during the past year. Visual field examination reveals a bitemporal hemianopsia. Laboratory examination reveals an increase in serum prolactin, while serum luteinizing hormone (LH) and testosterone are decreased. Which of the following is the most likely diagnosis?
   a. Idiopathic panhypopituitarism
   b. Pituitary infarction
   c. Prolactinoma
   d. LH deficiency

Answer is C. Hyperprolactinemia is the most common hypothalamic-pituitary disorder. A tumor in the pituitary (prolactinoma) that secretes excessive prolactin is the most common functional pituitary tumor. The increase in serum prolactin suppresses the normal GnRH-gonadotropin-gonadal steroid axis. Hypogonadism, manifested as amenorrhea in females or loss of libido and/or impotence in males, is a prominent symptom. Blood levels of sex steroids are usually decreased. Although not present in this patient, galactorrhea may occur due to the action of prolactin on the mammary gland. Since the anterior pituitary is located just below the optic chiasm, space-filling tumors that compress this structure may produce visual field defects.

9. At 26 weeks of pregnancy, an unidentified infection greatly compromises the viability of a developing fetus. The level of which of the following hormones in the mother's blood is most likely to be affected?
   a. Human chorionic gonadotropin
   b. Human chorionic somatomammotropin
   c. Progesterone
   d. Estriol.

   Answer is D. Plasma levels of maternal estrogens during pregnancy are dependent on a functioning fetus. The fetal adrenal cortex and liver produce the weak androgens, DHEA-S and 16-OH DHEA-S, which are carried to the placenta by the fetal circulation. The placenta then desulfates the androgens and aromatizes them to estrogens (16-OH DHEA-S, estriol) prior to delivery to the maternal circulation. Estradiol and estrone increase approximately 50 fold during pregnancy, but estriol increases about 1000 fold. When estriol is assayed daily, a significant drop may be a sensitive early indicator of fetal jeopardy.

10. A patient with signs and symptoms consistent with hypothyroidism exhibits a decrease in both serum TSH and serum T_4. Injection of TRH fails to produce the expected increase in TSH. Which of the following is the most likely cause of the patient's hypothyroidism?
    a. Secondary hypothyroidism
    b. Hashimoto's thyroiditis
    c. Iodine deficiency
    d. Tertiary hypothyroidism.

    Answer is A. A decrease in both serum T_4 and TSH could result from either a pituitary defect or a hypothalamic defect. In the case of the hypothalamic defect, decreased secretion of TRH leads to decreased TSH secretion and, hence, decreased T_4 secretion. In secondary hypothyroidism, a decrease in TSH secretion due to a pituitary defect is responsible for the decreased T_4. The TRH stimulation test can be used to distinguish between these two possibilities. Failure of TSH to increase after injection of TRH indicates a pituitary defect.

10 UNIT Plasma Proteins

LEARNING OBJECTIVES

At the end of this unit, the learner should be able to understand:

- Different types of plasma proteins.
- Separation and identification of proteins.
- Different types of immunoglobulins and their role in the humans.
- Determination and normal ranges for various proteins.

INTRODUCTION

- Blood mainly consists of solid elements, such as red blood cells (RBC), white blood cells (WBC) and platelets, suspended in a liquid medium called plasma.
- About 55 to 60% of blood is made up of plasma.
- Plasma consists of water, electrolytes, metabolites, nutrients and the proteins.
- If the blood kept without adding any anticoagulants it will clot. The liquid portion without fibrinogen is serum. This means that plasma contains over 300 proteins.
- Many of these proteins have a specific biological role and organic diseases may result when their concentration in plasma is reduced.
- Other plasma proteins, including enzymes and tumor markers, have no known function in blood, and arise a result of cell death or tissue damage.
- Plasma proteins can be classified into three main groups namely albumin, globulin and fibrinogen. All the plasma proteins except the gamma globulins are synthesized in the liver.

Albumin

- The name is derived from the white precipitate formed when egg is boiled (albus = white).
- It is present in high concentrations that is about 60% of the total proteins is albumin.
- It has one polypeptide chain with about 585 amino acids and 17 disulfide bonds with a molecular weight of 69000.
- The liver produces 12 g of albumin per day.
- Albumin helps to maintain the intravascular colloidal osmotic pressure. This pressure prevents the flow of plasma into the tissue spaces by which the fluid volume inside the blood vessels is maintained.
- The decrease in albumin level leads to escape of fluid into the tissue spaces, resulting in edema. Albumin is the intravascular transporter protein for many hydrophilic substances, such as unconjugated bilirubin, fatty acids, minerals, drugs and vitamins.
- Albumin serves as a source of amino acids for tissue protein synthesis when it is broken down. Albumin shows maximum buffering capacity. The large number of histidine

residues present in albumin is responsible for the buffering action of albumin.
- The decrease in serum albumin is called hypoalbuminemia, seen in cirrhosis, nephrotic syndrome and malnutrition.

Globulins

- The different types of globulins present in plasma are α1, α2, β1, β2 and γ-globulins.
- These proteins are glycoproteins with the molecular weight ranging from 90,000–130,000.
- The α and β-globulins helps to transport proteins, hormones, vitamins, minerals and lipids.
- The γ-globulins are known as immunoglobulin and they provide immunity against infections.

Fibrinogen

- Fibrinogen is an acute phase protein (Acute phase proteins are a class of proteins that are synthesized in the liver in response to inflammation and this response is called the acute phase reaction).
- Fibrinogen is an essential factor in blood coagulation. The conversion of fibrinogen to fibrin occurs by cleaving the Arg-Gly peptide bonds of fibrinogen.
- It is synthesized in the liver.
- The fibrin monomers aggregate and precipitate to form a clot.

Different types of plasma proteins and their concentration in the blood is as follows:

Plasma protein	*g/dL*	*%*
Total protein	6.0–8.0	100%
Albumin	3.5–5.0	60%
Globulins	2.5–3.0	40%
α1		3%
α2		11%
β		11%
γ		15%
Fibrinogen	0.2–0.4	

Q. Why fibrinogen is an acute phase protein?

Ans. Fibrinogen is a coagulation factor that is converted to fibrin and is essential for the formation of a clot. Inflammation and coagulation are tightly linked, and as such the fibrinogen level will rise in the presence of acute inflammation.

Separation of Plasma Proteins

Chemical and immunological methods are available that can quantify the concentration of a specific plasma protein with a high degree of specificity.

Less commonly electrophoresis is used to provide a semiquantitative estimate of the pattern of serum proteins.

Plasma proteins can be separated by different techniques, which mainly depend on certain properties of proteins.

i. Charged groups, which are present in the protein.
ii. Molecular weight of the protein.
 Gel filtration: Columns, which are packed with gel, are used to separate the proteins. The proteins are separated depending on their molecular weight.
iii. Precipitation of proteins by salts (salt fractionation).
 Albumin is soluble in water, whereas globulins are less soluble in water. All proteins are soluble in dilute salt solutions. As the concentration of the salt increases, proteins get precipitated from their solution.
 For example, when ammonium sulfate is added to a solution of a protein until it completely saturates, the availability of water molecules for the protein is decreased, causing the proteins to precipitate. This process is called **salting out.** Albumin is precipitated at full saturation with ammonium sulfate. Since albumin hydrophilic, it requires a higher concentration of salt to get precipitated. At full saturation, all the proteins are precipitated. Globulins are precipitated at half saturation with ammonium sulfate.

Solutions of sodium sulfite (21–28%) are also used to precipitate globulins.

iv. Precipitation by organic solvents.
Organic solvents like methanol, ethanol, acetone, etc. are dehydrating agents, which cause the precipitation of proteins. These solvents reduce the amount of water required to keep protein in solution. This results in precipitation. The protein may be denatured in this process. Hence, this process is usually carried out at 0°C.

Electrophoresis

- Electrophoresis separates the proteins into five broad fractions - albumin, α1, α2, β1, β2, and γ-globulins. Each of the globulin fractions consists of a mixture of several proteins.
- Electrophoresis is the migration of a charged molecule in an electric field.
- Negatively charged particles (anions) move towards anode (positively charged electrode). Positively charged particles (cations) move towards cathode (negatively charged electrode).
- Proteins in solution or plasma can be separated from one another by electrophoresis, because they are charged molecules.
- Proteins contain charges due to the presence of the amino group (NH_3^+) and the carboxyl group (COO^-). The presence of a larger number of negative charges depends on the number of COO^- groups.
- If a protein has more NH_3^+ group, it will have more positive charges.
- At acidic pH, the proteins will have more positive charges so proteins will be positively charged and move towards the negative electrode in an electric field.
- At alkaline pH, the proteins have more negative charges. Hence the protein will be negatively charged and move towards the positive electrode in an electric field.
- At isoelectric pH, the number of positive charges is equal to the number of negative charges. At this pH the net charge on the protein is zero and it is electrically neutral.
- Each protein has its own isoelectric pH.
- For example: Albumin has isoelectric pH of 4.7, globulin has one of 5.8–7.3.

Principle

Protein electrophoresis is performed usually at pH 8.6. At this pH, all the proteins are negatively charged and they move towards the anode in an electric field.

The rate of migration depends on the charge on the protein molecule. If the charge is greater, the protein moves faster.

Albumin has the highest number of negative charges and lower molecular weight, hence it moves at a greater speed, and is separated first. The high molecular weight globulins move according to their charge content with lesser speed. Therefore, albumin is followed by $\alpha_1\alpha_2$, β_1,β_2 ,and γ-globulins. The gamma globulins move very slowly and they remain almost at the point of application.

The movement of the proteins is also influenced by the molecular weight of the protein. The increase in the molecular weight reduces the movement of proteins in an electric field.

Buffer: Barbitone buffer with pH 8.6 with an ionic strength 0.05 is preferred.

Support media: The support media used for electrophoresis are agarose gel, starch gel, agar gel, acrylamide gel and cellulose acetate strips. Agarose is the most commonly used media which, after boiling with buffer and the semisolid gel, is spread on the glass slide.

Stains: Amido Schwartz 10B (Amido black) is the most commonly used dye for staining proteins. Bromophenol blue can also be used.

Reagents

1. *Buffer, pH 8.6, ionic strength 0.05:* Dissolve 10.3 g of sodium barbitone and 1.84 g of diethyl barbituric acid in about 900 mL water. Adjust the pH and make up to one liter.
2. *Staining solution:* Dissolve 500 mg of amidoschwarz 10 B in 40 mL of methanol, 10 mL of glacial acetic acid and 50 mL of water.
3. *Acetic acid 3% (v/v):* 3 mL glacial acetic acid in 97 mL water.
4. *Agarose solution:* Add 11 mL of barbitone buffer (pH 8.6) to 100 mg of agarose. Place the tube in a boiling water bath till agar dissolves completely.
5. Absolute alcohol.

Procedure

Fill the electrode vessels of the cabinet with enough buffers. Spread 1.3 to 1.4 mL of hot agar solution on a clean microscopic slide uniformly and allow it to stand for 3 to 5 minutes. Now apply serum on to agar plate by soaking a small piece of filter paper (Whatman No, 1 is suitable) in serum. Then, transfer the slide to the electrophoresis cabinet and contact the slide with buffer by means of filter paper at both ends. Close the lid. Adjust current at 3 milli amperes per slide and run the slide for about 2 hours.

Fixation is done by placing the slide in a Petri dish containing alcohol for 10 minutes. Then dry the slide. Spread a convenient amount of dye over the slide and it for about 5 minutes. Wash with 3% acetic acid and observe the pattern.

Interpretation of Separation

- This is done through visual inspection of the bands.
- Quantization of each band can be done with a densitometer.
- On electrophoresis plasma proteins get separated as distinct bands namely Albumin, $\alpha1$, $\alpha2$, $\beta1$, $\beta2$, fibrinogen and γ globulins.
- Electrophoresis of a serum sample will show all the bands, except fibrinogen **(Fig. 10.1)**.

Estimation of Plasma Proteins

Determination of serum protein, albumin, globulin and their ratio by Biuret method.

Principle

Proteins react with the Biuret reagent to form a violet colored complex, which has a maximum absorbance at 540–560 nm. Biuret reagent consists of cupric ions (Cu^{2+}) which react with the N atoms of the peptide bonds of peptides and proteins, in an alkaline medium (presence of peptide bonds is the minimum requirement). The density of the purple color is directly proportional to the concentration of protein.

The name "Biuret reaction" is given due to the fact that a substance named "Biuret" also gives the same color with Cu^{2+} ions.

Biuret reagent consists of copper sulfate, sodium hydroxide, sodium potassium-tartrate and potassium iodide.

- The NaOH provides alkalinity to the solution
- Sodium potassium tartrate keeps the Cu^{2+} ions in solution.
- The conversion of Cu^{2+} to Cu^{+} ions is prevented by potassium iodide.

Reagents

1. *Sodium chloride, 0.9%:* Dissolve 900 mg of sodium chloride in 80 mL of water and make up to 100 mL.
2. *0.2 N sodium hydroxide:* Dissolve 8 g of sodium hydroxide in about 400 mL of water in a liter flask. Make up to one liter.
3. *Biuret reagent:* Dissolve 45 g of sodium potassium tartrate in 400 mL of 0.2 N

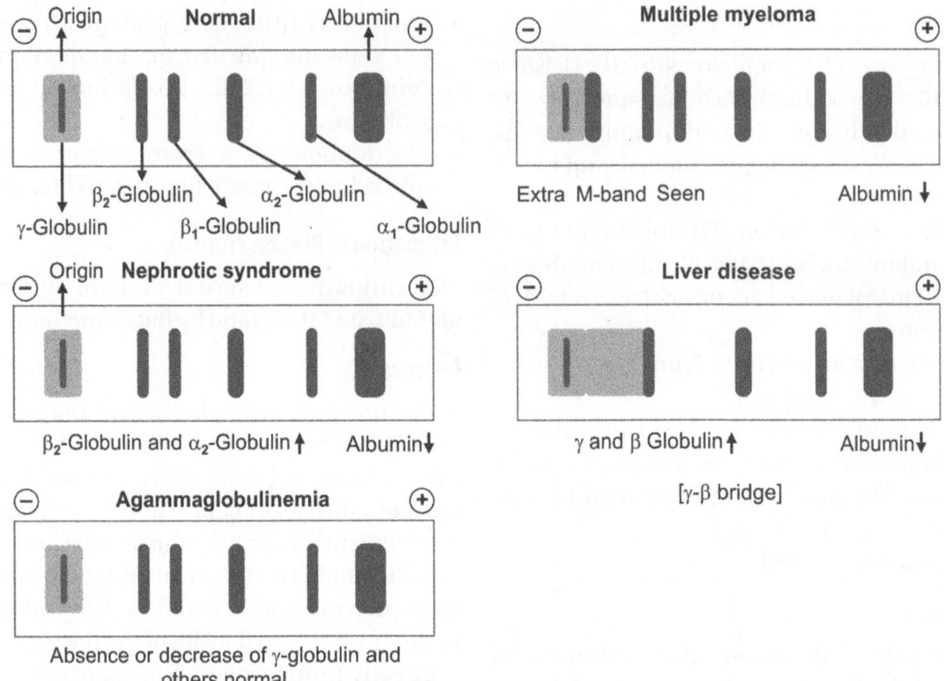

Fig. 10.1: Electrophoretic patterns of serum protein in normal and in certain clinical conditions.

sodium hydroxide (Reagent 2). Add 15 g of copper sulfate stirring continuously. Add 5 g of potassium iodide.
Dissolve and make up to one liter with 0.2 N sodium hydroxide. This is the stock Biuret reagent. Store in a polythene bottle. It is stable for months.

4. 0.2 N sodium hydroxide containing 5 g of potassium iodide per liter. Add 5 g of potassium iodide per liter to reagent 2 and dissolve.
5. *Biuret reagent for use:* Dilute 50 mL of stock Biuret reagent (Reagent 3) to 250 mL with 0.2 N sodium hydroxide containing 5 g potassium iodide per liter (Reagent 4).
6. *Standard protein solution 6 mg/mL:* Dissolve 714.3 mg of Bovine albumin and 100 mg of sodium azide used as preservative in 100 mL water. Store at 4°C.
7. Sodium sulfite 28%.
   Dissolve 28 g of anhydrous sodium sulfite in about 70 mL of water. Make up to 100 mL.
8. Ether, AR grade.

Calculation

G of total proteins/100 mL =

$$\frac{T-B}{S-B} \times \frac{100}{\text{serum}} \times \text{Concentration of standard}$$

$$\text{G of TP/100 mL} = \frac{T-B}{S-B} \times \frac{100}{0.1} \times 6 \times \frac{1}{1000}$$

taken

G of albumin/100 mL =

$$\frac{T-B}{S-B} \times \frac{\text{Total solution}}{\text{Taken solution}} \times \text{Concentration} \frac{100}{\text{Serum taken}}$$

Procedure

Reagents	B	S	A	Tp
Sodium sulfite, 28%	—	—	5.8 mL	
Serum	—	—	0.2 mL	
Ether	—	—	2.0 mL	
Mix gently, centrifuge for 5 minutes. Aspirate and discard the ether layer. Pipette the lower layer for albumin estimation				
Supernatant	—	—	3.0 mL	—
Sodium chloride, 0.9%	3.0 mL	2.0 mL	—	2.9 mL
Serum (mL)	—	—	—	0.1
Standard protein solution	—	1.0 mL	—	—
Biuret reagent for use (mL)	3.0	3.0	3.0	3.0
Mix. Stand for 10 minutes OD at 540 nm or green filter				

$$= \frac{T-B}{S-B} \times \frac{6}{3} \times 6 \times \frac{100}{0.2} \times \frac{1}{1000}$$

Globulins = Total proteins - Albumin.

A: G ratio is obtained by dividing albumin by globulin level.

For example, Albumin = 4 g% , Globulin = 2 g% Then, A:G Ratio = 4/2 = 2:1

Note: When calculating for A: G ratio always globulin is always considered as one.

Standard Graph

Stock: Bovine serum albumin—2 g/100 mL (store in refrigerator).

Working test for albumin—5.8 mL sodium sulfite + 0.2 mL serum + 2 mL ether, invert the tube 20 times gently. Centrifuge and use the lower layer.

0.30 OD corresponds to 9.2 mg

0.1 mL serum contains 9. 2 mg

100 mL contains 9.2 g/dL

Moisture content of the standard protein (albumin) is 15%.

$$\text{Correction factor} = \frac{9.2 \times 15}{100} = 1.38$$

The total protein in the given sample

= 9. 2 - 1. 38

= 7. 82

Albumin

0.11 OD corresponds to 3.2 mg of albumin

2 mL contains 3.2 mg

$$6\text{ mL contains} = \frac{6 \times 3.2}{2} = 9.6$$

0.2 mL serum contains 9.6 mg

$$100\text{ mL contains} = \frac{100 \times 9.6}{0.2} = 4.8\text{ g}$$

$$\text{Correction factor} = \frac{4.8 \times 15}{100} = 0.72$$

4.8 - 0.72 = 4.02

Globulin = Total protein - Albumin = 7.82 - 4.02 = 3.8 g%

A: G ratio 4.02/3.8 = 1.9: 1

Note:

- Ether is used to separate the globulin layer.
- Mixing is very important to precipitate globulin. Vigorous mixing may precipitate albumin also. Too gentle mixing may result in incomplete precipitation of globulin.

Reagents	*B*	S_1	S_2	S_3	S_4	S_5	S_6	S_7	*Tp*	*Alb*
Volume of standard (mL)	–	0.1	0.2	0.3	0.4	0.5	0.6	0.7	–	–
Concentration of standard (mg)	–	2	4	6	8	10	12	14	–	–
Serum									0.1	–
0.9% NaCl (mL)	2	1.9	1.8	1.7	1.6	1.5	1.4	1.3	1.9	–
Lower layer (albumin)										2.0
Biuret reagent (mL)	5	5	5	5	5	5	5	5	5	5
Mix and incubate at room temperature for 15 minutes										
Read at 540 nm	0.05	0.06	0.12	0.18	0.24	0.30	0.36	0.42	0.35	0.16

- Globulins may be removed by filtering through Whatman No. 44 filter paper, in which case ether is not required.
- Keep away from flames, as ether is inflammable.
- Albumin concentration per gram of bovine albumin is better determined by Kjeldahl method.

Estimation of Albumin by Dye-binding Method

Determine the total protein using the Biuret method and then albumin by dye-binding method.

Principle

Bromocresol green (BCG) is the dye used in this method. Albumin is positively charged at pH 4.2 and it binds with the negative charges of the bromocresol green forming a complex. The albumin-BCG complex is green in color and has a maximum absorbance at 628 nm. The color formed is proportional to the concentration of albumin present in the serum.

Succinate buffer of pH 4.0 is used to provide the required pH.

Brij-35 is used to prevent turbidity of the dye solution and reduces the blank value.

The amount of globulin is calculated by taking the difference between the values of total protein and albumin. A/G ratio is calculated using the albumin and globulin values.

Reagents

For total proteins, biuret method is used.

For Albumin

1. *Succinate buffer, 0.1 M, pH 4.0:* Dissolve 11.9 g of succinic acid in about 800 mL of water, adjust the pH to 4.0 with 1 N NaOH and dilute to one liter with water. Store at 4°C. Sodium azide (100 mg/L) is added to buffer stable for one month.
2. *Bromocresol green (dye solution): Stock solution, 0.6 nM:* Dissolve 419 mg of BCG in 10 mL of 0.1 N NaOH solution in one liter flask. Dilute to one liter with water. Store at 4°C. The dye solution is stable for a month.
3. *Working dye solution:* Dilute 250 mL of stock BCG solution to one liter with 0.1 M succinate buffer. Add 8.0 mL of 15% Brij-35. Store at room temperature. Prepare fresh every week.
4. *Standard protein solution, 6 mg per mL:* Dissolve 714.3 mg of bovine albumin (protein content remove determined by Kjeldahl method), add 100 mg of sodium azide and make up to 100 mL with water. Store at 4°C. The reagent is stable.
5. NaCl solution 0.9% (9 g of NaCl in 1 liter).

Procedure

Into the test tube pipette 5.8 mL of 0.9% NaCl and 0.2 mL of serum. Mix and centrifuge if required. Transfer 0.5 mL from this to a test tube labeled Test (T).

In another test tube, pipette 2.5 mL of 0.9% NaCl and 0.5 mL of standard protein solution. Mix and transfer 0.5 mL from this to a test tube labeled Standard (S).

To the third tube deliver 2.5 mL of 0.9% NaCl and 0.5 mL of water. Transfer 0.5 mL of this to a tube labeled blank.

Add 5 mL bromocresol green to each of B, S and T. Mix and stand at room temperature for 10 minutes.

Read the absorbance at 630 nm setting the colorimeter to zero with water.

Calculation

$$\frac{T-B}{S-B} \times \frac{\text{Total solution}}{\text{Taken solution}} \times \text{concentration of standard} \frac{100}{\text{Serum volume}}$$

$$\text{Albumin g/dL} = \frac{T-B}{S-B} \times \frac{6}{0.5} \times 0.5\,\text{mg} \times \frac{100}{0.2}$$

$$= \frac{T-B}{S-B} \times 6 \times \frac{100}{0.2} \times \frac{1}{1000}\ \text{g\%}$$

$$= \frac{T-B}{S-B} \times 3$$

Note: Standard albumin contains 15% moisture content, so during the calculation of total protein and albumin correction factor 15 is applied.

Total protein – Albumin = Globulin.

e.g., TP = 7, Alb = 4, Glb = 3

A/G = 4/3 = 1.3:1

Normal values

Total protein = 6.0–8.0 g/dL

Albumin = 3.5–5.0 g/dL

Globulin = 2.5–3.0 g/dL

A/G = 1.2:1–2.5:1 or 1.2–2.5

From the graph

0.066 OD corresponds to 0.23 mg of albumin.

Therefore, 0.1 mL diluted serum contains 0.23 mg of albumin.

Dilution factor 20, 20 × 0.23 = 4.6 mg

0.1 mL contains 4.6 mg,

$$100\text{ mL contains} = \frac{100 \times 4.6}{0.1} = 4.6\,\text{g\%}$$

Determination of Globulin by Kunkel Method

Principle

Globulin of the serum proteins produces turbidity when mixed with buffered zinc sulfate solution.

Sample: Serum.

Reagents

1. *Buffered zinc sulfate solution:* Dissolve 24 mg of zinc sulfate, 210 mg of sodium barbitone and 280 mg of barbitone in

Standard graph for albumin estimation by dye binding method
Serum is diluted to 1 in 20 with saline. Standard: Dissolve 250 mg of albumin in 100 mL of H_2O

Reagents	*B*	S_1	S_2	S_3	S_4	S_5	S_6	*T*
Standard (mL)	–	0.1	0.2	0.3	0.4	0.5	0.6	–
Concentration (mg)		0.25	0.5	0.75	1.0	1.25	1.50	
Water (mL)	1.0	0.9	0.8	0.7	0.6	0.5	0.4	0.8
Serum	–	–	–	–	–	–	–	0.2
Dye (mL)	5.0	5.0	5.0	5.0	5.0	5.0	5.0	5.0
Keep at room temperature for 15 minutes								
Absorbance at 630 nm	0.02 > 0	0.069	0.135	0.209	0.267	0.338	0.393	0.066

CO_2-free water (double distilled water) and make up to one liter. Check the pH. It should be around 7.45, if not adjust by adding either barbitone or sodium barbitone solution.
2. *Barium chloride solution:* Dissolve 1.15 g of barium chloride in water and make up to 100 mL. Dilute 3 mL of this with 0.2 N sulfuric acid to 100 mL. The turbidity of this ($BaSO_4$ solution) is equivalent to 20 Kunkel units.

Procedure

Pipette 0.1 mL of serum to 6 mL of buffered zinc sulfate solution. After mixing, keep it for 30 minutes at room temperature. Shake and read the turbidity using red filter. Read the turbidity of $BaCl_2$ with 0.2 N sulfuric acid in the same way.

Calculation

$$\text{Zinc sulfate turbidity} = \frac{T}{S} \times 20 \text{ units}$$

Clinical Significance

The change in the plasma protein value takes place either due to change in albumin or the globulin fraction. A reduced plasma protein level is mainly due to a decrease in albumin levels. Whereas, increased total protein is usually due to an increase in the globulin levels.

The conditions in which albumin is reduced are:

1. Nephrotic syndrome (more protein is excreted in urine)
2. Burns (dehydration)
3. Severe blood loss.
4. Reduced synthesis of proteins in liver diseases, such as cirrhosis of liver, hepatitis.
5. Impaired digestion and absorption of proteins as in peptic ulcer, carcinoma of stomach, cancer of pancreas and intestinal diseases, etc.
6. Increased breakdown of proteins as seen in fever, acute infections, untreated diabetes mellitus and hyperthyroidism.
7. Due to protein malnutrition (Insufficient dietary protein intake).
8. In liver diseases, such as cirrhosis, albumin is decreased and globulin is increased.
9. Increased globulin levels are seen in few conditions, such as multiple myeloma, infections (which leads to an increase in the total protein levels).

In multiple myeloma, increase in globulin accompanied by a slight decrease in the albumin or it may be normal some times. Hence, the estimation of total protein alone is not useful in the detection of the disease. The condition in which increased albumin is seen in dehydration. In this case, there is marginal increase in both albumin as well as globulin.

Presence of albumin in urine is called albuminuria.

A large quantity of albumin appears in urine in nephrotic syndrome.

Small quantities in urine in acute nephritis and other inflammatory conditions of urinary tract. Microalbuminuria or minimal albuminuria or pauci-albuminuria (paucity = small quantity) is seen in urine. It is clinically important because it predicts future renal diseases.

Proteins belong to different globulins

There are different types of globulins and each of them consists of mixture of several proteins.

α1-Globulin

1. α1-antitrypsin
2. α1-acid glycoprotein
3. α1-lipoproteins
4. Thyroxin binding globulin (TBG)

α1-Antitrypsin

- It is an acute phase reactant (APR) and protease inhibitor present in the extracellular fluid throughout the body.
- The class of certain proteins in blood may increase up to 1000 fold in several

inflammatory and neoplastic conditions. Such proteins are called as acute phase proteins.

- It neutralizes lysosomal elastase, which is released during phagocytosis of particles by polymorphonuclear leukocytes. Thus, α1-antitrypsin has a protective role in the body.
- The α1-antitrypsin level is increased during any infection or inflammation because of this protective role. Hence, it is known as an acute phase reactant.
- α-1-antitrypsin levels are found to be low in patients with genetic disease. These patients suffer from respiratory diseases, such as emphysema or liver damage.
- Decreased α1-antitrypsin leads to the loss of elasticity of lung tissue which results in emphysema with impaired ventilation and vulnerability to serious respiratory infections.

Reference Value

Newborn = 145–270 mg%,
Adult = 78–200 mg%

Estimation of α-1-antitrypsin and α-1-antichymotrypsin in Serum

Principle: The proteolytic enzymes (trypsin and chymotrypsin) hydrolyze casein with the formation of smaller peptides. The enzyme reaction after a suitable interval of time is arrested by the addition of TCA, which precipitates the proteins, but the peptides are soluble in the acid. The TCA soluble fragments are a measure of proteolytic activity of these enzymes. When the inhibitor (present in serum or urine) is added to the preincubation mixer, it prevents the release of peptides by the proteolytic enzymes. Thus, estimation of TCA-soluble components in the presence and absence of inhibitor is a measure of inhibitory activity against proteolytic enzyme.

The TCA soluble fragments were analyzed by the method of Lowry et al. The final color formed is a result of biuret reaction of the peptide with copper ions in alkali and reduction of phosphomolybdic phosphotungstic reagent by the presence of tyrosine and tryptophan present in the treated peptide.

Reagents

1. Casein 2%, 2 g of casein dissolved in 40 mL of 0.1 N NaOH by heating at 80°C for 10 minutes cooled and 11 mL of 0.1 N HCl is added so that final pH is 7.6. The volume is made up to 100 mL by adding 0.2 M phosphate buffer, pH 7.6 stored at 4°C. Stable for 6 days.
2. *Phosphate buffer, 0.2M, pH 7.6:*
   - Disodium hydrogen phosphate 0.2 M–87 mL
   - Sodium dihydrogen phosphate 0.2 M–13 mL
3. *Folin and Ciocalteu reagent:* 100 g sodium tungstate, 25 g sodium molybdate is dissolved in 700 mL water. Add 50 mL of 85% phosphoric acid and 100 mL of conc. HCl. Reflux for 10 hours. Cool and add 150 g of lithium sulfate, 50 mL water and a few drops of bromine. The solution is boiled to remove the excess bromine. Make up to 1 liter.
   For use: Dilute 1:2 (1N Folin's required).
4. *Alkaline copper reagent:*
   - *Solution A:* 30 g of sodium carbonate 4 g NaOH in 1 liter of water. To this 400 mg of sodium potassium tartrate dissolved in 10 mL of water is added.
   - *Solution B:* Copper sulfate 2%
   - *Working solution for use:* 1 mL of solution B to 100 mL solution A.
5. TCA: 5%.
6. *Trypsin enzyme:* 10 mg trypsin/mL of 0.001 M HCl.
   For use: Dilute with 0.001 M HCl with 300 fold.
7. *Chymotrypsin enzyme:* 10 mg/mL of 0.001 M HCl.
   For use: Dilute with 0.001 M HCl 250 fold. Dilute the sample with 1:100.

Procedure

	Test blank	Enzyme control	Enzyme blank	Test I
Buffer	0.5	0.5	0.5	0.5
Water	0.4	0.3	0.5	0.2
Enzyme (trypsin or chymotrypsin)	—	0.2	—	0.2
Diluted sample	0.1	—	—	0.1

Preincubate the mixtures at 37°C for 10 minutes. The enzyme reaction is started by the addition of 1 mL of 2% casein. After 20 minutes incubation at 37°C, the enzyme reaction is arrested by the addition of 3 mL 5% TCA. After standing for 30 minutes, centrifuge for 15 minutes.

To 1 mL of the supernatant 1 mL water, 4 mL of alkaline copper reagent is added. Wait for 10 minutes and 0.4 mL of Folin reagent is added. After 30 minutes the blue color is measured at 540 nm.

The inhibitor concentration is calibrated in terms of mg of trypsin or chymotrypsin inhibited, from the differences in the enzyme activity and without sample. One unit of inhibitor is defined as 1 mg of enzyme (trypsin or chymotrypsin) inhibited under the assay condition.

Calculation

OD differences for 0.1 mL × 600 units/100 mL (i.e., control - test).

Note: For serum dilute 1:100 and use (1 mL serum + 99 mL water).

For urine put up urine blank (C- T × 600)

α2-Globulins

Important proteins under this group are:

1. *α2-macroglobulin:*
   - It has protective role in the body.
   - It is synthesized by hepatocytes.
   - It inactivates all the proteases, therefore, it is considered as an in vivo anticoagulant.
2. *Haptoglobin:* This binds with hemoglobin and helps in the breakdown of hemoglobin to bilirubin.
3. *Ceruloplasmin:*
   - It is a copper containing protein in the plasma.
   - It is known to have antioxidant property.
   - It is thought that ceruloplasmin is involved in iron metabolism.
   - It is an acute phase reactant protein.
   - Its level is increased in the plasma in infections and malignant conditions, especially in Hodgkin's disease.
   - Ceruloplasmin level is decreased in Wilson's disease and used in the diagnosis of this disease.

Wilson's Disease (Genetic Disorder)

- It is an inherited autosomal recessive disorder.
- It is a disease of copper metabolism where Cu^{2+} is accumulated in liver tissue, brain cornea and kidney tubules. This results in liver damage, mental and retardation, and blindness.
- The peculiar finding of this disorder is that copper deposits as a green or golden-pigmented ring around the cornea: This is also called as Kayser- Fleischer ring.
- Renal failure may be observed in the patient because of copper deposition in the kidney.
- Plasma copper and ceruloplasmin levels are low in this condition.
  Normal serum value = 25–50 mg/dL

Estimation of Ceruloplasmin

Reagents

1. *Acetate buffer, pH 5.6:* Glacial acetic acid 1.34 mL, sodium acetate trihydrate 26.44 g make up to liter with double distilled water. Check the pH and keep in the refrigerator.

2. *Substrate:* Prepare before use—(very sensitive to light)—36 mg p-phenylene diamine hydrochloride make up to 25 mL with acetate buffer.
3. Sodium azide 3%—3 g of sodium azide and make up to 100 mL with double distilled water. Keep in the refrigerator.

Procedure

Acid washed tubes are used for the assay.

	Blank	*Test*
Substrate	3.0 mL	3.0 mL
Sodium azide	0.6 mL	—
Serum	0.06 mL	0.06 mL
Incubate at 37°C for 15 minutes		
Sodium azide		0.6 mL
Incubate for 15 minutes and read at 546 nm.		

Calculation

Concentration of ceruloplasmin= 237 × (OD T – B) = mg%

β Globulins

Important proteins of this class are:

1. *Transferrin:*
   - It is a transport protein for iron in the plasma.
   - It is a negative acute phase protein because its level decreases in some inflammatory conditions.
2. β-*lipoproteins:* Carries LDL cholesterol in the plasma from the liver to peripheral tissue.
3. C-Reactive protein: (β_2-microglobulin).

C-reactive Protein

- C-reactive protein (CRP) is an acute phase reactant.
- CRP is released in response to acute injury, infection, or other inflammatory stimuli.
- Recent development of a high sensitivity assay for CRP has enabled investigation of this marker of systemic inflammation.
- It consists of five identical nonglycosylated polypeptide subunits non-covalently linked to form a disc-shaped cyclic polymer.
- This consists little or no carbohydrate and migrates both on cellulose or agarose electrophoresis anywhere from γ to β region.

Clinical Significance

- Its level rises more than 6 hours after triggering stimulus.
- Peaks within 48 hours
- Short half-life of 5–7 hours (rapidly declines after condition resolves).

Indications

Detection, monitoring and differentiating conditions of:

- Systemic lupus erythematosus (SLE)
- CRP higher in rheumatoid arthritis
  Crohn's disease
  Ulcerative colitis
- Pyelonephritis
- The plasma CRP level increases after stress, trauma, inflammation, infections, myocardial infarction and neoplastic disease.
- The determination of CRP level is clinically useful:
  - For screening of organic disease.
  - Assessing the activity of an inflammatory diseases, such as rheumatoid arthritis,
  - For detecting intercurrent infections in systemic lupus erythematosus, leukemia and after surgery.
  - For detecting renal transplant rejection.
  - For managing neonatal septicemia and meningitis.

Analysis

Radial immunodiffusion (RID), RIA, nephelometry, homogeneous FIA.

Reference Interval

As per RID and rate nephelometry, it is 80–800 mg/dL.

Immunoglobulin (Ig)

The defense strategies of the body are collectively known as immunity.

Two types of immunity identified:

1. *Cellular immunity:* This is mediated by T-lymphocytes or T-cells (thymic origin)
2. *Humoral immunity:* Mediated by a specialized group of proteins known as immunoglobulins or antibodies.
   - The B-lymphocytes or B-cells (mature in bone) are responsible for the production of immunoglobulins.
   - The immunoglobulins are also known as γ globulins.
   - Protective in function,
   - Function as antibodies.
   - Synthesized in response to a foreign substance called an antigen.
   - Provide immunity.
   - Five different types of immunoglobulins.
   - They are IgA, IgG, IgM, IgD and IgE (remember it as Government (IgG) MADE or GAMED).

Structure

- All the immunoglobulin molecules consist of two identical Heavy (H) chains MW = 53000–75000 and two identical Light (L) chains MW = 23,000
- They are held together by disulfide bridges
- Heavy chains of immunoglobulins are linked to carbohydrates, hence immunoglobulins are glycoproteins
- Each chain (L or H) of Ig has two regions (domains), namely the constant and the variable
- At the amino terminal, half of the light chain is the variable region (VL)
- At the carboxyterminal, half is the constant region (CL)
- There are 5 types of heavy chains—γ, α, μ, δ and ε.
- Light chains are of 2 types—kappa (K) and lambda (λ)
- One-quarter of the amino terminal region of heavy chain is variable (VH). The remaining three-quarters is constant (CH1, CH2, CH3)
- The amino acid sequence of variable regions of light and heavy chains is responsible for the specific binding of immunoglobulin (antibody) with antigen
- There are certain hypervariable regions within the variable regions of VL and VH
- Light chains have 3 hypervariable regions
- Heavy chains have 4 hypervariable regions
- The hypervariable regions more specifically determine the antigen binding site.

Type	*Heavy chains*	*Light chains*	*Serum concentration mg%*	*Placental transfer*
IgG	γ	κ or λ	800–1500	+
IgM	μ	κ or λ	50–200	–
IgA	α	κ or λ	150–400	–
IgD	δ	κ or λ	1–10	–
IgE	ε	κ or λ	0.02–005	–

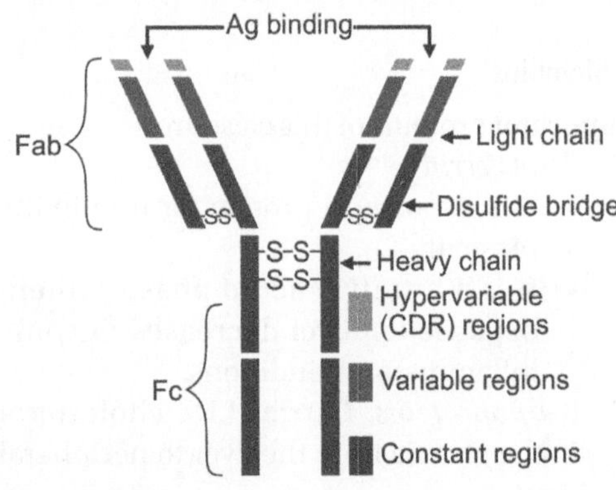

Ag = antigen

Functions

IgG

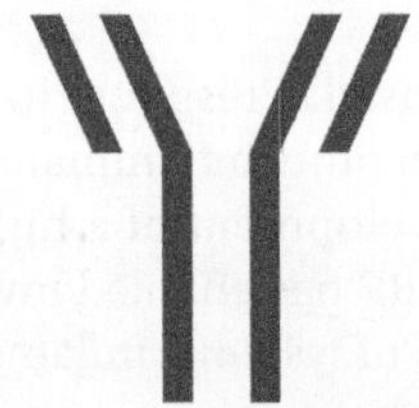

- Composed of a single unit (monomer).
- Major immunoglobulin present in the highest amount in plasma (75–80%).
- Produced in response to various infections and protects the body against infections.
- IgG, can cross the placenta from the mothers blood to the fetus and provide immunity to the fetus.
- Triggers foreign cell destruction mediated by complement system.

IgA

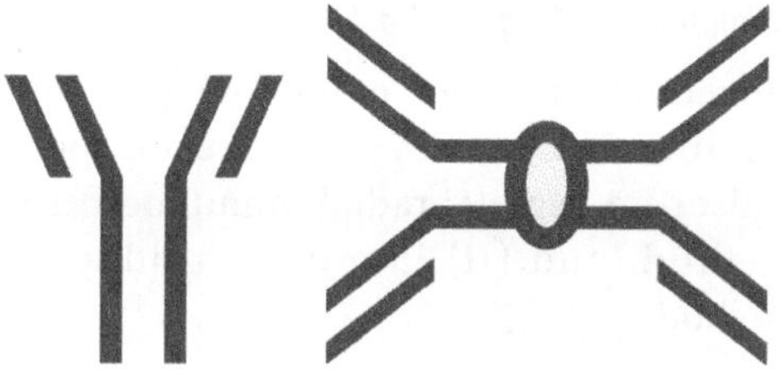

- Occurs as a single (monomer) or double unit (dimer) held together by J chain.
- Produced by the secretary cells of the respiratory tract, digestive tract, urinary tract, etc., and is present in the mucus secretions of these cells.
- It prevents the entry of bacteria into the body through these cells.

IgM

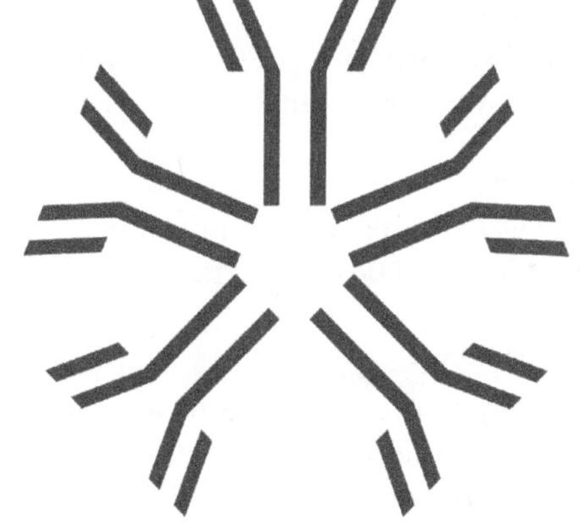

- Largest immunoglobulin composed of 5-Y shaped units held together by a J polypeptide chain
- Cannot traverse blood vessels, hence, it is restricted to bloodstream
- It is the first antibody to be produced whenever bacteria or virus attack the body
- It is also produced in the fetal stage itself.

IgD

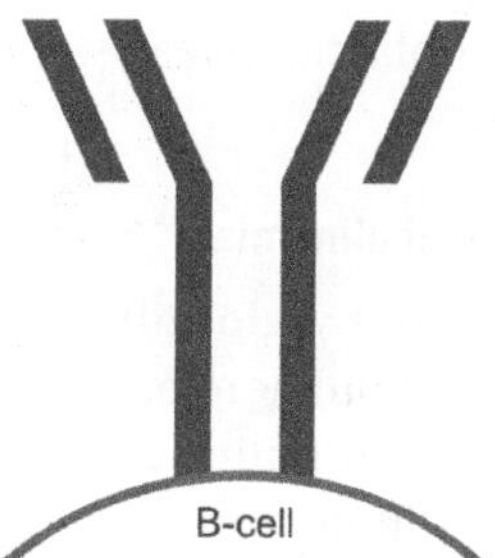

- Composed of single Y-shaped monomer
- IgE molecules tightly bind with mast cells which release histamine and cause allergy
- It is produced by the plasma cells of the respiratory tract
- Increases in allergic diseases.

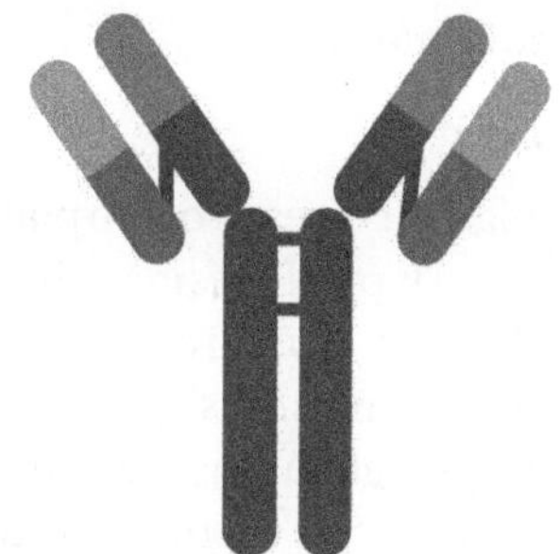

Immunoglobulin E is a type of antibody that has been found only in mammals. IgE is synthesized by plasma cells. Monomers of IgE consist of two heavy chains and two light chains, with the ε chain containing four Ig-like constant domain.

High level of IgE seen in some kind of allergy. But the results of a total IgE test do not show what the type of allergy. A specific IgE test result that is high means that one may be allergic to the allergen that was tested.

Variations in the upper limit of normal total serum IgE have been reported—they can range from 150 to 1,000 UI/mL; but the usually accepted upper limit is between 150 and 300 UI/mL

Diseases which cause the elevation of serum IgE levels include atopic diseases (asthma, allergic rhinitis, atopic dermatitis, urticaria), parasitic diseases, cutaneous diseases, neoplastic diseases, and immune deficiencies.

Hypergammaglobulinemia

Increased serum γ-globulin level is called hypergammaglobulinemia.

Increased γ-globulin level is seen in the following conditions:

1. Infections from foreign bodies
2. *Chronic liver disease:* There is a generalized increase in the γ-globulins. On electrophoresis the γ- globulins give diffused but deep stained band
3. Multiple myeloma
4. Waldenström's hypergammaglobulinemia: Increase in IgM only.

Multiple Myeloma

This is a malignant disease of the plasma cell. In this case, one type of plasma cell multiplies abnormally and produces one type of immunoglobulin in excessive quantities and the other immunoglobulins are decreased.

The electrophoresis of such a serum shows a thick deeply stained protein band in the γ-globulin region. This band is called 'M' band. This type of increase is known as monoclonal gammopathy.

Biochemical Findings

The biochemical findings of multiple myeloma are increased total proteins, decreased albumin and increased globulins and Ca^{++} levels in plasma. Some cases of multiple myeloma patients excrete light chains of immunoglobulins in the urine, which are known as Bence-Jones proteins. One type of immunoglobulin is increased in excess and the other types are decreased.

Hypogammaglobulinemia

Plasma globulin levels are decreased in the following conditions:

1. Congenital defect in the synthesis of γ-globulins
2. Leukemia
3. Protein loosing diseases, such as nephrotic syndrome.

Estimation of IgG, IgA and IgM

Individual estimation of immunoglobulins is done by Immunoassay methods using specific antiserum, e.g., (i) radial immunodiffusion method, and (ii) immunoturbidimetric method.

Determination of Plasma Fibrinogen

Procedure

1. 250 μL plasma + 250 mL $CaCl_2$ (25 g/L) + 7 mL distilled H_2O in a centrifuge tube. Mix and keep overnight at room temperature.
2. Centrifuge and discard the supernatant.
3. Add 2.5 mL of 0.2 N NaOH to the precipitate.
4. Keep in hot water for 5 minutes and mix to dissolve.
5. Add 1 drop of 10 N H_2SO_4 to neutralize and mix. Analyze protein by Micro-TP method.

Calculation

Fibrinogen: Autoanalyzer value × 10
Normal range 200–400 mg/dL.

Proteins in Urine

Normally urine contains of a very small amount of proteins. This is because the normal glomerulus does not allow high molecular weight protein including albumin to filter. Only low molecular weight proteins are allowed to pass through. The proteins, which are present in urine normally, are α and β-globulins of low molecular weight.

Proteins in Urine in Disease Condition

Increased excretion of proteins in urine than the normal is known as **proteinuria.**

The proteins, which are seen in urine, may be albumin, hemoglobin, or myoglobin depending on the state of the disease.

Albumin

- Albumin is the most common protein, which is excreted in urine under diseased conditions.
- Pathological conditions associated with albumin in urine are nephrotic syndrome and glomerular nephritis. In both cases, there is damage to the glomerular membrane causing proteins to be filtered into the urine.
- Physiological conditions where albumin is excreted are pregnancy and orthostatic proteinuria (due to prolonged standing).

Blood and Hb

- Excretion of blood in urine is known as **hematuria.**
- When renal tubules, bladder or glomeruli are severely damaged, blood is passed into the urine.
- Presence of free hemoglobin without RBC is known as **hemoglobinuria.**
- Hemoglobin is mainly excreted in urine when there is severe intravascular hemolysis mainly in mismatched blood transfusions, or some infectious diseases.

Myoglobin

- Myoglobin is a protein formed in the muscle cells.
- Its structure is similar to that of hemoglobin, which is present in muscle cells, and it is found in urine when there is severe muscle cell break down.

Qualitative Test for Urinary Proteins

Heat and Acetic Acid

A sample of freshly collected urine is mixed with 3% acetic acid and heated over a flame to boiling. Turbidity or cloudy precipitate indicates the presence of proteins, mainly albumin. Normal urine gives a negative test.

Sulfosalicylic Acid Test

To 5 mL clear urine, 0.5 mL of sulfosalicylic acid is added.

White precipitate or turbidity is formed if proteins present.

Dip Stick Test

The plastic strip with a cellulose area contains the dye and the buffer, which reacts with albumin and gives color.

Note: If the urine is acidified, test may become false negative; if the urine is alkaline, the test may become false positive.

Semiquantitative Determination of Microalbumin

This test is based on the principle of an immunochemical reaction. Hence, this test is very specific for albumin and very sensitive. The test strip contains the specific antibodies for albumin, a substrate and an enzyme. When the strip is dipped in urine, albumin reacts with the antibody of the strip and forms a complex. This complex reacts with the substances and forms a red color. This test is useful for the early detection of albuminuria, especially in diabetic nephropathy and hypertensive patients. If the result is positive by the qualitative test, then a quantitative estimation is recommended.

Estimation of Protein in Urine by Biuret Method

Reagents

1. *Biuret reagent:* Same as in serum protein estimation.
2. *TCA 20%:* 20 g of TCA dissolved in 100 mL of water.

3. *NaOH 1N:* 4 g of NaOH dissolved in 100 mL of water.
4. *Standard BSA:* 600 mg of BSA in 100 mL water.

Procedure

Contents	Blank	Standard	Test
Water (mL)	—	1.0	—
Standard 6 mg/mL	—	0.5 mL	—
Urine (mL)	—	—	1.5
20% TCA (mL)		1.5	1.5
Mix and Keep at room temperature for 10 minutes centrifuge and discard the supernatant			
1N NaOH (mL)	1.5	1.5	1.5
Biuret reagent	1.5	1.5	1.5
Mix and keep at room temperature for 15 minutes and read at 540 nm			

Calculation

Protein in mg/100 mL =

$$\frac{T-B}{S-B} = \frac{\text{concentration}}{\text{total volume}} \times 100$$

$$= \frac{T-B}{S-B} \times \frac{6}{3} \times 100$$

Micro-TP (Total Protein) Method (Pyrogallol Red)

The reagent consists of a pyrogallol red-molybdenum complex. The complex reacts with proteins forming a purple colored complex, which has a maximum absorption at 600 nm.

Introduction

The determination of total protein content in urine is important in the evaluation of kidney function and in the diagnosis of kidney diseases; nephritis, nephrosis and diabetic nephropathy. In the diagnosis of meningitis, cerebral hemorrhage and others, the determination of total protein content in cerebrospinal fluid is beneficial, along with the quantitation of glucose and chloride.

Principle

The pyrogallol red is combined with molybdenum acid forming a red complex with a λ maximum of 470 nm. When this complex is combined with protein under acidic conditions, its maximum absorption is shifted to a longer wavelength and if develops a blue purple color (λ max = 600 nm). The concentration of the total protein in the sample can be obtained by measuring the absorbance of colored solution at 600 nm.

Reagents

- Color reagent (pH 2.2):
- Glycine buffer solution 0.1 mol/L
- Pyrogallol red 0.067 mmol/L
- Ammonium molybdate 0.026 mmol/L
- Surfactant
- Standard: Albumin 100 mg/dL

Specimen Collection and Preservation

- Either a random or a 24 hours urine sample is collected with toluene as the preservative.
- Cerebrospinal fluid sample is collected without any contamination by blood components. Samples may be stored for 3 months.
- Hemoglobin shows about one-half the color of albumin.
- Hematuria presents a falsely high value.
- Copper and iron ions cause errors in measurement; special care should be taken to avoid contamination of the apparatus.

Be sure to filter or centrifuge turbid samples before performing measurements.

Procedure

- Wavelength 600 nm
- Temperature; 37°C

Measure the absorbance of Test (T) and standard (S) against blank (B) at 600 nm within one hour.

Reagents	Blank (B)	Standard (S)	Test (T)
Sample (mL)	—	—	10
Standard (mL)	—	10	
Water (mL)	10	—	—
Reagent (mL)	1.0	1.0	1.0
Mix well and incubate for 10 minutes read at 600 nm			

Concentration in the Test (Manual Procedure)

Glycine buffer solution 99 mmol/L,
Pyrogallol red 0,066 mmol/L,
Ammonium molybdate 0,026 mmol/L.

Calculation

$$\text{Micro TP (mg/dL)} = \frac{T-B}{S-B} \times 100$$

Note: When micro-TP value exceeds 330 mg/dL, dilute sample 1+1 with saline or distilled water, repeat the assay and multiply the result by 2.
Normal value = 25–180 mg/day.

Test for Hemoglobinuria

Principle

Heme proteins (hemoglobin, myoglobin) react with benzidine in presence of H_2O_2 forming colored products. Heme of Hemoglobin decomposes H_2O_2. The liberated oxygen oxidizes benzidine to a green colored product, which is unstable.

Hb + Benzidine + H_2O_2 ⟶ Benzidine (black)
(heme protein) (reduced (oxidized)
colorless)

Procedure

- Mix 3 drops of benzidine solution and 3 drops of H_2O_2.
- Add 3 drops of the above mixture to 2 mL of urine.
- Immediate blue or green color is obtained if urine contains blood or hemoglobin and disappears in a few seconds, leaving a stable brown color finally.
- This method is very sensitive and it can detect even 2 mg Hb/100 mL.
- If the test is negative it means that RBC or Hb is absent.
- If the test is positive, the patient may have hemoglobinuria or hematuria or myoglobinuria.

Note: False positive result may occur in the case of contamination of the urine container with hypochlorite or by bacteria.

Differentiation of hematuria and hemoglobinuria is done by microscopic examination of RBC.

Test for Myoglobin

Myoglobin in urine is determined by immunochemical methods (radial immuno-diffusion method).

Bence-Jones Proteins (BJP)

- Bence-Jones proteins are light chain fragments of immunoglobulins, which are excreted in urine, in some cases of multiple myeloma.
- It was discovered in the urine by its characteristic behavior on heating.
- Bence-Jones proteins precipitate between 40–60°C. But as the temperature increases above 60°C the protein redissolves. Again on cooling the protein gets precipitated.

Tests for Bence-Jones Protein

Bradshaw's Test

- This is a preliminary test for BJP.
- Concentrated HCl is taken in a test tube to which the urine is added drop by drop. If a white ring is formed at the junction of the two fluids, it indicates the presence of BJP.
- If albumin is high then also a ring is formed this is false positive test.
- So, to confirm the presence of Bence-Jones protein the heating test is performed.

The Heating Test

- The urine is acidified with few drops of 33% acetic acid and heated up to boiling.
- If a precipitate is formed at boiling temperature, it is due to albumin, filter it when it is hot.
- The filtrate is allowed to cool.
- If Bence-Jones proteins are present, it will be precipitated and will remain even if the filtrate reaches the room temperature.

Proteins in Cerebrospinal Fluid

Cerebrospinal fluid (CSF) is produced in the ventricles of the brain and passes on to the space around the spinal cord. The spinal cord ends near the 1st lumbar and the fluid accumulated below this is known as lumbar fluid. This is the portion of the CSF, which is examined in routine cases.

It is obtained by passing a needle between the L_3 and L_4. The total volume of CSF is about 130 mL. The normal lumbar CSF has the following characteristics:

1. Protein concentration is 15–45 mg/dL
2. Glucose concentration is about 20 mg less than plasma glucose
3. Chloride is about 120–130 mEq/L.

Methods for CSF Protein Estimation

1. *Micro-TP method* can be employed to estimate CSF proteins.
   The protein concentration of CSF increases in meningitis, some types of brain tumors, etc.
2. *Biuret method:* This method detects even small amount of protein.
3. Lowry's method.
4. Meulemans method.

Principle

Trichloroacetic acid at 3% concentration produces turbidity with proteins in CSF which is compared with the standard in a colorimeter.

Reagents

1. *Trichloroacetic acid 3% (w/v):* Dissolve 30 g of TCA in water and dilute to one liter.
2. *Stock protein standard—5 mg/mL:* Dissolve 595.25 mg of bovine albumin (whole nitrogen content is determined by Kjeldhal method) and 100 mg of sodium azide in water and make up to 100 mL. Store at 4°C in a refrigerator.
3. *Working standard protein solution, 50 mg/dL:* Dilute 10 mL of the stock standard to 100 mL with 0.9% NaCl solution. Store in a freezer. Prepare fresh every week.

Procedure

Contents	*Blank*	*Standard*	*Test*
CSF			0.5 mL
Standard		0.5 mL	
TCA 3%	4.0 mL	3.5 mL	3.5 mL
Kept at room temperature for 10 minutes Read the absorbance at 450 nm			

Calculation

$$\text{CSF protein in mg/100 mL} = \frac{T-B}{S-B} \times 50$$

Sulfosalicylic Acid Method

Principle

1. *Turbidimetric method:* Proteins in CSF are precipitated using sulfosalicylic acid. The turbidity produced is measured in a spectrophotometer at 660 nm. The extent of turbidity is proportional to the protein content. This method is very sensitive and rapid.

Reagents

1. *Sulfosalicylic acid, sodium sulfate reagent, 3%:* Dissolve 3 g of sulfosalicylic acid and 7 g sodium sulfate in 100 mL of distilled water.
2. Standard solution (1 mg/mL).

Dissolve 100 mg of bovine albumin in 100 mL of water. Store at 4°C in a refrigerator.

Procedure

Contents	Blank (B)	Standard (S)	Test (T)
Standard	—	0.5 mL	—
CSF (if turbid centrifuge)	—	—	0.5 mL
3% sulfosalicylic acid	4 mL	3.5	3.5
Mix and read after 10 minutes at 660 nm			

Calculation

$$\text{mg total protein per 100 mL CSF} = \frac{T-B}{S-B} \times 100$$

Note: If the CSF protein content is very high, it is better to estimate with Biuret method.

Interpretation

Normal CSF has a protein content of 15 to 45 mg per 100 mL.

It is elevated in meningeal inflammations, brain tumors and subarachnoid hemorrhage.

Color Reactions of Proteins

Proteins are made up of amino acids joined by peptide bonds. So, peptide bonds and different amino acids present in the proteins give colored products when they react with variety of reagents. These tests are very important in the detection of amino acids in the biological fluids. Some of the tests are also useful in the quantitative determination of proteins and amino acids also. Collectively these tests are called color reactions of proteins. A few tests are as given below:

Biuret Test

Principle: This test mainly detects the presence of peptide bonds in the proteins. The cupric ion in alkaline condition forms a violet colored complex with the peptide bond nitrogen of protein. The reaction name is dependent on the positive reaction given by the biuret reagent.

Procedure: Unknown solution 1 mL + 1 mL 5% NaOH + few drops of copper sulfate and mix. Violet color appears if the solution contains protein.

Ninhydrin Test

The free alpha amino group of protein reacts with ninhydrin and gives blue color.

Procedure: Sample 1 mL + 10 drops of ninhydrin. Boil it strongly, and observe for the color. A blue color appears if the solution contains proteins with free alpha amino groups.

Xanthoproteic Acid Test

The aromatic amino acids, such as tyrosine and tryptophan react with nitric acid and give a yellow color.

Procedure: Sample 2 mL + 1 mL concentrated nitric acid, boil for a minute and cool under running water. Observe for the color, yellow color immediately appears if the sample contains either tyrosine or tryptophan. There is a further specific test for individual aromatic amino acids.

Millon's Test (Cole's Test)

Tyrosine gives a red color when it reacts with mercuric sulfate and sodium nitrite.

Procedure: Sample 1 mL + 1 mL mercuric sulfate + 1 mL concentrated sulfuric acid, appearance of red color indicates the presence of tyrosine.

Aldehyde Test

The test is specific for tryptophan, which contains an indole ring.

Procedure: Sample 1 mL + drop of 0.2% formalin + 1 drop of mercuric sulfate, add concentrated sulfuric acid from the side of the tube. A violet ring appears at the junction of two layers if the solution contains tryptophan.

Sakaguchi Test

This test is specific for arginine, which contains the guanidino group.

Procedure: To 3 mL of unknown solution add 3 drops of 40% NaOH, 5 drops of alpha naphthol and few drops of bromine water. Red color appears if the solution contains arginine.

Sulfur Test

Sulfur containing amino acids, such as cysteine and cystine are the answer of this test.
Procedure: Unknown sample 2 mL + 2 mL 40% NaOH, boil strongly, cool under tap water then add few drops of lead acetate and mix properly. A brown color appears if the solution contains sulfur containing amino acids.

Pauly's Test

This test detects the presence of tyrosine and histidine.
Procedure: 0.5 mL sulfanilic acid + 0.5 mL of 0.5% $NaNO_2$ add 1 mL unknown solution after 1 or 2 minute mix and add 10% sodium carbonate. Mix again, and observe for the color. A red color appears if the unknown solution contains tyrosine or histidine.

Molisch's Test

The albumin is known to be a glycoprotein, contains carbohydrate and a protein portion. As this test is specific for carbohydrates, the sulfuric acid dehydrates carbohydrate to give a furfural derivative, which condenses with alpha naphthol to give the colored compound.
Procedure: Albumin solution 1 mL + 2 drops of alpha naphthol, mix and add concentrated sulfuric acid from the side of the test tube and observe for the reddish violet ring at the junction of two layers.

SELF TEST

1. Name the plasma proteins.
2. Explain the functions of albumin.
3. Write a note on albumin.
4. What is the normal level of albumin?
5. Name the conditions in which hypoalbuminemia are seen.
6. Explain gamma globulins.
7. Write the structure of gamma globulins.
8. Name the classes of globulins.
9. What are the classes of gamma globulins?
10. Write a note on transport proteins.
11. What are acute phase proteins?
12. Add a note on alpha 1 antitrypsin.
13. Write a note on ceruloplasmin.
14. Explain briefly the condition of emphysema.
15. Write a note on CRP.
16. Explain the term multiple myeloma and mention the technique used to identify it from the blood.
17. Give an account on Bence-Jones proteins and state the tests used to detect them in the urine.
18. Name the methods of protein estimation.
19. Write a note on fibrinogen.
20. Name the buffer used in protein electrophoresis.
21. What are the methods for the estimation of proteins in serum?
22. Explain the method of protein electrophoresis.
23. Name the different types of bands in the nephrotic syndrome and give the other biochemical findings.
24. Explain the clinical significance of protein electrophoresis.
25. Draw the electrophoretic pattern of multiple myeloma.
26. Write the electrophoretic pattern of normal serum.
27. Write the principle of benzidine test.
28. Which test is used as a general test for protein?
29. Which bond mainly stabilizes the primary structure of protein?
30. Give an example of a phosphoprotein.
31. Name the plasma protein, which provides immunity to our body.
32. What is the important function of albumin?
33. How many polypeptide chains are present in the hemoglobin molecule?

34. Give an example of the tertiary structure of a protein.
35. Name the sulfur containing amino acids.
36. What is the isoelectric pH of casein?
37. Name the urine protein, which helps in the diagnosis of multiple myeloma.
38. Give an example of acute phase proteins.
39. What are the causes for Wilson's disease?

MULTIPLE CHOICE QUESTIONS

1. **Albumin is synthesized by:**
   a. Intestine
   b. Kidney
   c. Liver
   d. Pancreas
2. **The normal range for total protein is:**
   a. 6.5 to 8.0 g%
   b. 5.0 to 6.0 g%
   c. 8.00 to 9.0 g%
   d. 4.00 to 7.0 g%
3. **Serum total protein can be estimated by:**
   a. Jaffe's method
   b. Molish's test
   c. Biuret method
   d. Dye binding method
4. **Number of polypeptide chains present in an immunoglobulin is:**
   a. 6
   b. 3
   c. 4
   d. 1
5. **The protein excreted in multiple myeloma is:**
   a. Globulin
   b. Myoglobin
   c. Myeloma protein
   d. Bence-Jones proteins
6. **Presence of hemoglobin in urine without RBC is known as:**
   a. Hematuria
   b. Hemoglobinuria
   c. Myoglobinuria
   d. Proteinuria
7. **The following are the properties of proteins at isoelectric pH (pI), *Except:***
   a. Proteins will have maximum solubility at pI
   b. Proteins possess equal number of positive and negative charges
   c. Proteins exist in zwitterionic form
   d. Below the isoelectric point they possess a net positive charge
8. **Which one of the following proteins is not a conjugated protein?**
   a. Egg albumin
   b. Hemoglobin
   c. Serum albumin
   d. Casein
9. **Which of the following statements is false regarding the structure of a protein?**
   a. Immunoglobulins possess quaternary structure
   b. Upon denaturation, primary structure is broken
   c. Proteins lose their biological activity if their secondary, tertiary and quaternary structures are damaged
   d. Hydrogen bonds are predominant forces stabilizing the α-helix and β-pleated sheets
10. **Which of the following proteins is absent in a normal person's serum?**
    a. Albumin
    b. γ-globulin
    c. Fibrinogen
    d. $\alpha 2$-globulin
11. **The following are examples of globular proteins, *Except:***
    a. Hemoglobin
    b. Collagen
    c. Albumin
    d. Myoglobin

11 UNIT Tumor Markers

Learning Objectives

At the end of this unit, the learner should be able to understand:
- The clinical significance of tumor marker determination.
- The various types of tumor markers and their clinical significance.

INTRODUCTION

- A tumor marker is a substance produced by a tumor or by the tissue containing the tumor. Measurement of such substances in the tissue or in the body fluids is helpful to detect the presence of cancer.
- These substances can be found in the blood, urine, stool, tumor tissue, or other tissues or bodily fluids of some patients with cancer.
- These are present in higher quantities in cancer tissue or in the blood of cancer patients.
- Normally, its concentration is low.
- Some tumor markers are specific for one type of cancer; while others are seen in cancer of different organs.
- Many of the well-known markers are seen in non-cancerous conditions as well as cancer.
- There are only a handful of well-established tumor markers that are being routinely used by physicians.
- Many other potential markers are still being researched.
- Although an elevated level of a tumor marker may suggest the presence of cancer, this alone is not enough to diagnose cancer. Therefore, measurements of tumor markers are usually combined with other tests, such as biopsies, to diagnose cancer.
- The goal is to be able to screen for and diagnose cancer early, when it is the most treatable and before it has had a chance to grow and spread.
- So far, the only tumor marker to gain wide acceptance as a general screen is the prostate specific antigen for men.
- Other markers are either not specific enough or they are not elevated early enough in the disease process.

The detection of tumor markers is clinically useful to:

Screen

- Most markers are not suited for general screening, but some may be used in those with a strong family history of a particular cancer.
- In the case of genetic markers, they may be used to help predict risk in family members; PSA testing for prostate cancer is an example.
- Help to diagnose.
- In a patient that has symptoms, tumor markers may be used to help identify the source of the cancer, such as CA-125 for ovarian cancer and to help differentiate it from other conditions.

- Tumor markers cannot diagnose cancer themselves but aid in this process.

Stage

- If a patient does have cancer, tumor marker elevations can be used to help determine how far the cancer has spread into other tissues and organs.
- Determine prognosis.
- Some tumor markers can be used to help doctors, determine how aggressive a cancer is likely to be.

Guide Treatment

Some tumor markers will give doctors information about what treatments their patients may respond to.

Monitor Treatment

- Tumor markers can be used to monitor the effectiveness of treatment, especially in advanced cancers.
- If the marker level drops, the treatment is working; if it stays elevated, adjustments are needed.
- The information must be used with care, however.
- Carcinoembryonic antigen (CEA) for instance, is used to monitor colorectal cancer but not every colorectal cancer patient will have elevated levels of CEA.
- If the marker level is not initially elevated with the cancer, it cannot be used later as a monitoring tool.

Determine Recurrence

- Currently, one of the biggest uses for tumor markers is to monitor for cancer recurrence.
- If a tumor marker is elevated before treatment, low after treatment, and then begins to rise over time, then it is likely that the cancer is returning (if it remains elevated after surgery, then chances is that not all of the cancer was removed.

TYPES OF TUMOR MARKERS

The important tumor markers are **(Fig. 11.1)**:

1. Alkaline phosphatase (ALP)
2. Lactate dehydrogenase (LDH)
3. Prostatic acid phosphatase (PAP)

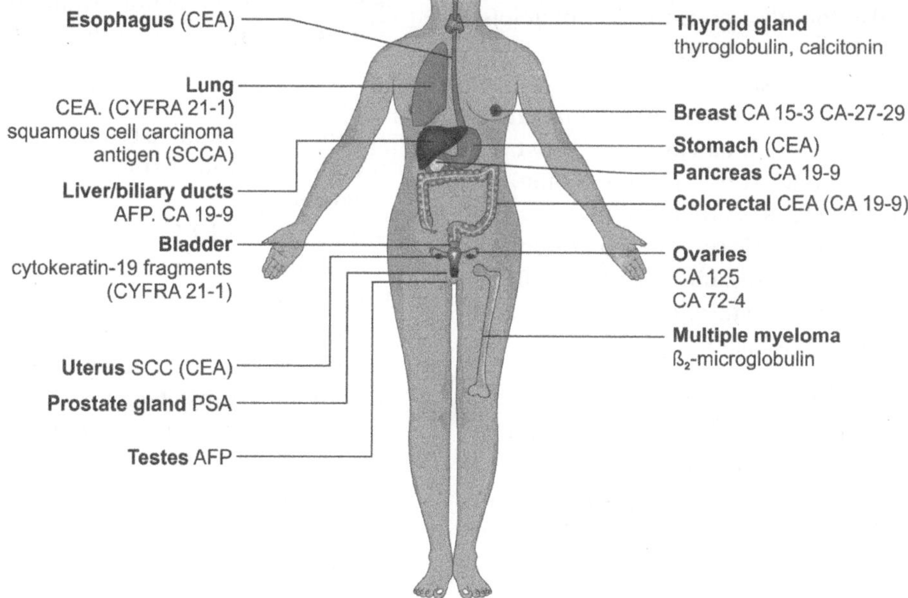

Fig. 11.1: Chart showing the tumor markers for the various tumors.

4. Prostate specific antigen (PSA)
5. Human chorionic gonadotropin (hCG)
6. Alpha-fetoprotein (AFP)
7. Carcinoembryonic antigen (CEA)
8. CA-15-3—marker for breast carcinomas
9. CA-125—marker for ovarian and endometrial carcinoma
10. Calcitonin (secreted by cells of thyroid gland. It is increased in medullary tumor of thyroid gland).

Carcinoma: Cancer arising from epithelial tissue.

Sarcoma: Cancer from connective tissue.

Alkaline Phosphatase (ALP)

Alkaline phosphatase elevated in:

- Primary or secondary liver cancer
- Secondary bone cancer
- Lung cancer
- Cancer of GIT and ovary
- Hodgkin's disease.

Prostatic Acid Phosphatase (PAP)

- PAP is produced mainly by the prostate gland.
- It is also found in erythrocytes, platelets, leukocytes, bone marrow, liver, spleen, kidney and intestine.
- Serum PAP level is increased in malignant conditions, such as cancer of prostate, multiple myeloma, osteogenic sarcoma and bone metastasis of other cancers.
- It may be elevated in some benign conditions such as benign prostatic hypertrophy (BPH) or enlarged prostate, osteoporosis and hyperparathyroidism.

Clinical Application

- It is not a sensitive marker for screening or for the early detection of cancer.
- It is useful in staging of prostate cancer (prognosis of the disease) and cancer therapy.

Prostate Specific Antigen (PSA)

- The major site of PSA production is the glandular epithelium of the prostate.
- A major function of PSA is the proteolytic cleavage of gel forming proteins and increases sperm motility.
- It is used as a marker for prostate cancer.
- Certain procedures involving prostate gland, such as transrectal biopsy, prostatectomy and conditions, such as prostatitis and acute urinary retention, BPH and cancer of prostate will cause an increased PSA.

Clinical Application

a. *Early detection of cancer:*
    - PSA is specific for prostatic tissue but not for prostate cancer.
    - PSA level alone will not detect cancer in early stages.
    - PSA level is highest even in BPH. Serum PSA value together with digital rectal examination, transrectal ultrasonography is useful in the early detection of prostatic cancer.
    - Early detection is important because prostatic cancer can be detected in the early stage.

b. *Staging of prostatic cancer:*
    - PSA level is found to be correlated well with the clinical stages of prostatic cancer.
    - Elevation of PSA level is seen in advanced stages of cancer.

c. *Monitoring treatment:*
    - PSA level is useful in monitoring the definitive treatment of prostatic cancer.
    - After radial prostatectomy or radiation therapy PSA level should decrease or should fall below the detection limit of the assay. High PSA levels even after prostate removal indicates the presence of residual tumor.

Methods for PSA Estimation

Most of them are immunoassay methods, such as:

- Radioimmunoassay (RIA)
- Enzyme-linked immunosorbent assay (ELISA)
- Fluoroimmunoassay (FIA)
- Microparticle enzyme immunoassay (MEIA)
- Chemiluminescent assay

Principle of MEIA

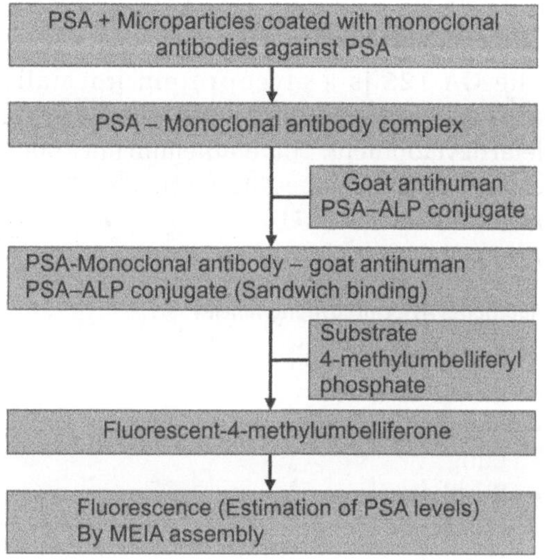

Normal range: 0 – 4 ng/mL
Specimen: Serum.
Storage: At 2 – 8°C, stable for 24 hour and stable for 3 days at 0°C.

Fluorescent Polarization Immunoassay

Principle

- Fluorescent polarization immunoassay is a type of homogenous competitive fluoroimmunoassay. Generally, the total assay time is less than one minute.
- Fluoroimmunoassay is widely used to detect drug levels in the serum.
- The principle is based on the increase of polarization of the fluorescence of small fluorescent labeled hapten (tracer) when bound by specific antibody.
- If the sample contains unlabeled analyte tracer will compete for binding with antibody and the polarization signal will decrease.

$$\underset{\text{(fast rotation)}}{\underset{\text{Low polarization}}{\text{FAg + Ab}}} \xrightarrow{+\text{Ag}} \underset{\text{(slow rotation)}}{\underset{\text{High polarization.}}{\text{Ab: Ag + Ab: Ag-F}}}$$

The polarization of the fluorescent antigen conjugate is determined by its state of rotation during the lifetime of the excited state in solution. A small rapidly rotating fluorescein antigen conjugate has a low degree of polarization, however binding to a large antibody molecule slows down the rate of rotation and increases the degree of polarization and a homogenous assay is possible.

Human Chorionic Gonadotropin (hCG)

- It is secreted by syncytiotrophoblast cells of the normal placenta.
  - Physiologically, hCG appears to maintain the corpus luteum, thereby allowing synthesis of progesterone and estrogens, which supports the endometrium.
  - The placental hormone, hCG is similar to LH, FSH and TSH. All these are glycoproteins contains two non-covalently bound dissimilar subunits, alpha and beta with carbohydrate side chains.
  - It increases normally in pregnancy and also in trophoblastic disease and germ cell tumors.

Clinical Applications

- It is an excellent marker for early confirmation and monitoring of pregnancy.
- Aiding in the detection of ectopic pregnancy.
- hCG is useful in identifying patients with trophoblastic tumors.

- Along with AFP, it is useful in the detection of non-seminiferous testicular tumor where hCG levels correlate well with tumor volume of prognosis.
- High levels of hCG even in CSF indicates brain metastasis, hCG is used to monitor the therapy of patients with CNS metastasis.
- Its level is useful in monitoring treatment and progression of trophoblastic disease.
- During chemotherapy and after remission, periodic levels are measured to detect the relapse.

Methods of Assay

Immunometric assays, such as RIA, ELISA, and FIA.
Specimen: Serum
Normal value: < 5.0 mIU/mL

CA 15-3/CA-27.29 CA 72-4

Primary tumor: Breast cancer
Additional Associated Malignancies

- Colon
- Gastric
- Hepatic
- Lung
- Pancreatic
- Ovarian and prostate cancers.

Benign Conditions

Breast, liver, kidney disorders and ovarian cysts.

Normal value: 38 units/mL

Level above which benign is >100 units per mL.

Sensitivity

Elevated in about 33% of early-stage breast cancers and about 67% of late-stage breast cancers.

CA-19.9

Primary Tumor(s): Pancreatic and Biliary Tract Cancers

Additional associated malignancies in which the level exceeds are:

- Colon
- Esophageal
- Hepatic cancers.

Benign Conditions

- Pancreatitis
- Biliary disease and cirrhosis.

Normal value: 37 units/mL

Level above which benign is more than 1,000 units per mL

Sensitivity

Elevated in 80 to 90% of pancreatic cancers and 60 to 70% of biliary tract cancers.

Cancer Antigen 125 (CA-125)

The CA 125 is a glycoprotein normally expressed in coelomic epithelium during fetal development. This epithelium lines body cavities and envelopes the ovaries.
Normal values: < 35 U/mL.
Primary tumor (s): Ovarian cancer.

Additional Associated Malignancies

- Endometrial
- Fallopian tube
- Breast
- Lung
- Esophageal
- Gastric
- Hepatic
- Pancreatic cancer.

Benign Conditions

- Menstruation
- Pregnancy
- Fibroids
- Ovarian cysts
- Pelvic inflammation
- Cirrhosis
- Pleural pericardial effusions
- Endometriosis.

Level above which benign >200 units per mL.

Sensitivity

Elevated in about 85% of ovarian cancers; elevated in only 50% of early-stage ovarian cancers.

Calcitonin

Thyroid medullary carcinoma
Normal ranges:
$\leq$ 0.155 ng/mL for men
$\leq$ 0.105 ng/mL for women.

ONCOFETAL ANTIGENS

Oncofetal antigens are proteins produced during fetal life. These proteins are present in high concentration in the sera of fetuses and decrease to low levels or disappear after birth. These proteins reappear in cancer patients. The production of these proteins demonstrates that certain genes are reactivated as the result of the malignant transformation of cells. There are several examples for oncofetal antigens; AFP, CEA, β oncofetal antigens, and pancreatic oncofetal antigen.

Alpha-fetoprotein (AFP)

- Alpha-fetoprotein is the best example for oncofetal antigen.
- It is a marker for hepatocellular and germ cell carcinoma.

Clinical Application

- For detecting fetuses with neural tube defect.
- Screening of hepatocellular carcinoma.
- Prognosis and monitoring the therapy of the patients.
- Along with hCG, it is used in classifying and staging germ cell tumors into a single type or a mixture of seminoma, yolk sac choriocarcinoma, teratoma (skin cancer).
- Increased AFP is considered as yolk sac tumor.
- Increased hCG indicates choriocarcinoma.
- Increase in both hCG and AFP indicates embryonal carcinoma.
- These markers correlate with tumor volume and prognosis of the disease.
- hCG-AFP combination is also useful in monitoring patients with germ cell tumors.
- The decreased levels indicate the success of therapy and increased levels indicates recurrence or metastasis.

Methods of Assay: Immunometric Assays, such as FIA, RIA and ELISA
Normal levels: 0–15 ng/mL.

Carcinoembryonic Antigen (CEA)

It is a marker for:
- Colorectal cancer
- Gastrointestinal cancer
- Lung cancer
- Breast carcinoma.

Clinical Applications

- It is elevated in the benign conditions, such as cirrhosis, pulmonary emphysema, rectal polyps, benign breast diseases and ulcerative colitis.
- It also increases in colorectal, lung, gastric, breast, pancreatic, ovarian, and uterine cancers. Moreover, CEA is not a marker in these cases because of the elevations associated with benign disease of the number of tumors that do not produce CEA.
- The CEA is used as an adjuvant in clinical staging. If CEA increases 5–10 times than the normal, it may be a colon cancer, or may be associated with other cancers.
- If 28% increased than the normal it may be a colorectal cancer of stage A. If it is 45% more, it is colorectal cancer of stage B.
- In the prognosis of the development of the metastasis.
- Monitoring the therapy of colorectal cancer.
- Monitoring breast, lung, gastric, and pancreatic carcinomas.
- Monitoring metastatic colon cancers.

Methods of Assay

Immunoassays, such as RIA, FIA and ELISA
Normal level: 0–4 ng/mL
For smoker: 0–5 ng/mL.

Immunoglobulins

Production of a monoclonal immunoglobulin molecule is characteristic of multiple myeloma. These paraproteins are usually complete antibody molecules but may be isolated light chains or, rarely, heavy chains. They may be lambda or kappa light chains and of any immunoglobulin subtype.

Immunoglobulins are valuable in the staging and treatment of myeloma, the amount of paraprotein serving as an index of tumor volume. Response to treatment is indicated by a fall in paraprotein production, whereas a rise points to relapse.

SELF TEST

1. Define tumor markers.
2. State the clinical importance of tumor marker estimation in the laboratory.
3. Name any 4-tumor markers.
4. Which marker is used to find out the tumor of the prostate gland?
5. Write the clinical significances of PSA estimation.
6. Write the normal value for the following:
   a. PSA
   b. AFP
   c. CEA
7. Write the clinical applications of β-hCG estimation.
8. What are oncofetal antigens, give one example?
9. In which tumor the CA-125 increases?
10. Mention the other associated benign conditions in which CA-125 increases.
11. State the conditions associated with AFP increase.
12. Write the clinical applications of CA-27.29 estimation in the laboratory.

MULTIPLE CHOICE QUESTIONS

1. The specific tumor marker for prostate is —
   a. Prostatic acid phosphatase
   b. Prostate specific antigen
   c. Carcinoembryonic antigen
   d. Lactate dehydrogenase

2. The β-hCG secreted from:
   a. Adrenal medulla
   b. Syncytiotrophoblastic cells of placenta
   c. Prostate gland
   d. Ovarian follicles

3. The following are the examples for oncofetal antigens, *Except:*
   a. hCG
   b. CEA
   c. AFP
   d. α-Oncofetal antigens

4. CEA is not a marker for:
   a. Colorectal cancer
   b. Gastrointestinal cancer
   c. Lung cancer
   d. Liver cancer

5. Which of the following does not have AFP as a marker:
   a. For detecting fetuses with neural tube defect
   b. Screening of hepatocellular carcinoma
   c. Yolk sac tumor
   d. Colon cancer

12 UNIT Lipids

LEARNING OBJECTIVES

At the end of this unit, the learner should be able to understand:

- Lipids and its classification.
- Know about the determination of bile acids and merits and demerits of its determination.
- Know about the synthesis and determination of cholesterol.
- Different types of lipoproteins and its clinical significance.
- Causes and symptoms of fatty liver.
- Causes and concerns of atherosclerosis.

INTRODUCTION

Lipid or fat is characterized by their physical property. With water, it says, "touch me not" but it goes well into solution with organic solvents. To the tongue, it is tasteful; within limits, it is good for the life but makes it danger when it is in excess.

Lipids constitute a heterogeneous group of compounds relatively insoluble in water and freely soluble in organic solvents, such as chloroform, ether, alcohol and acetone. They are classified into three classes:

1. **Simple lipids**:
   For example, fats and waxes
   Fats: Esters of fatty acids with glycerol. A fat in the liquid state is known as oil. Fat is also called as triglyceride or triacylglycerol
   Triacylglycerol (Triglyceride):
   - Nearly all the commercially important fats and oils of animal and plant origin consist almost exclusively of the simple lipid class triacylglycerols (often termed "triglycerides").
   - They consist of a glycerol moiety with each hydroxyl group esterified to a fatty acid. In nature, they are synthesized by enzyme systems, which determine that a center of asymmetry is created about carbon-2 of the glycerol backbone, so they exist in enantiomeric forms, i.e., with different fatty acids in each position.
   - They are esters of fatty acid with the trihydric alcohol glycerol.
   - The glycerol with one molecule of fatty acid is called monoacylglycerol.
   - The glycerol with two molecule of fatty acid is called diacylglycerol.
   - The glycerol with three fatty acid is called triglyceride.

$$\begin{array}{l} \alpha_1 CH_2-OH \\ \beta_1 CH-OH \\ \alpha_1 CH_2-OH \\ \text{Glycerol} \end{array} + 3 \text{ fatty acids} \rightarrow \begin{array}{l} \alpha_1 CH_2-O-CO-R_1 \\ \beta CH-O-CO-R_2 \\ \alpha_1 CH_2-O-CO-R_3 \\ \text{Triacylglycerol} \end{array}$$

R_1, R_2 and R_3 indicate the fatty acids. The fatty acids may be same or different type. Usually, R_2 is an unsaturated fatty acid.

Waxes: Esters of fatty acids with monohydric long chain alcohols.

2. **Compound lipids:**
   They are esters of fatty acid with one of the various alcohols and in addition, it contains other groups (non-lipid component).
   For example, phospholipids, glycolipids and lipoproteins.
3. **Derived lipids:**
   Substances derived from above groups by hydrolysis.
   For example, fatty acid, glycerol, alcohol and cholesterol.

FATTY ACID

Fatty acids are aliphatic monocarboxylic organic acid with chain length usually ranging from C-4 to C-24 and it is a constituent of lipid. The fatty acids have the general formula R-CO -OH.

Fatty acids are classified into saturated and unsaturated fatty acids.

Saturated fatty acid does not have double bond.

For example, acetic acid (2 carbon atoms), butyric acid (4 carbon atoms), palmitic acid (C16), stearic acid (C18) and lignoceric acid (C24).

Unsaturated fatty acids have double bonds.

They are further classified into monounsaturated (one double bond) fatty acid [MUFA].

For example, Palmitoleic acid (C16, Δ^9), Oleic acid (C18, Δ^9).

Polyunsaturated fatty acids (with more than one double bond) [PUFA].

For example, Linoleic acid, linolenic acid and arachidonic acid.

Functions of Fatty Acids

1. Essential fatty acids are involved in the esterification of cholesterol and thus help in its transport and metabolism. So, essential fatty acid lowers cholesterol level and hence decreases the risk of heart disease.
2. Essential fatty acids are constituent of the cell membrane and membranes of cell organelle (e.g., mitochondria).
3. They are essential for maintaining normal growth and health.
4. Fatty acids are components of simple and compound lipids, which are present in various tissues like adipose tissue.
5. They are responsible for the hydrophobic nature of the compounds contains them. They provide energy when they are oxidized in human body.
6. The prostaglandins and leukotrienes are formed from PUFA (arachidonic acid). They act as local hormones.
7. They protect the liver from accumulation of fat (prevent fatty liver).
8. Essential fatty acids help to prevent skin disease.

CHOLESTEROL

Cholesterol is an extremely important biological molecule that has roles in membrane structure as well as being a precursor for the synthesis of the steroid hormone and bile acids. Both dietary cholesterol and that synthesized de novo are transported through the circulation in lipoprotein. The synthesis and utilization of cholesterol must be tightly regulated in order to prevent over-accumulation and abnormal deposition within the body.

The OH group present in the 3rd position can get esterified to fatty acids to form cholesterol esters **(Fig. 12.1)**. This esterification occurs in the body by transfer of PUFA moiety by **Lecithin cholesterol acyl transferase.** This step is important for the regulation of cholesterol level.

If cholesterol increases in the blood the condition is called hypercholesterolemia. The accumulation of cholesterol in the human body leads to several disturbances. The estimation of cholesterol in the blood helps to detect the disorder and treat the person in a right time.

Fig. 12.1: Structure of cholesterol.

The cholesterol is converted to **bile acids** and excreted.
Cholesterol is mainly excreted in the form of bile salts in stool.

Metabolic Fate of Cholesterol

Cholesterol is converted into the following compounds:

Acetyl-CoA→ Cholesterol →	Steroid hormone (Testosterone, estrogens progesterone, gluco-corticoids mineralo-corticoids) Vitamin D_3 Bile salts, Bile acids

BILE ACID SYNTHESIS AND UTILIZATION

- The end products of cholesterol are the bile acids, synthesized in the liver.
- Synthesis of bile acids is one of the predominant mechanisms for the excretion of excess cholesterol. However, the excretion of cholesterol in the form of bile acids is insufficient to compensate for an excess dietary intake of cholesterol.
- The most abundant bile acids in human bile are:
  - Chenodeoxycholic acid (45%) and
  - Cholic acid (31%). These two are referred to as the primary bile acids.
- Before secretion, they will be conjugated with either glycine or taurine, which increases their polarity and water solubility.
- This mechanism of conjugation leads to the formation of four bile acids, within cholesterol.
  - Glycocholic acid (GCA)
  - Taurocholic acid (TCA)
  - Glycochenodeoxycholic acid (GCDCA)
  - Taurochenodeoxycholic acid (TCDCA).
- Within the intestines, the primary bile acids are acted upon by bacteria and converted to the secondary bile acids, identified as deoxycholate (from cholate) and lithocholate (from chenodeoxycholate).
- Both primary and secondary bile acids are reabsorbed by the intestines and delivered back to the liver via the portal circulation.

Clinical Significance of Bile Acid Synthesis

Bile acids perform four physiologically significant functions:

1. Synthesis and subsequent excretion in the feces represent the significant mechanism for the elimination of excess cholesterol.
2. Bile acids and phospholipids solubilize cholesterol in the bile, thereby preventing the precipitation of cholesterol in the gall-bladder.
3. They facilitate the digestion of dietary triglycerides by acting as emulsifying agents that render fats accessible to pancreatic lipases.
4. They facilitate the intestinal absorption of fat-soluble vitamins.

Merits of Serum Bile acid Measurement

1. *Endogenous excretion:* The measurement of serum bile acid is the best method of reflecting the extent of liver function reserve, and with much less side effects as compared with dye excretion test
2. *Enterohepatic circulation:*

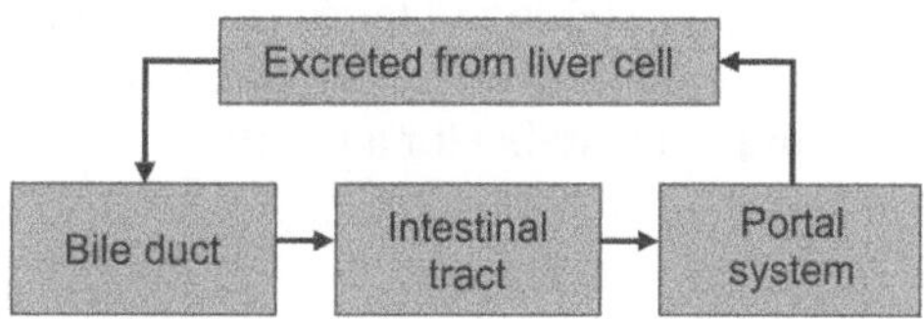

3. The 95% of excreted bile acids are reabsorbed from gastrointestinal tract
4. Frequency of enterohepatic circulation—4 ~ 10 times/day
5. Amount of bile acids excreted out of the human body per day—3 to 5% of the total amount of body bile acids
6. Useful for evaluation of the extent of reservation of liver cell function of chronic hepatitis and cirrhosis.

Demerits of Bile Acid Measurement

- The bile acid measurement is of no use for differential diagnosis of liver diseases.
- It is elevated in the presence of portacaval shunt and cholestasis.

The list of tests to be done when a request made for lipid profile are:

- Total cholesterol
- Triglyceride
- LDL cholesterol
- HDL cholesterol
- VLDL
- Total cholesterol/HDL cholesterol ratio
- Lipoprotein electrophoresis.

Determination of Serum Cholesterol by Zak's Ferric Chloride Method

Principle

Cholesterol in acetic acid reacts with ferric chloride and sulfuric acid to produce a red color. The absorbance of the red colored solution is read at 560 nm.

Specimen: Serum.

Reagents

Analytical grade (AR) chemicals should be used.

1. Glacial acetic acid.
2. Ferric chloride, 0.05% reagent.
   Dissolve 500 mg of ferric chloride in one liter glacial acetic acid. Store in brown bottle. It is stable for a month.
3. Sulfuric acid, AR grade.
4. *Stock cholesterol standard solution:* 100 mg per 100 mL in acetic acid. Dissolve exactly 100 mg cholesterol in 100 mL glacial acetic acid. Keep in a cool, dark place. Reagent is stable for one month.
5. Working standard cholesterol solution 0.04 mg per mL:

Dilute 4 mL of stock standard cholesterol solution to 100 mL with ferric chloride reagent (Reagent 2). Keep in cool, dark place.

Calculation

$$\text{mg \% of cholesterol /100 mL} = \frac{T}{S} \times \text{Conc} \times \frac{\text{Total sol}}{\text{Taken sol}} \times \frac{100\text{ mL}}{\text{Serum taken}}$$

$$\text{Mg cholesterol / 100 mL} = \frac{T}{S} \times 0.2 \times \frac{10}{5} \times \frac{100\text{ mL}}{0.1}$$

$$= \frac{T}{S} \times 400$$

Note: Transfer concentrated sulfuric acid from autodispenser in a fume hood.

Standard Graph

1. *Cholesterol standard (stock):* 100 mg of cholesterol in 100 mL of glacial acetic acid is prepared fresh and stored in cool dark place.
   Working standard 1 mL of stock + 24 mL of 0.05% $FeCl_3$.
2. *NaCl 0.9%*: 0.9 g NaCl in 100 mL water.

Calculation

OD of 0.23 corresponds to 100 μg from graph

5 mL of supernatant contains = 100 μg

10 mL diluted sample contains =

$$\frac{100 \times 10}{5} = 200\ \mu g$$

0.1 mL of undiluted sample contains = 200 μg

100 mL contains =

$$\frac{200}{0.1} \times 100 = 200000\ \mu g = 200\text{ mg/dL}$$

Reagents	Blank (B)	Standard (S)	Test (T)
Ferric chloride reagent	—	—	10.0 mL
Serum	—	—	0.1 mL
Mix Stand for 10 minutes and centrifuge			
Supernatant	—	—	5 mL
Working standard cholesterol	—	5 mL	—
Ferric chloride reagent	5 mL	—	—
Sulfuric acid	3 mL	3 mL	3 mL
Mix and incubate for 30 minutes at room temperature Read absorbance at 560 nm			

Clinical Significance

- Normal serum cholesterol ranges from 150 to 200 mg/dL.
- This may be slightly higher in middle age and pregnancy.
- Cholesterol has a sterol ring.
- In plasma, about 2/3rd esterifies with fatty acids to form cholesterol esters and remaining is free. The total cholesterol value is helpful for the clinical purposes.
- Increased levels of cholesterol in serum is called **hypercholesterolemia**. This is seen in the following cases:
  - Nephrosis
  - Nephrotic syndrome
  - Obstructive jaundice
  - Myxedema
  - Xanthochromatosis
  - Glomerulonephritis (slight increase)
  - Acute nephritis (marked increase in subacute stage)
  - Coronary artery thrombosis and angina pectoris.
- Decreased level is called **hypocholesterolemia** and seen in the following cases:
  - Hyperthyroidism
  - Pernicious and other anemia
  - Malabsorption syndrome
  - Severe wasting and acute infections
  - Hemolytic jaundice.

Procedure for standard graph

Contents	*B*	S_1	S_2	S_3	S_4	S_5	*T*
Volume of standard (mL)	—	1	2	3	4	5	—
Conc of standard (µg)	—	40	80	120	160	200	—
Volume of serum (mL)	—	—	—	—	—	—	10 mL 0.05% $FeCl_3$ + 0.1 mL serum and centrifuged
Volume of 0.05% $FeCl_3$ in CH_3COOH (mL)	5	4	3	2	1	—	—
Supernatant (mL)	—	—	—	—	—	—	5
0.9% NaCl (mL)	0.05	0.05	0.05	0.05	0.05	0.05	
Concentrated H_2SO_4 (mL)	3	3	3	3	3	3	3
Mixed and kept at room temperature for 30 minutes							
Absorbance at 560 nm	0.002	0.06	0.17	0.247	0.34	0.42	0.23

Cholesterol Estimation by Enzymatic Method

Principle

Cholesterol esters $\xrightarrow{\textit{Cholesterol esterase}}$ Cholesterol + free fatty acids

Cholesterol + O_2 $\xrightarrow{\textit{Cholesterol oxidase}}$ Chol. 4-ene 3-one + 2 H_2O_2

2 H_2O_2 + 4 -aminoantipyrine +p-HBS $\xrightarrow{\textit{Peroxidase}}$ Quinonimine dye + $2H_2O_2$

Reagents

4-aminoantipyrine:	0.6 mmoL
Sodium cholate:	8.0 mM
Cholesterol esterase:	≥ 150 u/L
Cholesterol oxidase:	≥ 200 u/L
Horseradish peroxidase:	≥ 1500 u/L
p-hydroxybenzenesulfonate:	20 mM

Surfactant, Buffer pH 7.2, and sodium azide.

Specimen: Non-hemolyzed fasting serum sample is recommended, stable for a month if the serum is frozen.

Procedure

Wavelength 520 nm
Temperature; 37°C
Prepare reagents according to the instructions

Reagents	Blank (B)	Standard (S)	Test (T)
Working sol (mL)	1.0	1.0	1.0
Prewarm the reagents for 5 minutes			
Sample (mL)	—	—	10
Standard (mL)	—	10	—
Water (mL)	10	—	—
Mix well and incubate for 5 minutes and measure the absorbance at 520 nm			

Calculation

$$\frac{T-B}{S-B} \times \text{Concn. of standard mg/dL}$$

= Cholesterol mg/dL

Triglyceride Estimation by Glycerophosphate Oxidase Method (GPO-PAP)

Introduction

Triglycerides have been commonly determined by methods that liberated and then measured glycerol. Liberation has been performed either by enzymatic hydrolysis or with the use of an alkali. The first fully enzymatic method was described by Bucolo and David in 1973. This method was modified to a colorimetric test by Megraw et al in 1979.

Reagents

Pipes buffer: pH 7.2	50 mmol/L
P-chlorophenol:	2 mmol/L
Lipoprotein lipase:	150000 u/L
Glycerokinase:	800 u/L
Glycerol 3-P-oxidase:	4000 u/L
Peroxidase:	440 u/L
4-Aminoantipyrine:	0.7 mmol/L
ATP:	0.3 mmol/L

Standard: Glycerol equivalent to 200 mg/L

Principle

Triglycerides $\xrightarrow{\textit{Lipase}}$ Glycerol + Free FA

Glycerol +ATP $\xrightarrow{GK}$ G_3P+ADP

$G_3P + O_2$ $\xrightarrow{GPO}$ DAP+H_2O_2

H_2O_2 + 4-aminoantipyrine + p-chlorophenol $\xrightarrow{\textit{Peroxidase}}$ Quinoneimine dye + $4H_2O_2$

Triglycerides in the samples are hydrolyzed by lipase to glycerol and fatty acids. The glycerol is then phosphorylated by adenosine -5-triphosphate (ATP) to glycerol -3- phosphate (G_3P) and adenosine-5-diphosphate in a reaction catalyzed by glycerol kinase (GK). Glycerol-3-phosphate is then converted to dihydroxyacetone phosphate (DAP) and hydrogen peroxide by glycerophosphate oxidase (GPO). The hydrogen peroxide then reacts with 4-Amino-antipyrine (4-AAP) and p-chlorophenol [or 3-hydroxy-2, 4, 6-tribromobenzoic acid (TBHB)] in a reaction catalyzed by peroxides to yield a red colored quinoneimine dye. The intensity of the color produced is directly proportional to the concentration of triglycerides in the sample when measured at 540 nm.

Specimen Collection and Storage

1. Specimens from fasting individuals are recommended.
2. Serum, EDTA, or heparinized plasma samples can be used.
3. The plasma treated with citrate, oxalate or fluoride should not be used.
4. The hemolyzed or icteric specimens are not recommended.
5. The triglycerides of serum are stable for several days when stored at 2–8°C.
6. Do not store samples at room temperature as phospholipids may hydrolyze, releasing free glycerol and falsely elevating triglyceride values.

Procedure

Wavelength 540 nm
Temperature; 37°C
Prepare reagents according to the instructions.

Calculation

Abs = Absorbance

$$\frac{\text{Abs Test}}{\text{Abs Std.}} \times \text{concentration of standard (mg/dL)}$$

Sample calculation: If Abs of Test = 0.300, Abs. of standard = 0.200,
Concentration of standard = 200 mg/dL

Reagents	*Blank (B)*	*Std (S)*	*Test (T)*
Working sol (mL)	1.0	1.0	1.0
Prewarm the reagents at least for 5 minutes			
Sample (mL)	—	—	10
Standard (mL)	—	10	—
Water (mL)	10	—	—
Mix well, incubate for 5 minutes, and measure the absorbance at 520 nm			

$$\frac{0.300}{0.200} \times 200 \text{ mg/dL}$$

Triglyceride = 300 mg/dL

LIPOPROTEINS

These are conjugated proteins, composed of core and surface **(Fig. 12.2)**.

- Lipoprotein core consist of:
  - Triglycerides
  - Cholesterol esters.
- Lipoprotein surface consists of:
  - Phospholipids
  - Proteins
  - Cholesterol.
- Lipids are water insoluble
- Present in the blood in the form of lipoproteins, which are water soluble
- They have an outer polar surface, which makes them water soluble
- They are mainly responsible for transport of lipid
- These lipoproteins circulate in blood
- The specific proteins that bind with lipids are called apolipoproteins
- There are various apolipoproteins, such as Apo-A, Apo-B, Apo-C, Apo-E, and a minor fraction Apo-D.
- The lipoproteins are synthesized either in the intestine or by the liver.

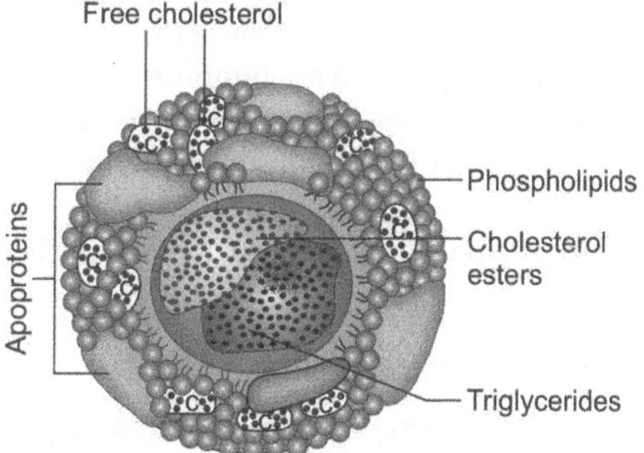

Fig. 12.2: Structure of lipoprotein.

- The lipoproteins from intestine are mostly exogenous and are dietary in origin (chylomicron).
- Those synthesized by the liver are of endogenous origin.
- After the lipoproteins are released to bloodstream, their composition may be altered by the action of some of the enzyme. The resulting fragments are taken up by the receptor cells.
- Apoproteins play a major role in the metabolism of lipoprotein.
- The density of lipoprotein is mainly due to the protein content.
- Depending on the density or on the electrophoretic mobility, the lipoproteins are classified into five major classes, they are **(Fig. 12.3)**:
  a. Chylomicrons (d <0.96)
  b. Very low density lipoproteins (VLDL) (d = 0.96–1.006)
  c. Low density lipoproteins (LDL) (d= 1.006–1.063)
  d. Intermediate density lipoproteins (IDL) and
  e. High density lipoproteins (HDL) (d = 1.063–1.21).

Separation of these lipoproteins from the serum is achieved through ultracentrifugation using solutions of different densities in which the plasma is suspended.

When plasma is centrifuged in a solution, the lipoproteins with density less than 0.91 float, is chylomicrons.

After the removal of chylomicron, the same solution is centrifuged the lipoproteins having density 0.91 to 1.006 separates out, is VLDL.

At a density of 1.006 to 1.063 LDL separates out.

The density of 1.063 to 1.21, the HDL separates out.

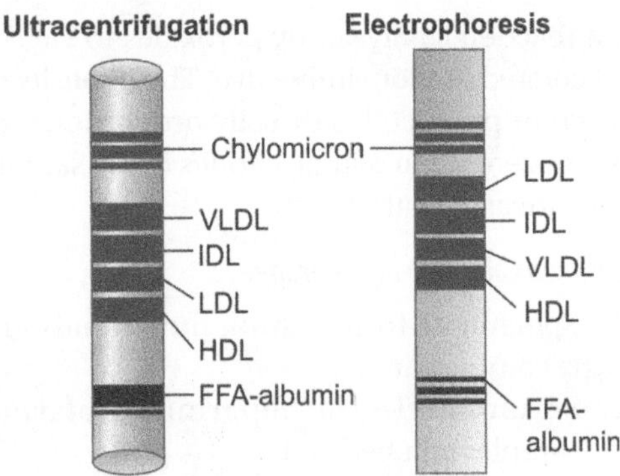

Fig. 12.3: Separation of lipoprotein.

Characteristics and composition of lipoproteins (Fig. 12.4)

Characteristic	*Chylomicron*	*VLDL*	*LDL*	*HDL*
1. Density				
2. Electrophoretic mobility	Origin	Pre β	β	α
3. % composition				
Protein	2%	10%	22%	40%
Cholesterol	8%	22%	46%	30%
TAG	83%	50%	10%	8%
PL	7%	18%	22%	29
4. Apoproteins	A,B,C,E	B,C,E	B	A and E

Chylomicrons (Fig. 12.5)

Synthesized in small intestine (mucosal cells)

- To mobilize dietary lipids
- Transport dietary lipids
- About 98% lipid, large sized, lowest density
- *Apo B-48:* Receptor binding
- *Apo C-II:* Lipoprotein lipase activator
- *Apo E:* Remnant receptor binding
- Nascent chylomicron (apo-B-48, apo-A) before they enter circulation
- Mature chylomicron (+apo C and apo E)
- Lipoprotein lipase found on the surface of endothelial cells lining the capillaries in muscle and adipose tissues removes the fatty acids of triglycerides
- Chylomicron remnant
- Apo-C removed in the liver
- Substantial portion of the phospholipid, apo-A and apo-C are transferred to HDLs during the process of fatty acid removal

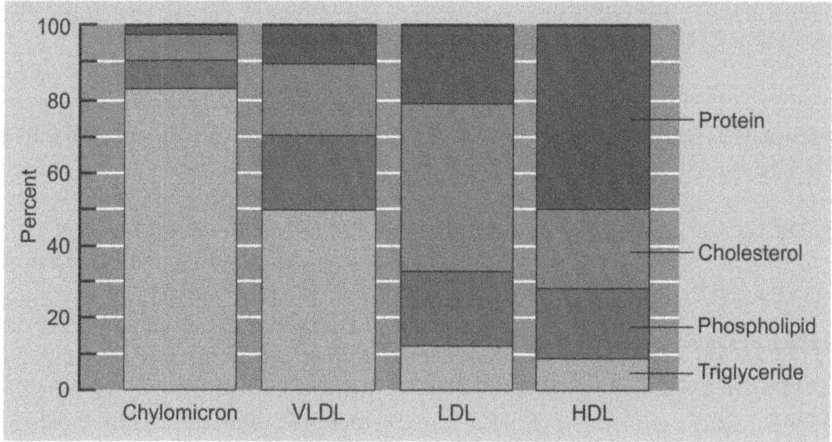

Fig. 12.4: Composition of lipoproteins.

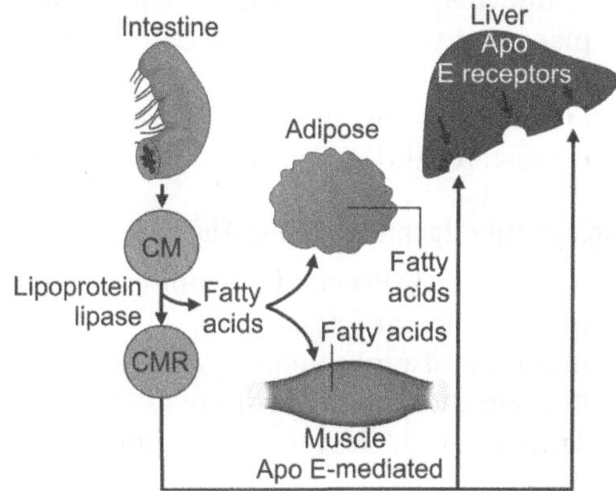

Fig. 12.5: Chylomicron metabolism.

- Chylomicron remnant containing primarily cholesterol
- Apo-E and apo-B-48 are taken up by the liver though the interaction with the chylomicron remnant receptor.

Very Low Density Lipoprotein (VLDL) (Fig. 12.6)

- Synthesized in liver
- Transport endogenous triglycerides (liver to peripheral tissues)
- Contains 90% lipid, 10% protein
- *Apo B-100:* Receptor binding
- *Apo C-II:* LPL activator liberates free fatty acids that are taken up by the adipose tissue and muscle

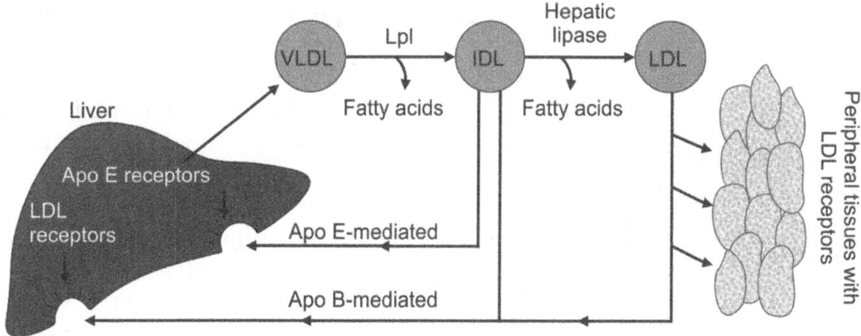

Fig. 12.6: Very low density lipoprotein metabolism.

- Apo E: Remnant receptor binding
- Nascent VLDL (B-100) + HDL (apo C and E) = VLDL
- LPL hydrolyzes TG forming IDL
- IDL loses apo C-II (reduces affinity for LPL)
- 75% of IDL removed by liver
- Apo E and Apo B mediated receptors
- 25% of IDL converted to LDL by hepatic lipase
- Loses apo E to HDL.

Intermediate Density Lipoprotein (IDL)

- Synthesized from VLDL during VLDL degradation
- Triglyceride transport and precursor to LDL
- *Apo B-100:* Receptor binding
- *Apo C-II:* LPL activator
- *Apo E:* Receptor binding.

Low Density Lipoprotein (LDL) (Fig. 12.7)

- Synthesized from IDL
- Half-life of LDL in blood is 2 days

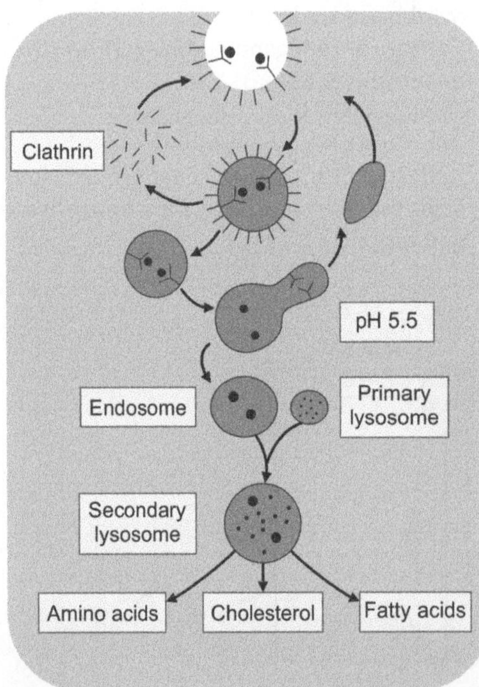

Fig. 12.7: Low density lipoprotein metabolism.

- Transport cholesterol from liver to peripheral tissues
- About 75% of the plasma cholesterol is incorporated into the LDL particles are derived from VLDL, a small part is directly released from liver
- About 78% lipid (58% cholesterol and CE)
- *Apo B-100:* Receptor binding
- Interaction of LDL with LDL receptor
- This is a bad cholesterol
- LDL receptor-mediated endocytosis
- About 75% of LDL are taken up by the liver, adrenal and adipose tissue cells by LDL receptor mediated endocytosis
- LDL receptors on 'coated pits', Clathrin: a protein polymer that stabilizes pit
- Endocytosis, loss of clathrin coating takes place and uncoupling of receptor, returns to surface
- Fusing of endosome with lysosome frees cholesterol and amino acids.

High Density Lipoprotein (HDL) (Fig.12.8)

- Synthesized in liver and intestine as protein-rich discoid particles
- Reservoir of apoproteins
- Reverse cholesterol transport
- Transport cholesterol from peripheral tissues to liver
- About 52% protein, 48% lipid, 35% C and CE
- *Apo A:* Activates lecithin-cholesterol acyl-transferase (LCAT)
- *Apo C:* Activates LPL
- *Apo E:* Remnant receptor binding
- Apoprotein exchange and provides apo C and apo E from VLDL and chylomicrons
- Reverse cholesterol transport takes place
- Discoid HDLs are converted into spherical lipoprotein through the accumulation of cholesterol ester
- Uptake of cholesterol from peripheral tissues (binding by apo-A-I)
- Esterification of HDL-C by LCAT
  LCAT activated by apoA1
- Transfer of CE to lipoprotein remnants (IDL and CR) by CETP

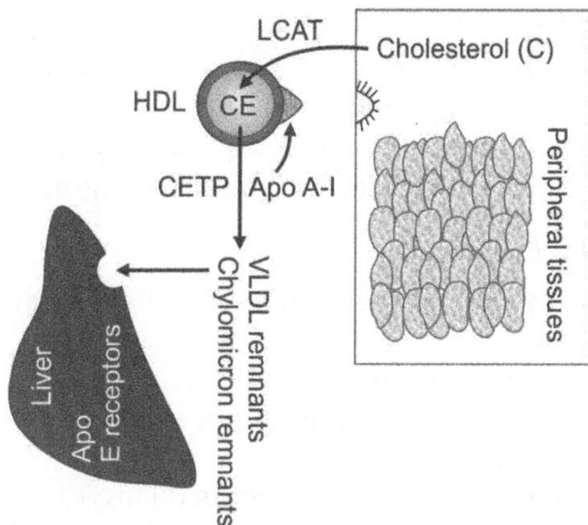

Fig. 12.8: High density lipoprotein metabolism.

- Removal of CE-rich remnants by liver, converted to bile acids and excreted
- This is considered as the beneficial one to the human body:

Lipoprotein Electrophoresis on Agar Gel

Serum lipoproteins get separated into four fractions on agar gel electrophoresis:

1. Alpha-lipoproteins (HDL)
2. Pre-beta lipoproteins (VLDL)
3. Beta-lipoproteins (LDL)
4. Chylomicrons.

These bands can be visualized by staining them with Sudan black. Alteration in any of these fractions in various diseased conditions can be viewed by the visual observation of the band thickness.

Sample

Fasting blood sample without any anti-coagulant

Serum is used for electrophoresis.

Reagents

1. Barbitone buffer, pH 8.6 (1 N): Dissolve 20.6 g sodium barbitone, 3.68 g barbituric acid and 1.0 g sodium azide in deionized water and make up to 1 liter.
2. Working buffer: Dilute 1:1 with water to get 0.05 N.
3. Staining solution: 100 mg Sudan black in 100 mL of 60% ethanol.
4. Fixative: 3% acetic acid
5. Agar gel preparation:
   a. 50 mg of agarose + 5 mL of working buffer. Boil the contents in a water bath to dissolve completely.
   b. Dissolve 50 mg of bovine albumin in 5 mL of working buffer in another test tube.

   Cool solution (a) to 50°C and then add solution (b) mix. Pour 1.4 mL of this mixture on a glass slide (2.5 × 7 cm) in to a thin uniform film, using a pipette.

Procedure

1. Cut the Whatman No. 3 paper into strips of 2 cm × 10 mm dimension and dip it in the serum sample for 1 minute.
2. Drain the excess sample from the strip.
3. Place the strip on the slide at one-third distance from one end. Strip should be placed before the gel becomes hard.
4. Keep the slides in the electrophoresis chamber containing the working buffer.
5. Connect the slides to the buffer using Whatman No.1 paper wicks of the same width as the slide.
6. Equilibrate chamber along with the slides for 30 minutes in the tank.
7. Then apply a current of 200 volts for 2 hours approximately 4 milliamps/slide.
8. The direction of current flow is from cathode to anode.
9. After 2 hours remove the slide and fix, with 3% acetic acid for 30 minutes in a Petri dish.
10. Remove the slides from acetic acid; dry the slides at 60° to 80°C in the incubator approximately for 20 minutes until the agar gel appears in the form of a thin film.
11. Immerse the slides in a Petri dish containing Sudan black solution (15 mL/slide). Keep for 1 hour.

12. Then wash the slide with running tap water to remove excess stain.

Note

1. Buffer used in the electrophoresis chamber can be reused for about 15 to 20 times.
2. Duration of the run should be more if the buffer becomes old.
3. Buffer should be discarded when it becomes turbid on usage.
4. The serum applied approximately amounts to 10 mL.
5. The serum should be absorbed uniformly by the filter paper strip.
6. Albumin mixed with gel facilitates the movement of lipoproteins through the gel and hence causes better separation. The mobility of lipoproteins on electrophoresis mainly depends on their protein content. The lipoprotein with higher protein content moves faster towards the anode and those with lesser protein moves slow. The VLDL with less protein than LDL moves in front of LDL this is due to the nature of the apoprotein present. The pattern of separation is shown in **Figure 12.9**.

Apoproteins

The protein part of the lipoprotein is called as apoprotein or apolipoprotein. The following types of apoproteins are found in blood.

- Apo A-I
- Apo A-II
- Apo B-100
- Apo B-48
- Apo C-I
- Apo C-II
- Apo C-III
- Apo D
- Apo E
- Apo J

Apo A-I

- It is synthesized in the intestine and liver.
- It is a component of HDL-2.
- It is antiatherogenic since it activates LCAT.
- Normal blood level is about 150 mg/dL.

Apo A-II

- It is also synthesized in the intestine and liver.
- It is a component of HDL-3.
- It stimulates hepatic lipase and inhibits LCAT.
- Normal blood level is about 30 mg/dL.

Apo B-100

- It is synthesized in liver.
- It is a component of VLDL and LDL.
- It binds to LDL receptors.
- Normal level in blood is about 100 mg/dL.

Apo B-48

- It is synthesized in the intestine.
- It is a component of chylomicron.
- It has 48% size of apo B-100.

Apo C-I

- It is synthesized in liver.
- It is a component of chylomicron and VLDL.
- It activates LCAT.
- Normal level in blood is about 10 mg/dL.

Apo C-II

- It is synthesized in liver.
- It is a component of chylomicron and VLDL.
- It activates lipoprotein lipase in vessel wall of adipose tissues and skeletal muscles. Due to its action, triglycerides from chylomicrons and VLDL are broken down to give fatty acids and glycerol.
- Normal level in blood is about 5 mg/dL.

Apo C-III

- It is synthesized in liver.
- It is a component of chylomicron and VLDL.
- It is antiatherogenic.

- It inhibits lipoprotein lipase.
- Normal level in blood is about 10 mg/dL.

Apo D

- It is a component of HDL-3.
- It transfers cholesterol from tissues to HDL.

Apo E

- It is synthesized in liver.
- It is a component of chylomicron, VLDL and IDL.
- It acts as ligand for hepatic uptake.
- Normal level in blood is about 2 mg/dL.

Apo J

- It is synthesized in liver.
- It is a component of HDL-2.
- It is antiatherogenic.
- It inhibits macrophage mediated cell damage.
- Normal level in blood is about 10 mg/dL.
- The lipoproteins of plasma are separated and characterized by electrophoresis. By the position they occupy, they are characterized as α, β or pre β lipoproteins. HDL cholesterol is also known as α-lipoprotein, LDL as β-lipoprotein, and VLDL as pre β -lipoprotein.

Hyperlipoproteinemia

A common abnormality in humans is the presence of excessive amounts of lipoproteins, such as VLDL, LDL, or chylomicrons in the plasma following a 10 to 12 hours of fasting. This is called as hyperlipoproteinemia.

Fredrickson's Classification of Hyperlipoproteinemias (Fig. 12.9)

Type I hyperlipoproteinemia

- It is characterized by the presence of chylomicrons, which contains **high TG.**
- This type arises because of the absence of **lipoprotein lipase** in blood.

Type II a hyperlipoproteinemia

- It is characterized by the presence of high LDL, which contains **high cholesterol.**

Type II b hyperlipoproteinemia

- It is characterized by high LDL and VLDL, which contains **high cholesterol and triglyceride** respectively.
- It is due to overproduction of apo B.

Type III hyperlipoproteinemia

- Broad beta band is observed in electrophoretic pattern and so it is called broad beta disease.
- In this type, IDL and LDL levels are increased.

Type IV hyperlipoproteinemia

- It is characterized by the high-level of VLDL (high-level of cholesterol and triglyceride).
- It is due to the overproduction of endogenous triacylglycerol.
- It is observed in secondary conditions, such as:
  - Diabetes mellitus
  - Obesity
  - Chronic alcoholism and renal failure.

Type V hyperlipoproteinemia

- Both chylomicrons and VLDL levels are increased
- In this type triglyceride is high
- It is commonly seen in conditions, such as:
  - Obesity
  - Diabetes mellitus
  - Alcoholism
  - Nephrotic syndrome.

Lipoprotein (a) and its Importance in Cardiovascular Diseases

- A lipoprotein (a) is a heterogeneous macromolecule associated with early myocardial infarction, coronary artery disease, and stroke.
- It composes 27% protein, 65% lipid and 8% carbohydrates.

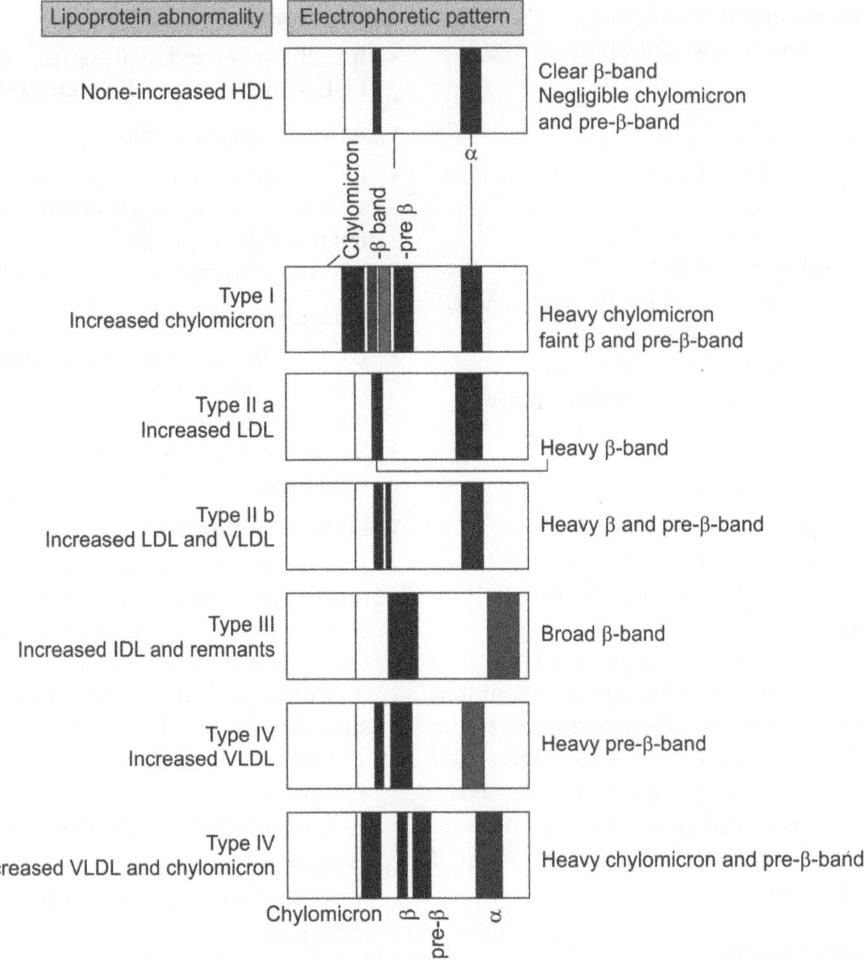

Fig. 12.9: Pattern of lipoprotein separation in normal and abnormal conditions.

- Its composition is similar to that of LDL, but is usually present in much lower concentration.
- The structure of Lp (a) consists of an apolipoprotein (a) molecule linked to apolipoprotein B-100 on a lipid-rich LDL core.
- Its electrophoretic mobility is in the pre-beta region.
- Although similar to LDL, Lp (a) is not affected by dietary factors.
- The Lp (a) determination is being recognized as a significant independent marker for assessment of the risk of coronary heart disease.
- The levels of Lp (a) is genetically controlled.
- It has a strong structural homology to plasminogen.

FATTY LIVER

What is fatty liver?

- Fatty liver, also known as fatty liver disease (FLD), is a reversible condition wherein large vacuoles of triglyceride fat accumulate in liver cells via the process of steatosis.

- Accumulation of fat (triacylglycerol) may also be accompanied by a progressive inflammation of the liver (hepatitis) called steatohepatitis. By considering the contribution by alcohol, fatty liver may be termed alcoholic steatosis or non-alcoholic fatty liver disease (NAFLD) and the more severe forms as alcoholic steatohepatitis (part of alcoholic liver disease), and nonalcoholic steatohepatitis (NASH).
- Fatty liver occurs when excess triacylglycerol accumulates inside liver cells. This means normal, healthy liver tissue becomes partly replaced with fatty tissue. The fat starts to invade the liver, gradually infiltrating the healthy liver areas, so that less healthy liver tissue remains. The fatty liver has a yellow greasy appearance and is often enlarged, and swollen with fat. This fatty infiltration slows down the metabolism of body fat stores, which means that the liver burns fat less efficiently, resulting in weight gain and inability to lose weight. However, some people can have a fatty liver without being overweight.
- Fatty liver is slightly enlarged and yellow in color, and 'shiny' or 'greasy' in appearance because it is congested with fat **(Fig. 12.10)**.
- *Severe fatty liver **(Fig. 12.11)**:* The condition is more severe degree of fatty liver and is more often due to incorrect diet, alcohol excess or obesity.

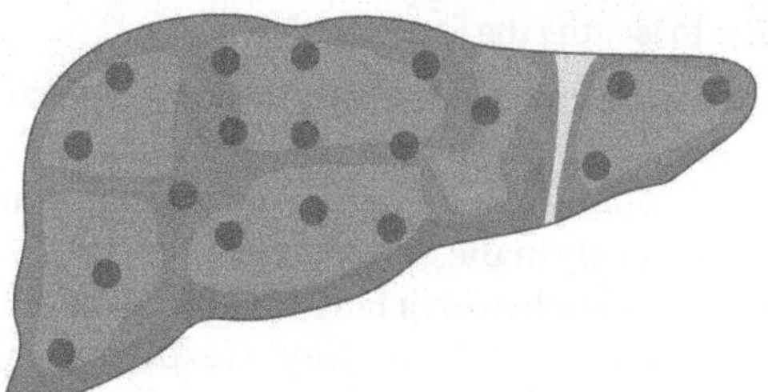

Fig. 12.10: Fatty liver.

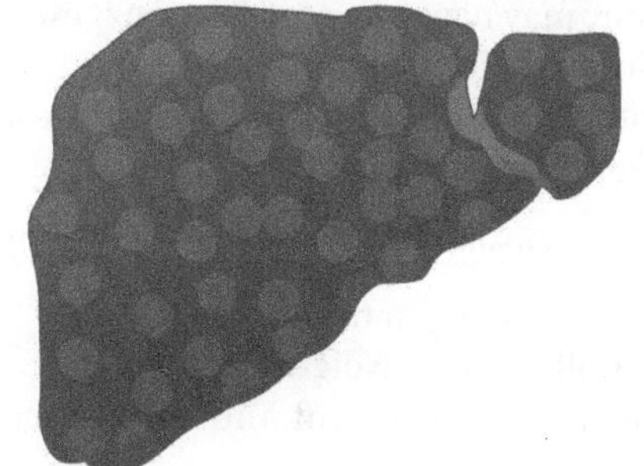

Fig. 12.11: Severe fatty liver.

What Causes Fatty Liver?

- *Increased synthesis of triacylglycerol:* Mobilization of free fatty acids from adipose tissue and their entry into liver is higher than utilization. This leads to overproduction of triglyceride (TG) and their accumulation in liver. The conditions in which increased mobilization of fatty acids takes place are diabetes mellitus, starvation, obesity and alcoholism.
- *Impaired synthesis of lipoproteins:* The synthesis of very low density lipoprotein (VLDL) takes place in liver and its formation requires phospholipids and apolipoprotein (ApoB). Fatty liver due to impaired lipoproteins synthesis may be due to:
- A defect in phospholipids synthesis.
- A block in apoprotein formation.
- Failure in the formation/secretion of lipoprotein.
- Fatty liver due to impairment in phospholipids is associated with the dietary deficiency of lipotropic factors, such as choline, betaine, inositol, etc. Deficiency of essential fatty acids leads to decreased formation of phospholipids.
- Some chemicals, such as puromycin, ethionine, carbon tetrachloride (CCL4), chloroform and lead that inhibit protein synthesis cause fatty liver. This is due to blockage in the synthesis of ApoB required for VLDL production.
- Certain hormones, such as adrenocorticotropic hormone (ACTH), insulin, thyroid, adrenocorticoids promote deposition of fat in liver.

How to Identify the Fatty Liver?

- Many people with a fatty liver are unaware that they even have a liver problem, as the symptoms can be vague and non-specific, especially in the early stages.
- Most people with a fatty liver feel generally unwell, and find they are becoming increasingly fatigued and overweight for no apparent reason.
- They may have elevated liver enzymes on a blood test for liver function.
- Fatty liver is diagnosed with a blood test and liver ultrasound scan.

Possible Symptoms of Fatty Liver (NASH or NAFLD)

- Weight excess in the abdominal area
- Inability to lose weight
- Elevated cholesterol and/or triglyceride levels
- Fatigue
- Nausea and/or indigestion
- Overheating of the body
- Excessive sweating
- Red itchy eyes
- Discomfort over the liver area.

Familial Hypercholesterolemia

Familial hypercholesterolemia (FH) is a genetic disorder characterized by high cholesterol levels, specifically very high levels of low-density lipoprotein, in the blood and early cardiovascular disease.

- Many patients have mutations in the *LDLR* gene that encodes the LDL receptor protein (which normally removes LDL from the circulation), or apolipoprotein B (ApoB), which is the part of LDL that binds with the receptor.
- Patients who have one abnormal copy (heterozygous) of the *LDLR* gene may have premature cardiovascular disease at the age of 30 to 40. Having two abnormal copies (*homozygous*) may cause severe cardiovascular disease in childhood.

Physical Signs

- Normally, high cholesterol levels do not cause any symptoms. Cholesterol may be deposited in various places in the body that are visible from the outside, such as in yellowish patches around the eyelids (xanthelasma palpebrarum), the outer margin of the iris and in the form of lumps in the tendons of the hands, elbows, knees and feet.
- Past or present symptoms of recurrent Achilles tendonitis or arthritic complaints.

Cardiovascular Disease (CVD)

- Deposition of cholesterol in the walls of arteries leads to atherosclerosis, the underlying cause of cardiovascular disease. The most common problem in familial hypercholesterolemia is the development of coronary artery disease (atherosclerosis) at a much younger age than would be expected in the general population. This may lead to angina pectoris (chest pain) or heart attacks.

Pathophysiology

- *Normally:* LDL cholesterol circulates in the body for 2.0–2.5 days and subsequently binds to the LDL receptor on the liver cells, undergoes endocytosis, and is digested. Synthesis of cholesterol by the liver is suppressed in through HMG-CoA reductase pathway.
- In FH, LDL receptor function is reduced or absent and LDL circulates for an average duration of 4.5 days, resulting in significantly increased level of LDL cholesterol in the blood with normal levels of other lipoproteins. In mutations of *Apo B*, reduced binding of LDL particles to the receptor causes the increased level of LDL cholesterol

Plasminogen

- It is an **inactive precursor of plasmin.**

- It is present in plasma and is converted to plasmin by the action of an enzyme **urokinase**.
- Plasmin is a proteolytic enzyme with a high specificity for fibrin and the particular ability to **dissolve fibrin clots**.
- Lp (a) because of significant homology with plasminogen, interferes with plasminogen activation and **imposes fibrinolysis**. This leads to unopposed intravascular thrombosis and possible myocardial infarction.
- **Interference with normal thrombolysis** may account for the association between elevated Lp (a) levels and **cardiovascular disease**.
- It has been suggested that Lp (a) binds to endothelial cells and provide a pathway by which cholesterol rich particles enter the arterial wall.
- Thus Lp (a) **has coronary atherogenic properties** and is associated with cerebrovascular disease and stroke.
- Alpha lipoprotein Lp (a) should not be confused with apo A.
- **Apo A is a constituent of HDL** and is seen in all persons, **while Lp (a)** is seen as a constituent **of LDL** in certain persons only.
- Lp (a) level associated with infarction and is sometimes called the little rascal.
- In 40% population, there is no detectable level of Lp (a) in serum.
- In 20% of population, the Lp (a) concentration in blood is **more than 30 mg/dL** and the persons are **susceptible for heart attack** at a young age.
- Its levels **more than 30 mg/dL** increase the risk three times and when increased Lp (a) is associated with increased LDL, the risk is increased six times.
- The identification of individuals at coronary heart disease risk through the diagnostic testing of Lp (a) can play a significant role in alarming such individuals for the need to eliminate or control other high-risk factors when possible.

Atherosclerosis and Coronary Heart Disease

Atherosclerosis (athero = organic matter schlero = deposit) is the condition where LDL cholesterol deposited in the subintimal regions of arteries causing obstruction to the flow of blood. This may lead to extra burden on the heart, which may be one of the reasons for hypertension. If this condition is neglected for long time, may lead to cardiac diseases and ischemia.

Atherosclerosis leads to coronary heart diseases (CHD) or coronary artery diseases (CAD) or (IHD). The deposited organic matter mainly composed of cholesterol and cholesterol ester. Hypercholesterolemia may be due to defects in transport, utilization and excretion. Most of the cholesterol is esterified, which only can conjugate with plasma protein making ease its transport.

The protein-cholesterol conjugate also takes up triacylglycerol (TAG) and phospholipids.

Risk Factors for Atherosclerosis

Serum Cholesterol Values

- Values **above 250 mg/dL increase the risk** and the person needs active treatment.
- Values **around 220 mg/dL** indicate **moderate risk**.
- Values **below 200 mg/dL are safer**.

Low Density Lipoprotein Cholesterol

- LDL cholesterol level is directly related to risk of atherosclerosis. So LDL is named as **bad cholesterol.**
- Values **above 160 mg/dL** indicate high-risk.
- Values **between 129–130 mg/dL** are in borderline risk.
- Values **below130 mg/dL** are safer.

High Density Lipoprotein Cholesterol

- HDL cholesterol is inversely related to the risk of atherosclerosis. So it is named as **good cholesterol.**
- HDL cholesterol values **above 60 mg/dL** indicate very low-risk for atherosclerosis.

- HDL **below 35 mg/dL** increases the risk of atherosclerosis. Below 35 mg/dL, with every 1 mg/dL decrease in HDL increase the risk of atherosclerosis by 3 percent.
- It is very important to note the ratio of total cholesterol to HDL cholesterol. It is important to maintain the normal **ratio of below 4.5.** Increase in ratio increases the risk of atherosclerosis.
- It is also important to note the ratio of LDL cholesterol to HDL cholesterol. It is important to maintain the normal ratio of less than 3.
- Women have higher HDL (due to the presence of estrogens) and so they are less prone to heart diseases compared to men.

Apoprotein Level

- It is important to maintain apoprotein level in normal range.
- Apo A1 is a measure of HDL cholesterol while Apo B is a measure of LDL cholesterol.
- Apo A1 is the most reliable index for predicting cardiac diseases.

Lp (a)

- Its level more than 30 mg/dL increases the risk of atherosclerosis by three times.
- If increased Lp (a) is associated with high LDL, the risk is increased six times.

Diabetes Mellitus

- Insulin deficiency produces large number of acetyl-CoA that may enter cholesterol synthesis and increases the risk of coronary artery disease.

Hypertension

- Atherosclerosis may lead to hypertension.
- Systolic blood pressure of more than 160 further increases the risk of coronary artery disease.

Serum Triglyceride Level

- Serum triglyceride level above 200 mg/dL increases the risk of atherosclerosis.

Cigarette Smoking

- Nicotine of cigarette increases lipolysis and so large number of acetyl-CoA are produced.
- These may channel into cholesterol synthesis.
- Nicotine has a role in transient constriction of coronary and carotid arteries.
- Chain smokers have high-risk of coronary artery disease.

Alcoholism

- Oxaloacetate is depleted during alcohol metabolism.
- This oxaloacetate is required for the conversion of acetyl-CoA in Krebs cycle.
- Depletion of oxaloacetate causes the conversion of acetyl-CoA into cholesterol.

Control of Atherosclerosis

- Consume of sufficient amount of polyunsaturated fatty acids (PUFA) for the excretion of cholesterol from the body.
- Normal diet consisting of cereals, pulses and vegetables provide about 10 g of PUFA per day, which is sufficient to maintain cholesterol level, and there is no need to take extra PUFA.
- Keep diabetes and hypertension under control.
- Check lipid profile once in every 6 months.
- Dietary control.
- Consume less oily food.
- Avoid sucrose since it increases triglyceride level.
- Take more green leafy vegetables. These contain fiber content, which increases the bowel motility in intestine and thus reduces the reabsorption of bile salts. It will helps in maintaining cholesterol level.
- Do moderate exercises.
- Avoid cigarette.
- Drugs such as clofibrate, nicotinic acid (not nicotine), lovastatin and mevinolin

decreases serum cholesterol level. Take the drug only with doctor's prescription.

Estimation of HDL Cholesterol

1. Methods available
   a. Enzymatic method
   b. Phosphotungstate/Mg^{2+} method
   c. Heparin/Mn^{2+} method.
2. Using Liebermann-Burchard reagent.

Enzymatic Method

Principle

Chylomicrons, VLDL, LDL present in serum are precipitated by polyions. Cholesterol esters left behind are hydrolyzed by cholesterol esterase to free cholesterol and fatty acids. Free and liberated cholesterol are oxidized by cholesterol oxidase to chol-4-ene-3-one and H_2O_2 is liberated. The H_2O_2 produced couples with 4-aminoantipyrine and phenol in the presence of peroxidase to form a colored compound. The intensity of the color developed is proportional to the concentration at 500 nm (490–550) or with green filter.

Reagents

1. *Phosphotungstic acid reagent:* 169 mg of phosphotungstic acid is dissolved in 50 mL of distilled water. To this 508 mg of $MgCl_2$ is added, mix and the volume is made up to 100 mL with distilled water and mix again.
2. *Enzyme reagent:* It contains 4-aminoantipyrine, phenol, peroxidase, cholesterol esterase, cholesterol oxidase and sodium azide in a powdered form in an amber colored bottle. The enzyme reagent is reconstituted by adding 20 mL of diluent reagent.

The solid given in the bottle is gently mixed, stored in the refrigerator after keep it at room temperature for 15 minutes.

Procedure

Serum 0.2 mL and 0.4 mL phosphotungstic acid reagent containing $MgCl_2$ is taken in a centrifuge tube and mixed in a vortex mixer for 10 seconds. Keep it in a room temperature for 20 minutes.

Then it is centrifuged at 1500 rpm for 30 minutes at room temperature. The supernatant is removed carefully avoiding mixing of the contents. If the supernatant is not clear, the contents are recentrifuged at high speed and if still slightly turbid the analysis is repeated on diluting with equal volume of the buffer. 0.2 mL of standard is also treated like test and the supernatant is taken. 25 µL of supernatant of test and 25 µL of cholesterol standard are taken in different tubes using an autopipette. 1 mL each of enzyme reagent (chromogen reagent) is added to standard and test and contents are mixed well and incubated at room temperature for 20 minute. Absorbance of test, standard and blank are read against distilled water at 546 nm or using green filter. Color developed is pink and is stable for one hour at room temperature and is protected from direct light (incubation can also be done for 5 minutes at 37°C).

Contents	*Blank*	*Standard*	*Test*
Standard cholesterol	—	25 µL	—
Sample	—	—	25 µL
Chromogen (mL)	1	1	1
Incubate at 37°C for 5 minutes			
O.D at 520 nm	0.08	0.226	0.123

Calculation

$$\frac{T-B}{S-B} \times \text{concentration of standard} \times \text{Dil factor}$$

$$= \frac{AT}{AS} \times 50\ \text{mg/dL} \times 3$$

$$= \frac{0.123-0.08}{0.226-0.08} \times 50 \times 3$$

$$= \frac{0.043}{0.146} \times 50 \times 3$$

$$= \frac{43 \times 50 \times 3}{146} = 44.1\ \text{mg/dL}$$

Clinical Significance

- The HDL or α-lipoproteins contain certain cholesterol and phospholipids as the main lipids.
- The HDL particles carry about 20% of the total plasma cholesterol and this cholesterol has a clinical implication.
- It has been observed that HDL-cholesterol is inversely associated with the development of ischemic heart diseases. Thus, persons with HDL-cholesterol elevated are less likely to develop ischemic heart disease.
- The main function of HDL-cholesterol is transport of cholesterol.
- The HDL serves in removing cholesterol from peripheral cells and transporting it back to the liver where most of the cholesterol excreted from the body is removed. So HDL is called as beneficial factor among the other lipoproteins concerned.

Normal Range

- Males 28–61 mg/dL
- Females 38–75 mg/dL

Reduced HDL seen in

1. Administration of androgens, propanol, neomycin
2. Maturity onset diabetes mellitus
3. Chronic renal dialysis
4. Nephrosis
5. Cystic fibrosis
6. Hepatocellular disease
7. Cigarette smokers.

LDL-Cholesterol

Estimation of LDL cholesterol by enzymatic method:

Specimen

Serum is preferred.

Principle

LDL-cholesterol is precipitated by heparin at their isoelectric pH. When the tube is centrifuged, LDL-cholesterol separates at the bottom. The supernatant contains HDL-cholesterol and VLDL-cholesterol. The supernatant is tested enzymatically for cholesterol concentration. Then LDL-cholesterol is calculated as LDL-cholesterol = Total cholesterol—cholesterol present in the supernatant.

Reagents

1. Precipitation reagent contains:
   - Heparin—50,000 IU/L
   - Sodium citrate—0.004 mol/L. pH 5.04.
   - The reagent is ready for use.
2. Cholesterol reagent—ready for use.
3. Cholesterol standard—200 mg/dL—ready for use.

Procedure

- Take 0.1 mL of serum in a centrifuge tube.
- To this add 1 mL of precipitation reagent.
- Mix and keep it for 10 minutes at room temperature.
- Then centrifuge at 4000 rpm for 15 minutes.
- The supernatant is used for cholesterol estimation.
- Take 3 test tubes and label them as B, S, and T.
- To the tube labeled B, add 0.05 mL of distilled water.
- To 'S' tube add 0.05 mL of cholesterol standard.
- To the 'T' tube add 0.05 mL of supernatant from the step 1.
- To all the tubes add 1 mL of cholesterol reagent.
- Mix and keep for 5 minutes at 37°C or 10 minutes at room temperature.
- Measure the absorbance of B; S and T at 505 nm.

Calculation

Cholesterol concentration in the supernatant

$$= \frac{T-B}{S-B} \times \text{Concentration of standard}$$

LDL cholesterol = Total cholesterol - cholesterol in the supernatant.

Clinical Significance

Increased LDL cholesterol increases the risk of coronary heart disease and atherosclerosis.
Normal range: 10–160 mg/dL

Estimation of LDL Cholesterol and VLDL Cholesterol

Commonly total cholesterol, HDL cholesterol and triglycerides are estimated.

The remaining two (VLDL and LDL) are calculated from the above values as follows:

$$\text{VLDL cholesterol} = \frac{\text{Serum triglycerides}}{5}$$

LDL cholesterol = Total cholesterol—(HDL cholesterol + VLDL cholesterol).

SELF TEST

1. What is cholesterol?
2. Mention the methods available for cholesterol estimation.
3. Write the principle of Zak's method of cholesterol estimation.
4. Write a note on bile acids.
5. Write the merits and demerits of bile acids.
6. Name some hormones synthesized from cholesterol.
7. Explain hypercholesterolemia.
8. When hypocholesterolemia is seen?
9. Define lipoproteins.
10. Classify lipoproteins.
11. Explain the metabolism of chylomicrons.
12. Write a note on VLDL.
13. What do you know about IDL?
14. What is the importance of LDL?
15. Why HDL cholesterol is considered as beneficial factor?
16. LDL cholesterol is called as a risk factor why?
17. State the clinical significance of HDL.
18. What do you know about hyperlipoproteinemias?
19. Explain the different types of hyperlipoproteinemias.
20. Discuss the plasminogen.
21. Explain the different apoproteins.
22. How do you estimate HDL cholesterol?
23. What is the principle of LDL cholesterol estimation?
24. Why is serum triglyceride estimation important?
25. Write a note on atherosclerosis.
26. Explain the risk factors in coronary artery disease.
27. What are the precautions to take to control atherosclerosis?
28. List the tests under lipid profile.
29. Why Lp (a) determination is important? Explain.
30. Why HDL cholesterol settles at the bottom? Explain with reason.
31. Classify lipids with an example.
32. Write the metabolic fates of cholesterol.
33. Write the formula to determine the LDL cholesterol.
34. Mention the role of plasminogen in the human body.
35. Highlight the risk factors for atherosclerosis.
36. State some controlling measures to prevent atherosclerosis.
37. Cholesterol above 250 mg/dL is bad. Explain.
38. In which form the cholesterol is present in the blood?
39. How the cholesterol is excreted?
40. Mention the functions of lipoproteins.

MULTIPLE CHOICE QUESTIONS

1. Cholesterol estimation done by:
   a. Zak's method
   b. Jaffes method
   c. Henry's method
   d. None of the above

2. The normal range for cholesterol is:
   a. 100–150 mg%
   b. 80–140 mg%
   c. 200–300 mg%
   d. 150–240 mg%

3. The protein part bound to lipid is called:
a. Apoproteins
b. Glycoproteins
c. Heme proteins
d. Phosphoproteins.

4. Lipoprotein with higher protein content:
a. Moves faster towards anode in electrophoresis
b. Moves slower towards anode in electrophoresis
c. Does not move towards anode in electrophoresis
d. Moves faster towards cathode in electrophoresis.

5. The cholesterol which is beneficial to human body is:
a. LDL
b. VLDL
c. HDL
d. Chylomicrons.

13

UNIT

Acid-Base Balance

LEARNING OBJECTIVES

At the end of this unit, the learner should be able to understand:
- The regulation of acid-base balance
- Role of bicarbonate buffer system in the regulation of acid-base balance
- Acid-base regulation by respiratory and renal mechanism
- Causes, biochemical findings, symptoms and compensatory mechanism of different types of acid-base disorders

INTRODUCTION

The human body can be described as a complex system, which consists of several levels and subsystems. At the chemical level, acids and bases are some of the essential compounds upon which all biochemical processes depend. The biochemical reactions, which are taking place in our body, are extremely sensitive to even small changes in the acidity or alkalinity of the environment. The acid-base homeostasis should be maintained for cellular viability, enzymatic reactions, protein conformation and CNS functions, etc. These functions are modified when there is change in the cellular and extracellular acid-base status. For these reactions, the acids and bases that are formed constantly should be kept in balance.

To understand acid-base homeostasis a definition of some of the terms needed are explained below.

Acids: Bronsted defined an acid as a chemical entity that donates protons in solution.

$HCl \longleftrightarrow H^+ + Cl^-$

$H_2CO_3 \longleftrightarrow H^+ + HCO_3^-$

$NH_4 \longleftrightarrow H^+ + NH_3$

$H_2PO_4 \longleftrightarrow H^+ + HPO_4$

Bases: Are those, which accept protons.

pH: Sorenson expressed pH as the negative log of H^+ concentration

$pH = - \log [H^+]$

Buffers

A buffer is a solution that resists changes in pH when a small quantity of acid or base is added. The effectiveness depends on its pK or (pKa) value. The pK is the pH at which the buffer is 50% ionized meaning that, the acid concentration is exactly equal to that of the conjugate base. The buffer is very efficient at a pH of $\pm$ 1 around its pK, e.g., phosphate buffer pK = 6.8. This buffer will have maximum buffer capacity between pH 5.8 and 7.8.

A buffer solution is a mixture of a weak acid and its base (Na or K salt).

Henderson-Hasselbalch Equation

$$pH = pKa + \log_{10} \frac{[Base]}{[Acid]}$$

This indicates the relationship between the pH, pK, of the buffer and the ratio of the conjugate base to the undissociated acid. It quantitatively regulates the changes in pH, [Acid] and [Base].

H^+ Balance

- In a healthy individual, the normal pH of arterial blood is 7.4 ± 0.05 and that of venous blood is 7.4 ± 0.02.
- When the arterial pH rises above 7.45 then the individual is considered to have alkalosis. If the pH is below 7.35 is the individual considered to have acidosis.
- In a healthy subject, the pH of blood is always between 7.35 and 7.45.
- The change in pH has serious effects and therefore the control of pH is necessary.
- There are two types of metabolic acids:

1. Fixed acids→ lactic acid, acetoacetic acid, β-hydroxy butyric acid, H_2SO_4 and H_3PO_4
   - The fixed acids H_2SO_4 and H_3PO_4 are the end product of the metabolism of sulfur containing amino acids. phospholipids, nucleic acids, phosphoproteins and phosphoglycerides.
   - The organic acids like lactic acid and β-hydroxy butyric acid are formed during the metabolism of carbohydrates and lipids.
   - Accumulation of lactic acid is called lactic acidosis.
   - Normally, lactic acid produced through anaerobic glycolysis is taken up by the liver and converted to glucose through a Cori's cycle.
   - Pyruvate and lactate accumulate in conditions like arsenic or mercury poisoning and also in thiamine deficiency.
   - Inherited enzyme pyruvate dehydrogenase deficiency also leads to lactic acidosis.
2. Volatile acids → CO_2
   - CO_2 is the major end product in the oxidation of carbohydrates, fats and amino acids. It has the ability to react with H_2O to form H_2CO_3 which further dissociate to H^+ and HCO_3^-.
   - The CO_2 can be regarded as an acid by virtue of its ability to react with H_2O to form H_2CO_3.
   - In vivo, it is the carbonic anhydrase in tissues of the liver and kidney, which catalyzes the following reaction either way depending on the blood pH.

$$CO_2 + H_2O \xleftrightarrow{\text{Carbonic anhydrase}} H_2CO_3$$

$$H_2CO_3 \xleftrightarrow{\text{Carbonic anhydrase}} H^+ + HCO_3^-$$

REGULATION OF ACID-BASE BALANCE

- The pH of plasma is 7.4 and is normally maintained within a narrow range of 7.35 to 7.45.
- The blood buffer system regulates small changes in pH.
- The respiratory system also does this by increasing the expulsion of the CO_2 (hyperventilation) or by conservation of CO_2 (hypoventilation) to regulate the blood pH.
- These two compensatory mechanisms cannot last for long. It is only temporary balance.
- The renal system maintains acid-base balance of blood by adjusting the rate of reabsorption and excretion of H^+ or HCO_3^- or HPO_3^- in addition to formation and excretion of NH_3 and NH_4^+.

Blood Buffer Systems

ECF Buffers

1. Carbonate-bicarbonate—HCO_3^-/H_2CO_3 (20:1).
2. Phosphate buffer—HPO_4^-/H_2PO_4 (4:1).
3. Basic proteins/acidic proteins.
4. Organic base/organic acid.

Bicarbonate Buffer System

- The most important buffer system in the plasma is the bicarbonate-carbonate system.
- It accounts for 60% of buffering action in plasma and 40% in the whole body.
- The bicarbonate (HCO_3^-) is regulated by the kidney; the acid part carbonic acid (H_2CO_3) is under respiratory control.
- The buffer is most active when the ratio of salt and acid are equal according to the Henderson-Hasselbalch's equation.
- The normal plasma bicarbonate level is 24 mmol/L.
- The normal pCO_2 of arterial blood is 40 mm of Hg.
- The normal carbonic acid level is 1.2 mmol/L.
- The pKa of carbonic acid is 6.1.
- Substituting these values in Henderson-Hasselbalch's equation:

$$pH = pK + \log_{10} \frac{[Base]}{[Acid]}$$

$$\text{pH of blood} = 7.4 = 6.1 + \log \frac{(HCO_3^-)}{(H_2CO_3)}$$

$$6.1 + \log \frac{24}{1.2}$$

6.1 + log 20 (antilog of 20 = 1.3)

6.1 + 1.3

So the ratio between (HCO_3^-) and (H_2CO_3) = 20:1

(HCO_3^-): (H_2CO_3) = 20:1

- Therefore, the ratio of HCO_3^- to H_2CO_3 at pH 7.4 is 20 in normal conditions.
- The bicarbonate represents the alkali reserve and it is sufficient to meet the acid load.
- During the process of compensatory mechanism, if (HCO_3^-) is 24, then (H_2CO_3) will be adjusted to 1.2. This is how compensatory mechanism operates to bring the ratio back to 20:1.
- Whenever metabolic acid is added to the blood it reacts with the basic component of the buffer system, producing salt and water and helps to prevent the fall in blood pH.
- Reversal of this mechanism takes place in the event of the addition of base by metabolic processes.

Phosphate Buffer System

- It is the main intracellular buffer system.
- The pKa value (6.8) of this is nearer to the physiological pH 7.4.
- When the equation is applied,

$$pH = pKa + \log \frac{[Base]}{[Acid]}$$

$$7.4 = 6.8 + \log \frac{[Base]}{[Acid]}$$

$$0.6 = \log \frac{[Base]}{[Acid]}$$

- Antilog of 0.6 is 4, therefore the ratio is 4.
- The phosphate buffer system is effective at wide range of pH, because of the more ionizable groups it has different pKa values.

$$H_3PO_4 \xleftrightarrow{pKa = 1.96} H + H_2PO_4^-$$

$$H_2PO_4^- \xleftrightarrow{pKa = 6.8} H + HPO_4^-$$

$$HPO_4^- \xleftrightarrow{pKa\,12.4} H + PO_4^{2-}$$

- The $Na_2HPO_4/NaH_2PO_4^-$ is an effective buffer system in the human body because of its pKa value nearer to the physiological pH.

Protein Buffer System

- The buffering action of protein mainly depends on the pKa value of its ionizable side chains.
- The effective group is the amino acid, histidine with a pKa value of 6.1.
- Therefore, the albumin and hemoglobin, which have more histidine residues play important role in buffering action in the body.

Isohydric Principle

The H^+ is common to the reactions of buffer systems of the body fluids. Whenever there is a change in the concentration of H^+ in ECF the balance of all the buffer systems changes at the same time. This phenomenon is called isohydric principle.

Respiratory Regulation of Acid-Base Balance

- The second line of defense against acid-base disturbance is through controlling the CO_2 level in the lungs by either increasing or decreasing the rate of respiration.
- The rate of respiration is known to be controlled by the receptors present in the respiratory center, which are very sensitive to the changes in pH and pCO_2 of blood.
- When there is a fall in plasma pH, the respiratory center is stimulated, resulting in hyperventilation, which eliminates more CO_2 thus lowering H_2CO_3 concentration in blood.
- In the same way whenever the blood pH increases the respiratory centers are inhibited so that elimination of CO_2 is decreased by hypoventilation until the blood pH comes to normal.
- Hemoglobin transports CO_2, which is formed in the tissues and it also serves to generate bicarbonate or alkali reserve by the activity of an enzyme, carbonic anhydrase (CA).

Renal Regulation of pH

- An important function of the kidney is to regulate the function by excreting either acidic or basic urine.
- The pH of urine ranges from 4.5 to 9.5, because the renal system plays a significant role in the long-term maintenance of the blood at pH 7.4 ± 0.05.
- This is possible by its capacity of reabsorption, secretion and excretion of the non-volatile acids like lactic acid, pyruvic acid, HCl, phosphoric acid and H_2SO_4, which are produced in the body cannot be excreted by lungs.
- The first mechanism for removal of acids from the body is by renal excretion.
- The major mechanisms by which the kidney regulates the level of HCO_3^- in plasma are:

1. Reabsorption of filtered HCO_3^-.
2. Generation of new HCO_3^- and by secreting HCO_3^- under condition of chronic alkalosis.
3. Excretion of H^+ ions.

The filtered HCO_3^- combines with H^+ forming H_2CO_3, carbonic anhydrase present in the brush border of the cell wall dissociate H_2CO_3 into H_2O and CO_2. The CO_2 diffuses into the cell. The CO_2 combines with H_2O to form H_2CO_3 again. This H_2CO_3 again ionizes to HCO_3^- and H^+ with the help of carbonic anhydrase. The H^+ diffuses into the lumen in exchange for Na^+, and HCO_3^- is reabsorbed into plasma along with Na^+. There is no net excretion of H^+ or generation of new HCO^-_3. So, this mechanism helps to maintain a steady state of acid-base balance **(Fig. 13.1)**.

Another function of the kidney is to buffer acids and thus to conserve fixed base through the production of NH_3 from amino acids with the help of an enzyme glutaminase. Whenever there is excess acid production, the NH_3 production is also increased which combines with H^+ to form NH_4^+, which is excreted as NH_4Cl. This occurs in the event of acidosis. When alkali is in excess, the H^+ is reabsorbed into the cell in exchange to Na^+/K^+.

Acid-Base Disorders

- Acid-base disorders result from a variety of pathological conditions.
- The normal pH of blood is referred as euphemia.
- If the pH of the blood is more than the normal range, it is termed as alkalemia and the condition is called alkalosis.

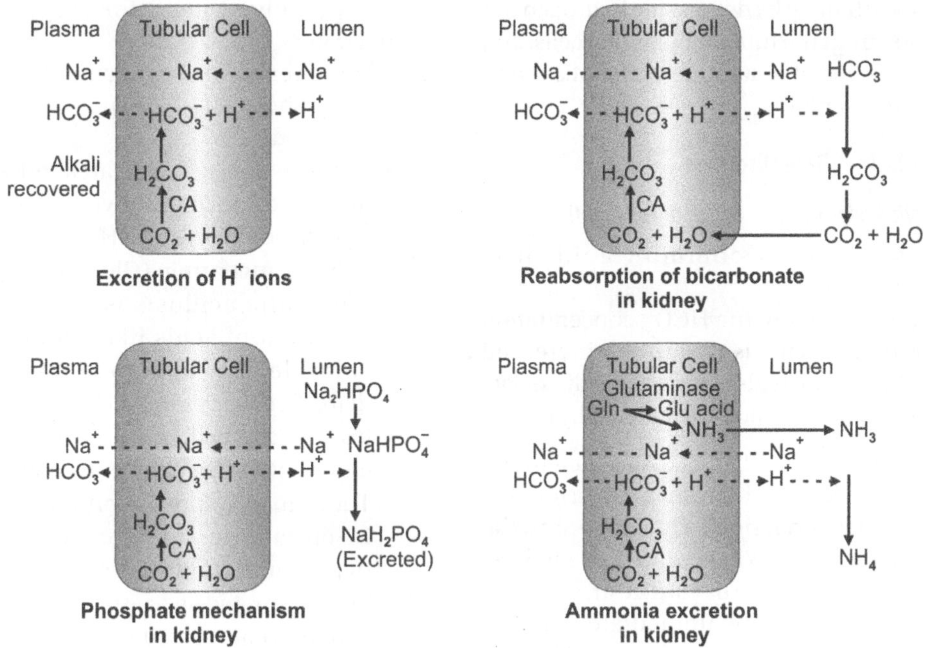

Fig. 13.1: Buffer mechanisms in the kidney.

- The pH lesser than the normal range, is called acidemia and the condition is called acidosis.
- There are two reasons for the pH abnormalities in blood, which are metabolic or respiratory causes.
- Metabolic causes are responsible for metabolic acidosis and alkalosis.
- The respiratory causes are mainly responsible for respiratory acidosis and alkalosis.

Compensation

The body's acid-base balance is tightly regulated. Several buffering agents exist, which reversibly bind hydrogen ions and slow down any change in pH. Extracellular buffers include bicarbonate and ammonia, while proteins and phosphate act as intracellular buffers. The bicarbonate buffering system is especially key, as carbon dioxide (CO_2) can be shifted through carbonic acid (H_2CO_3) to hydrogen ions and bicarbonate (HCO_3^-) as shown below.

$$HCO_3^- + H^+ \leftrightarrow H_2CO_3 \leftrightarrow CO_2 + H_2O$$

Acid-base imbalances that overcome the buffer system can be compensated in the short-term by changing the rate of ventilation. This alters the concentration of carbon dioxide in the blood. For instance, if the blood pH drops too low (*acidemia*), the body will compensate by increasing breathing, expelling CO_2.

The kidneys are slower to compensate, but renal physiology has several powerful mechanisms to control pH by the excretion of excess acid or base. In responses to acidosis, tubular cells reabsorb more bicarbonate from the tubular fluid, collecting duct cells secrete more hydrogen and generate more bicarbonate, and ammoniagenesis leads to increased formation of the NH_3 buffer. In responses to alkalosis, the kidney may excrete more bicarbonate by decreasing hydrogen ion secretion from the tubular epithelial cells, and lowering rates of glutamine metabolism and ammonia excretion.

Metabolic Acid-Base Disorders

Metabolic Acidosis (HCO_3^- Deficit or Fall in pH)

- It is the most common acid-base disturbance.
- In this condition, the HCO_3^- concentration is reduced. This is due to the increased production of acids. These acids dissociate to give H^+ ions, which are buffered by HCO_3^-.

Causes: (a) uncontrolled diabetes mellitus

1. Lactic acidosis: This results from a number of causes, particularly tissue anoxia. In acute hypoxia, condition such as respiratory failure or cardiac arrest, lactic acidosis develops immediately. Lactic acidosis may also be caused by liver disease. The presence of lactic acidosis can be determined by plasma lactate.
2. Diabetic ketoacidosis:
   Ketoacidosis is a metabolic state associated with high concentrations of ketone bodies, formed by the breakdown of fatty acids and the deamination of amino acids due to lack of insulin. The two common ketones produced in humans are acetoacetic acid and β-hydroxybutyrate
3. Ketoacidosis is most common in untreated type 1 diabetes mellitus, when the liver breaks down fat and proteins in response to a perceived need for respiratory substrate.
4. Chronic renal failure (accumulation of sulfates, phosphates, urea).
5. intoxication:
   - Organic acids (salicylates, ethanol, methanol, formaldehyde, ethylene glycol, paraldehyde, INH)
   - Sulfates, metformin (Glucophage)
   - Metabolic acidosis is also due to ingestion of acids like ammonium chloride. The ammonia part after detoxified, leaves behind the H^+.
   - It also occurs in diarrhea, which leads to loss of HCO_3^- from the intestinal fluid.
   - The primary compensatory mechanism in metabolic acidosis is through hyperventilation that removes CO_2. The deep, rapid and gasping respiratory pattern is known as Kussmaul breathing

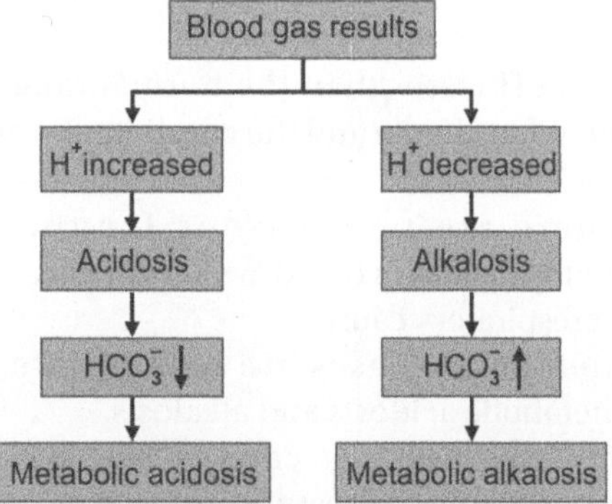

Laboratory findings in acid-base disturbances				
	pH	*pCO_2*	*HCO_3^-*	*HCO_3^-/H_2CO_3*
Normal	7.4 ± 0.05	40 mm Hg	20 mm Hg	20
Metabolic acidosis	Decreased	Normal	Decreased	Decreased
Metabolic alkalosis	Increased	Normal	Increased	Increased
Respiratory acidosis	Decreased	Increased	Normal	Decreased
Respiratory alkalosis	Increased	Decreased	Decreased	Increased

- There is also elimination of acids in the urine and the urinary ammonia is also increased.

For example, $[HCO_3^-] = 15$ mEq/L, $pCO_2 =$ 1.2 mEq/L

$pH = pKa + \log [HCO_3^-]/pCO_2$

6.1 + log15/1.2

6.1 + 12.5

6.1 + 1.2 = 7.3 (Anti log of 12.5 is 1.2)

Metabolic Alkalosis (*HCO_3^- Excess or Rise in pH*)

- This condition occurs due to the gain of more HCO_3^-.
- This occurs in; (a) Vomiting (loss of gastric HCl); (b) Ingestion of bicarbonate in the treatment of peptic ulcer; (c) Potassium depletion: Hypokalemic alkalosis is caused by the kidneys' response to an extreme lack or loss of potassium, which can occur when people take certain diuretic medications.
- The compensatory mechanism is through hypoventilation to prevent CO_2 loss. CO_2 is then consumed toward the formation of the carbonic acid intermediate, thus decreasing pH.
- The secondary compensatory mechanism by increasing the excretion of HCO_3^- by kidney.

For example, $[HCO_3^-] = 36$ mEq/L, $pCO_2 =$ 1.2 mEq/L

$pH = pKa + \log [HCO_3^-]/pCO_2$

6.1 + log 36/1.2 = 6.1 + 30 = 6.1 + 1.45 = 7.55

Respiratory Acid-Base Disorders

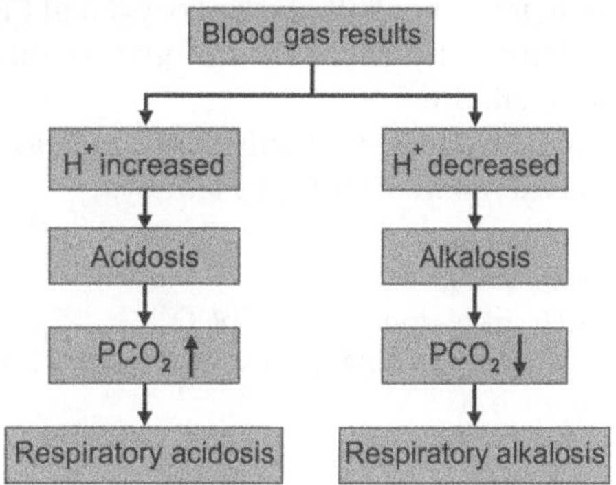

Respiratory Acidosis (Excess CO_2)

- The retention of CO_2 leads to change in HCO_3^-.
- The ratio of $[HCO_3^-]$: $[CO_2]$ decreases.
- This is caused by hypoventilation, which occurs due to an obstruction of respiration that is in pneumonia, emphysema, asthma and depression of the respiratory centers in morphine bicarbonate poisoning and alcohol ingestion.
- The primary compensatory mechanism is reabsorption of HCO_3^- from the kidney.

e.g., $[HCO_3^-] = 27$ mEq/L, $pCO_2 = 1.8$ mEq/L

$pH = pKa + \log [HCO_3^-]/ pCO_2$

6.1 + log 27/1.8 = 6.1+15 = 6.1 + 1.17 = 7.27

Respiratory Alkalosis (CO_2 deficit)

- This is caused by hyperventilation that leads to reduced concentration of CO_2.
- The HCO_3^- level also slightly varies.

Reference list for acid-base disturbances			
Disorders	*pCO_2*	*HCO_3*	*pH*
Respiratory acidosis	> 45 mm Hg	Varied	< 7.3
Respiratory alkalosis	< 35 mm Hg	Varied	> 7.4
Metabolic acidosis	< 22 m mol/L	Varied	< 7.3
Metabolic alkalosis	> 33 m mol/L	Varied	> 7.4

- This occurs when respiration is stimulated as in fever, hot bath, lack of oxygen at high altitude and increased environmental temperature.
- Compensatory mechanism is by increasing the excretion of HCO_3^- by kidney.

  For example, $[HCO_3^-]$ = 27 mEq/L, pCO_2 = 0.68 mEq/

  pH= pKa +log $[HCO_3^-]/pCO_2$

  6.1 + log 27/0.68 = 6.1 + 39.7 = 6.1 + 1.6 = 7.7.

Mixed Acid-Base Disorders

Mixed acid base disorders occur when there is more than one primary acid-base disturbance present simultaneously. They are frequently seen in hospitalized patients, particularly in the critically ill.

Mixed Acid-Base Disorder Occurs When

- The expected compensatory response does not occur.
- Compensatory response occurs, but level of compensation is inadequate or too extreme.
- Whenever the PCO_2 and $[HCO_3^-]$ become abnormal in the opposite direction (i.e. one is elevated while the other is reduced). In simple acid-base disorders, the direction of the compensatory response is always the same as the direction of the initial abnormal change.
- pH is normal but PCO_2 or HCO_3^- is abnormal.
- In anion gap metabolic acidosis, if the change in bicarbonate level is not proportional to the change of the anion gap. More specifically, if the delta ratio is greater than 2 or less than 1.
- In simple acid base disorders, the compensatory response should never return the pH to normal. If that happens, suspect a mixed disorder.

Mixed acid base disorders usually produce arterial blood gas results that could potentially be explained by other mixed disorders. Oftentimes, the clinical picture will help to distinguish. It is important to distinguish mixed acid-base disorders because management will depend on accurate diagnosis.

Chronic Respiratory Acidosis With Superimposed Acute Respiratory Acidosis

- Acute exacerbation of COPD secondary to acute pneumonia
- COPD patient with worsening hypoventilation secondary to oxygen therapy or sedative administration.

Chronic Respiratory Acidosis And Anion Gap Metabolic Acidosis

- COPD patient who develops shock and lactic acidosis.

Chronic respiratory acidosis and metabolic alkalosis

Example:

- Pulmonary insufficiency and diuretic therapy, or
- COPD patient treated with steroids or ventilation (important to recognize as alkalemia will reduce acidemic stimulus to breathe).

Respiratory alkalosis and metabolic acidosis

- Salicylate intoxication
- Gram-negative sepsis
- Acute cardiopulmonary arrest
- Severe pulmonary edema.

ANION GAP

- The sum of cations and anions in extracellular fluid is always equal to maintain the electrical neutrality.
- 95% of the cations were maintained by Na^+ and K^+.
- Chloride and HCO_3^- account for 86% of anions.
- These are the commonly measured electrolytes and hence there is a difference between cations and anions.

- The difference between cations and anions or the unmeasured anions constitutes the anion gap, which is due to the presence of Phosphorous, SO_4^-, PO_4^{3-} and organic acid salts.
- The difference between $Na^+ + K^+$ and $Cl^- + HCO_3^-$ is normally about 12 ± 5 mEq/L (m Mols/L).
- Measurement of anion gap is extremely useful in the clinical assessment with acid-base disorders.

Assessment of Acid-Base Analysis

The blood gas analyzers which measures pH, pCO_2 and pO_2 by means of electrodes is usually used to measure acid-base parameters of arterial blood. Heparinized blood is collected and directly introduced into the analyzer. The blood should be analyzed within 20 minutes of collection. There should not be any contact of collected blood with the external air during either collection or analysis.

Procedure

Usually, blood is taken from an artery. The blood may be collected from the radial artery in the wrist, the femoral artery in the groin, or the brachial artery in the arm.

The healthcare provider will insert a small needle through the skin into the artery. You can choose to have numbing medicine (anesthesia) applied to the site before the test begins.

After the blood is taken, pressure is applied to the site for a few minutes to stop the bleeding. The healthcare provider will watch the site for signs of bleeding or circulation problems.

The sample must be quickly sent to a laboratory for analysis to ensure accurate results.

There is no special preparation. If you are on oxygen therapy, the oxygen concentration must remain constant for 20 minutes before the test.

The test is used to evaluate respiratory diseases and conditions that affect the lungs. It helps determine the effectiveness of oxygen therapy. The test also provides information about the body's acid/base balance, which can reveal important clues about lung and kidney function and the body's general metabolic state.

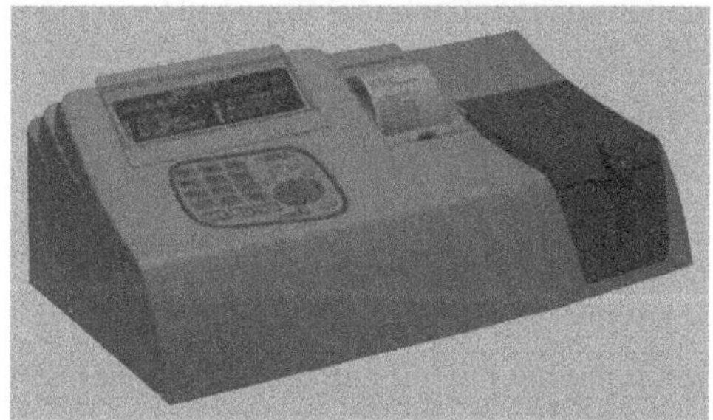

In absence of blood gas analyzer, venous blood may be collected under paraffin. Bicarbonate is estimated by titration to pH 7.4. If acid-base disturbance is suspected, the electrolytes should also be estimated. From the values of electrolytes and bicarbonate, the anion gap is calculated.

SELF TEST

1. Name the blood buffer systems.
2. Write about the role of bicarbonate buffer system in maintaining the acid base balance.
3. How does the renal mechanism help to maintain the acid base balance?
4. State the biochemical findings of metabolic acidosis and respiratory acidosis.
5. What is anion gap?

MULTIPLE CHOICE QUESTIONS

1. **Which one of the following is not a fixed acid?**
   a. Lactic acid
   b. Butyric acid

c. CO_2
d. Acetoacetic acid.

2. The following are the blood buffer systems EXCEPT:
a. Carbonate/bicarbonate
b. Protein
c. Phosphate
d. Acid/alkali.

3. The normal arterial blood pH is:
a. 7.7
b. 7.3
c. 7.4
d. 7.2.

4. The following are the findings of metabolic acidosis EXCEPT:
a. pCO_2 increased
b. HCO_3^- decreased
c. The HCO_3/H_2CO_3 decreased
d. pH decreased.

5. All the following are the biochemical findings of metabolic alkalosis EXCEPT:
a. Increased pH
b. Increased pCO_2
c. Increased HCO_3^-
d. Increased HCO_3^-/H_2CO_3

6. Excess CO_2 is found in:
a. Metabolic acidosis
b. Metabolic alkalosis
c. Respiratory acidosis
d. Respiratory alkalosis.

CASE STUDIES

1. A 23-year-old man was found to be cyanotic, apneic and unresponsive in the orthopedic surgery ward following reconstructive knee surgery. About 30 minutes earlier, he received 25 mg of intravenous (IV) morphine for pain relief. While he is being assessed and resuscitated, an arterial blood gas sample was taken, revealing the following:

pH	7.08
PCO_2	80 mm Hg
HCO_3	23 mEq/L (mmol/L)

i. Which of the following is TRUE?
a. A metabolic acidosis is present
b. This is a clinical picture compatible with acute respiratory acidosis
c. This is a clinical picture compatible with chronic respiratory acidosis
d. The patient is hypocarbic from hypoventilation
e. The patient has a low bicarbonate level.

Answer b

ii. Which of the following is FALSE?
a. A respiratory acidosis is present
b. The arterial PCO_2 is elevated
c. The 25 mg of intravenous morphine for pain relief was an overdose
d. The cyanosis was as a direct result of elevated arterial PCO_2 levels
e. The patient is hypercarbic from respiratory depression.

Answer d

2. A 5-week-old baby boy is admitted to hospital with history of projectile vomiting of several days duration. The following blood gases are obtained:

pH	7.50
PCO_2	49 mm Hg
HCO_3	37 mEq/L (mmol/L)

i. Which of the following is TRUE?
a. The primary disturbance here is an elevated pH
b. The primary disturbance here is an elevated PCO_2
c. The primary disturbance here is an elevated HCO_3
d. The data are not compatible with the Henderson-Hasselbalch equation
e. These are normal laboratory results for a 4-week-old baby.

Answer c

ii. Which of the following is FALSE?
a. The primary disturbance in this case is metabolic, with the HCO_3

being elevated. Since the PCO_2 is raised in the face of an alkalemia, there is not a primary respiratory disturbance —the raised PCO_2 merely indicates that respiratory compensation has occurred

b. The expected PCO_2 in metabolic alkalosis is $0.7 \times HCO_3 + 20$ mm Hg = $[0.7 \times 37] + 20$ = 46 mm Hg. Since the actual PCO_2 (49) and the expected PCO_2 (46) are approximately the same in this case, this suggests that respiratory compensation is appropriate for a setting of metabolic alkalosis

c. The laboratory and clinical information is compatible with the following diagnosis: metabolic alkalosis from persistent vomiting due to pyloric stenosis

d. The loss of gastric bicarbonate is the basis for the metabolic alkalosis in this setting

e. Pyloric stenosis is fixed with an operation called a pyloromyotomy, where the surgeon spreads open the muscle around the pyloric valve.

Answer d

3. Michael is undergoing treatment for frequent panic attacks. The attacks are accompanied by hyperventilation, a racing heartbeat (tachycardia), dizziness, feelings of "unreality" and tingling in the hands. In one particularly severe attack, when taken to the emergency department, an arterial blood-gas sample was taken, which revealed the following:

pH	7.52
PCO_2	26 mm Hg
HCO_3	22 mEq/L (mmol/L)

i. Which of the following is TRUE?

a. The primary disturbance here is an elevated pH

b. The primary disturbance here is a lowered PCO_2

c. The primary disturbance here is a lowered HCO_3

d. The data are not compatible with the Henderson-Hasselbalch equation

e. These are normal laboratory results.

Answer b

ii. Which of the following is TRUE?

a. The data indicate that the respiratory disturbance is acute

b. The data indicate that the respiratory disturbance is chronic

c. The data indicate that hypercarbia is present

d. Treatment with a respiratory depressant agent like morphine would be a clinically sensible means to treat the hyperventilation

e. A clinically sensible means to treat the hyperventilation would be to encase his whole head in a plastic bag so that he rebreathes his expired CO_2.

Answer a

4. A 31-year-old man presents with lethargy, weakness, labored respiration, and confusion. He has had diabetes for 15 years, and has been suffering from the "intestinal flu" for a day or so, for which he has been avoiding food to help prevent further vomiting and "make his stomach ache go away". Since he stopped eating, he thought that it would be a good idea to stop taking his insulin. When seen in the emergency department his urine dipped positive for both glucose and ketones and his breath had a strange sweet, fruity smell. The following arterial blood gas data was obtained:

pH	7.27
PCO_2	23 mm Hg
Sodium	132 mEq/L
Chloride	83 mEq/L

Potassium	4.9 mEq/L
HCO_3	10 mEq/L
Glucose	345 mg/dL

i. Which of the following is TRUE?
   a. The data indicate that hypercarbia is present
   b. The data indicate that hypoglycemia is present
   c. The data indicate that an alkalemia is present
   d. The anion gap is 19 mEq/L
   e. An elevated anion gap type metabolic acidosis is present.

   Answer e

ii. Which of the following is TRUE?
   a. The primary disturbance here is a lowered PCO_2
   b. The primary disturbance here is a lowered pH
   c. The potassium level is dangerously elevated
   d. The labored respiration, with increased depth and rate of breathing, occurs because the patient is hyperventilating to lower the PCO_2. This is known as "Kussmaul breathing", after Adolph Kussmaul, the 19th century German doctor who first noted it
   e. The fact that glucose was present in the urine is initiative of renal gluconeogenesis.

   Answer d

5. A 39-year-old woman had severe chronic back pain, which she treated aggressively with a variety of over the counter (OTC) nonsteroidal anti-inflammatory drugs (NSAIDs) for a number of years. At a routine clinical visit her blood pressure is found to be elevated at 155/95. Her urine dips 2+ positive for protein, and microscopic examination of her urine reveals 4-5 white blood cells per high-power field (4-5 WBC/hpf) with a specific gravity of 1.01 and a pH of 5.0. An arterial blood gas sample is as follows:

pH	7.31
PCO_2	33 mm Hg
HCO_3	15 mEq/L
Sodium	139 mEq/L
Potassium	5.3 mEq/L
Chloride	110 mEq/L

i. Which of the following is TRUE?
   a. The primary disturbance here is a lowered HCO_3
   b. The primary disturbance here is a lowered PCO_2
   c. The potassium level is dangerously elevated
   d. The anion gap is elevated
   e. An elevated anion gap metabolic acidosis is present.

   Answer a

ii. Which of the following is FALSE?
   a. The kidneys have been damaged, as evidenced by proteinuria and the fact that they are unable to secrete a normal hydrogen ion load
   b. This is likely a case of analgesic nephropathy resulting from chronic NSAID use
   c. This is a case of metabolic acidosis with normal (appropriate) respiratory compensation
   d. The renal toxicity of NSAIDs results from the blocking of prostaglandin formation, which can impair glomerular filtration
   e. Renal transplantation is indicated in this case

   Answer e

14

UNIT

Diagnostic Enzymes

LEARNING OBJECTIVES

At the end of this unit, the learner should be able to understand:
- The enzymes with its classification.
- About the functional and nonfunctional enzymes.
- The factors affecting the enzyme activity.
- The diagnostic significance of enzyme determination.

INTRODUCTION

- Enzymes are biological catalysts produced by the living cells and they catalyze several reactions in the body.
- They are protein in nature.
- They are specific in action, i.e., each enzyme can catalyze only one type of reaction.
- They are required in very small quantities.
- The loss of catalytic activity is observed when they are subjected to heat or strong acids or bases or organic solvents.
- The metabolic pathways in the human body are mainly catalyzed by enzymes.
- Enzyme deficiency leads to inborn errors of metabolism.
- Most of the enzymes are produced by the cells of a particular tissue and function within that cell. Such enzymes are called **intracellular enzymes.**
  Examples: Enzymes of glycolysis, TCA cycle and fatty acid synthesis.
- On the other hand, there are certain enzymes, which are produced by the cells of a particular tissue from where these are liberated for use in the other tissues. Such enzymes are called as **extracellular enzymes.**
  Example: Various proteolytic enzymes of the gastrointestinal tract (Trypsin, chymotrypsin).
  - The enzyme binds with its specific substrate and forms an enzyme-substrate complex. At the end of the reaction, the substrate is converted into the product and the enzyme remains unchanged.

E + S ⟶ ES ⟶ E + P

CHEMICAL NATURE OF ENZYMES

- Almost all enzymes are **proteins by nature.**
- Enzymes with two or more subunits (polypeptides) are called as **oligomeric enzymes.**
- Several enzymes occur in the form of the **multienzyme complex.**

For example, pyruvate dehydrogenase, fatty acid synthase complex.

- Some enzymes require the presence of certain additional organic or inorganic substances and are conjugated proteins. Such enzymes are called as **holoenzymes.** The protein part of the conjugated protein is called the **apoenzyme.** The nonprotein part is called the **prosthetic group.**
  Apoenzyme + Prosthetic group [coenzyme] →*Holoenzyme*

Coenzymes

These are dialyzable, thermostable, low molecular weight organic substances, which may be regarded as a cosubstrate or second substrate, required the reaction to complete.

For example, the thiamine pyrophosphate (vitamin B_6) derivative is required for the action of the pyruvate dehydrogenase enzyme.

NAD^+ is required for the activity of lactate dehydrogenase.

Metalloenzymes

Several apoenzymes require the presence of metal ions such as Mg^{2+} (for Hexokinase), Zn^{2+} (for the activity of carboxy peptidase). Such inorganic ions are called as **cofactors.** If the metal ion is the integral part of the enzyme, such enzymes are called as *metalloenzymes.*

Zymogens or Proenzymes

The protein digesting enzymes (proteolytic enzymes) of a gastrointestinal tract are produced in the form of a precursor. This is to prevent unwanted degradation of body self-protein. These precursor forms of enzymes (zymogen) are converted into active forms by HCl and trypsin.

For example, Pepsinogen → pepsin (HCl activates the pepsinogen).

Trypsinogen to trypsin (trypsin and enteropeptidase activate the enzymes)

Procarboxypeptidase,
Chymotrypsinogen

Classification of Enzymes

Based on the chemical reactions they catalyze, enzymes are classified into six classes:

1. *Oxidoreductases:* Catalyze the oxidation-reduction reactions
   For example, lactate dehydrogenase.
2. *Transferases:* Catalyze the transfer of groups from one substrate another
   For example, aspartate aminotransferase.
3. *Hydrolases:* Catalyze the breakdown of compounds by utilizing a molecule of water
   For example, glucose 6-phosphatase and trypsin.
4. *Lyases:* Catalyze removal of a group from a substrate without using a molecule of water
   For example, fumarase.
5. *Isomerases:* Catalyze the isomerization of substrates
   For example, epimerase.
6. *Ligases:* Which catalyze the reactions, which involve joining together of two substrates
   For example, DNA ligases.

Functional Enzymes of Plasma

Certain enzymes are normally present in the plasma and they have specific functions to perform. These enzymes are called *functional enzymes of plasma.* Generally, these enzyme activities are higher in plasma than in tissues. Mostly they are synthesized in liver and enter the circulation.

For example, Lipoprotein lipase, ceruloplasmin, clotting factors, etc.

Nonfunctional Enzymes of Plasma

Certain enzymes are present in very small quantities or even absent in plasma compared to their level found in some tissues. These enzymes do not have any function in plasma. These are called *non-functional enzymes of plasma.* These enzymes are commonly abbreviated with three letters.

For example, aspartate transaminase is called AST.

Alkaline phosphatase is called as ALP.

Creatine phosphokinase is called CPK.

These come out from the cells due to normal wear and tear of the cells. The normal serum level of these enzymes indicates the balance between its synthesis and release in the routine cell turnover. The increased enzyme levels in serum may be mainly due to cellular damage of the particular tissue in which the enzyme is present. So these enzymes can be used as markers for measuring the cellular damage of a particular tissue. So disease of the tissue can be diagnosed using these enzyme levels in serum.

For example, increased alanine amino transferase (ALT) generally indicates liver disease.

Enzyme Units

One international unit (one IU) is the amount of enzyme that will convert one micromole of the substrate per minute per liter of the sample and is abbreviated as U/L. The earlier unit is katal (SI unit). It is defined as number of moles of substrate transformed per second per liter of the sample. Katal is abbreviated as kat or k. 1 mkat = 60 U.

Isoenzymes

Different forms of the same enzyme catalyzing the same reaction are called isoenzymes or isozymes. Isoenzymes are differ in their physical and chemical properties, which include structure, electrophoretic mobility, etc.

For example, lactate dehydrogenase has 5 isoenzymes while gamma glutamyl-transpeptidase has 11 isoenzymes.

Factors Affecting the Enzyme Activity

1. pH
2. Temperature
3. Concentration of substrate
4. Concentration of enzyme.

Effect of pH (Fig. 14.1A)

Each enzyme has an optimum pH, at which the activity of the enzyme is maximum.

The decrease or increase in pH causes a decrease in enzyme activity.

For example:

1. Pepsin has an optimum pH of 1–2
2. Optimum pH for amylase is 6.8
3. Optimum pH for ALP is 9.0
4. Optimum pH for ACP is 5.0.

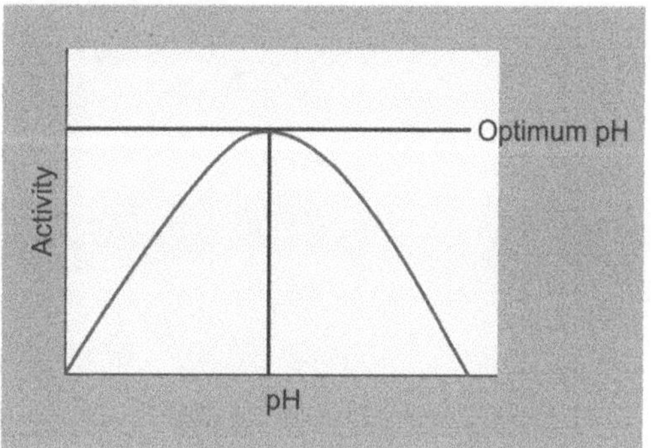

Fig. 14.1A: Effect of pH.

Effect of Temperature (Fig. 14.1B)

The temperature at which the enzyme activity is greatest is called optimum temperature. Any drastic change in the optimum temperature results in the loss of enzyme activity. Optimum temperature of enzymes in the human body is 37°C.

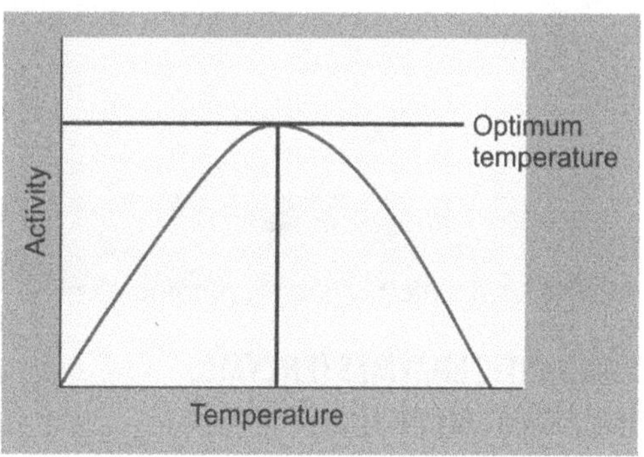

Fig. 14.1B: Effect of temperature.

Effect of Substrate Concentration

At low substrate concentrations enzyme molecules are free initially and the ES complex (ES = enzyme-substrate) formation is proportional to the substrate concentration **(Fig. 14.1C)**. At higher concentrations all the enzyme molecules are saturated with substrate. There is no change in the activity. Hence, in an enzyme reaction system more substrate is taken than required.

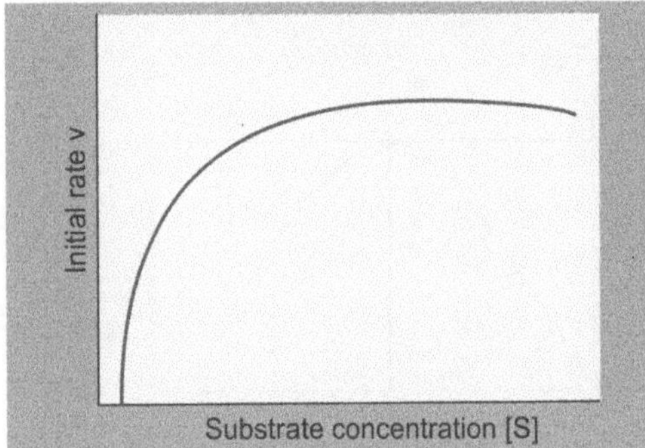

Fig. 14.1C: Effect of substrate concentration.

Effect of Enzyme Concentration

The velocity of the enzyme reaction is directly proportional to the enzyme concentration **(Fig. 14.1D)**.

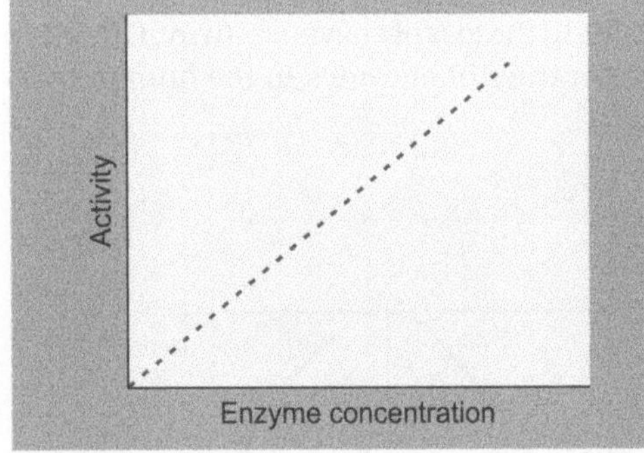

Fig. 14.1D: Effect of enzyme concentration.

DIAGNOSTIC ENZYMES (ENZYMES IN CLINICAL MEDICINE)

Enzymes are produced by the cells and they remain within the cells. Very small amounts of the enzymes are released into the bloodstream, due to the normal breakdown of the cells. Hence, the enzymes are present even in the blood in very small amounts under normal conditions. The levels of these enzymes are greatly increased in blood under certain disease conditions, which leads to breakdown of cells. Estimation of these enzyme levels in blood or plasma is useful in the diagnosis of disease and these indicate from which organ they are released.

Depending on this, it is easy to find out the organ, which is affected.

The diagnostic enzymes are grouped according to the organ they belong.

Important groups are as follows:

1. Liver enzymes (AST, ALT, ALP and GGT)
2. Cardiac enzymes (LDH, LDL, CK, CKMB, AST)
3. Muscle enzymes (CK, LDH, AST)
4. Pancreatic enzymes (Amylase, Lipase)
5. Bone enzymes (ALP and ACP)

Important enzymes to remember:

1. AST (Aspartate transaminase)
2. ALT (Alanine transaminase)
3. LDH (Lactate dehydrogenase)
4. CK (Creatine kinase)
5. ALP (Alkaline phosphatase)
6. ACP (Acid phosphatase)
7. GGT (Gamma glutamyltransferase)
8. Amylase
9. Lipase
10. Cholinesterase
11. Glucose-6 (P) DH.

Transaminases

1. Serum glutamate oxaloacetate transaminase or AST
2. Serum glutamate pyruvate transaminase or ALT.

The AST and ALT belong to the group of enzymes known as transaminases or aminotransferases. They catalyze the transamination reaction, which is very important in amino acid metabolism.

Aspartate Transaminase

The AST transfers the amino group from aspartate to α-ketoglutarate. As a result, aspartate is converted to oxaloacetate and α-ketoglutarate (α-KG) is converted to glutamate. This is a reversible reaction, it requires a coenzyme PLP (pyridoxal phosphate).

$$\text{L-aspartate} + \alpha\text{-ketoglutarate} \xrightleftharpoons[\text{PLP}]{\text{AST}} \text{Oxaloacetate} + \text{L-glutamate}$$

Sources of AST

- Heart
- Liver
- Skeletal muscle
- *RBCs:* This enzyme is specific for the heart.

AST increases in:

1. *Heart muscle diseases:* Myocardial infarction
2. *Liver disease*: Mainly viral hepatitis jaundice and cirrhosis of the liver
3. *Muscle diseases*: Muscular dystrophy.
   - In viral hepatitis, the serum level of AST increases 20–30 times more than the normal level.
   - In cirrhosis, a mild increase in its level seen.
   - The AST level increases 2–3 times more than normal in heart muscle diseases. Therefore, it is one of the enzymes included in the cardiac enzyme panel.

Alanine Transaminase

This enzyme catalyzes the transfer of the amino group from alanine to α-KG.

As a result, alanine is converted to pyruvate and α-KG is converted to glutamate.

$$\text{L-alanine} + \alpha\text{-ketoglutarate} \xrightleftharpoons[\text{PLP}]{\text{ALT}} \text{Pyruvate} + \text{L-glutamate}$$

Sources of ALT

- Liver is the major source
- The ALT level increases in all types of liver diseases, such as:
  - Viral hepatitis
  - Cirrhosis
  - Liver cancer
  - Drug induced jaundice
- In liver diseases, serum level of both AST and ALT elevated.
- ALT is specific for liver because it is present only in the liver and increased during liver disease.

Determination of Serum Transaminases

The methods available are:

a. Kinetic method
b. DNP method
c. Method of Reitman and Frankel
d. Sax and Moor method using disodium salt
e. Continuous monitoring method.

Kinetic Method

AST

$$\text{L-aspartate} + \alpha\text{-ketoglutarate} \xrightleftharpoons{\text{AST}} \text{Oxaloacetate} + \text{glutamate}$$

$$\text{Oxaloacetate} + \text{NADH}^+ \xrightleftharpoons{\text{Malate dehydrogenase}} \text{Malate} + \text{NAD}^+$$

- In the above reaction, the oxaloacetate produced is converted to malate with the help of malate dehydrogenase and NADH produced is converted to NAD^+ in the 2nd reaction.
- The NADH has the maximum absorbance at 340 nm and NAD^+ has less absorbance at 340 nm.
- So when the reaction continues the NADH is converted to NAD^+ and causing a decrease in the absorbance.
- The readings are measured for about 3 minutes and change in the absorbance per minute is calculated.
- The activity of the enzyme is calculated and is expressed as U/L.

ALT

$$\text{L-alanine} + \alpha\text{-ketoglutarate} \xleftrightarrow{\text{ALT}} \text{Pyruvate} + \text{Glutamate}$$

$$\text{Pyruvate} + \text{NADH} \xleftrightarrow{\text{Lactate dehydrogenase}} \text{Lactate} + \text{NAD}^+$$

- The pyruvate produced in the 1st reaction is converted to lactate in the presence of lactate dehydrogenase and NADH is converted to NAD^+ and the decrease in the absorbance is measured at 340 nm.
- The readings are measured for about 3 minutes and change in the absorbance per minute is calculated.
- The activity of the enzyme is calculated using Δ^A/minute. It is expressed as U/L.

Normal Value in Serum or Plasma

AST: 5–40 U/L
ALT: 5–40 U/L.
Use of hemolyzed samples is not recommended because the RBC, once broken, releases the AST to the medium.

Colorimetric Method
Using 2, 4 Dinitrophenylhydrazine

Serum Aspartate Transaminase

Principle

AST (or SGOT) is measured by oxaloacetate formed in the reaction.

$$\alpha\text{-KG} + \text{L-aspartate} \xleftrightarrow{\text{AST}} \text{L-glutamate} + \text{Oxaloacetate}$$

- Oxaloacetate produced in the above reaction is unstable and gradually converted to pyruvate with loss of CO_2.
- The pyruvate formed is measured colorimetrically at 520 nm and its hydrazone derivative after reaction with 2, 4 dinitrophenylhydrazine.

Serum Alanine Transaminase

- The activity of this enzyme is measured with the pyruvate formed in the reaction.

$$\alpha\text{-KG} + \text{L-alanine} \xleftrightarrow{\text{ALT}} \text{L-glutamate} + \text{Pyruvate}$$

- Pyruvate formed is measured colorimetrically at 520 nm as the hydrazone derivative after reaction with 2, 4, DNP hydrazine.

Reagents

1. *Buffer substrate* (100 mM/L).
2. *Phosphate buffer* 100 mM/L, 2 oxoglutarate 2 mM/L
3. *L-aspartate* 100 mM/L.
4. 1.7 g of Na_2HPO_4 (15 g of K_2HPO_4 and 2 g of KH_2PO_4) and 2.30 g of NaH_2PO_4 and 300 mg of 2-oxoglutarate dissolved in about 700–800 mL of water. Divide this buffer into two equal parts and add aspartate to one part and alanine to another part:
   a. For AST—6.65 g of L-aspartate is added.
   b. For ALT—8.901 g of L-alanine is added. Adjust the pH to 7.4 with 1 N NaOH and make up to 500 mL with water.
5. 2, 4 DNPH [1 mmol (200 mg)/lit] in 1 N HCl: 200 mg of 2, 4, DNPH dissolved in 1 N HCl and volume is made up to 1 liter with 1N HCl.
6. *NaOH 0.4 M/L:* 16 g NaOH dissolved in 1 liter of distilled water.
7. *Pyruvate 2 mM/L:* Sodium pyruvate, 22 mg in 100 mL of distilled water.

Procedure

a. *AST*: Buffer aspartate solution 1.1 mL is taken in two test, tubes control and test respectively. To the test 0.1 mL of serum is added and both the tubes are incubated at 37°C for 60 minutes. Sodium pyruvate 0.1–0.5 mL of solutions are added to different test tubes as standards (conc. ranging from 0.2–1 μmol). The volume of all the tubes are made up to 1.2 mL with buffer substrate solution. Buffer aspartate of 1.2 mL is taken as blank.

After incubation of the control and test at 37°C, add 1 mL of color reagent 2, 4 DNPH to all the tubes including standard and blank. Add 0.1 mL serum to control. Mix and keep tubes at room temperature for

Contents	B	S_1	S_2	S_3	S_4	S_5	C	T
Buffer	–	–	–	–	–	–	1.1	1.1
Preincubate at room temperature for 5 minutes								
Serum	–	–	–	–	–	–	–	0.1
Incubate for 30 minutes at 37°C								
Pyruvate	–	0.1	0.2	0.3	0.4	0.5	–	–
Concentration (μmol/ tube)	–	0.2	0.4	0.6	0.8	1.0	–	–
Buffer	1.2	1.1	1.0	0.9	0.8	0.7	–	–
Color reagent	1.0	1.0	1.0	1.0	1.0	1.0	1.0	1.0
Serum (mL)	–	–	–	–	–	–	0.1	–
Keep at room temperature for 20 minutes								
0.4N NaOH<—— 10 mL ——>								
Keep at room temperature for 5 minutes								
OD at 520 nm								
(ALT) Adjusted to 0	0	0.08	0.16	0.24	0.32	0.38	0.09	0.33
(AST) Adjusted to 0	0	0.08	0.16	0.24	0.32	0.36	0.09	0.40

20 minutes. Then add 10 mL of 0.4 N NaOH solutions to all the test tubes. The tubes are kept at room temperature for 5 minutes after proper mixing. The color development is read at 520 nm using a spectrophotometer.

b. *ALT:* The procedure is same as that for AST except the incubation time that is 30 minutes and alanine buffer is added to the tubes instead of aspartate buffer.

Calculation

ALT

C - T = 0.09–0.33 = 0.24

0.24 OD corresponds to 0.6 μmoLs.

∴ 0.1 mL of serum liberates 0.6 μmoL

$$1 \text{ mL of serum liberates} = \frac{0.6 \times 1}{0.1} = 6.0 \ \mu\text{moL}$$

∴ 1000 mL of serum liberates 6 × 1000 = 6000

So in 30 min, 6000 μmol of pyruvate is released from one liter solution.

$$\text{Therefore, in 1 min} = \frac{6000}{30} = 200 \text{ U/L}$$

AST

C - T = 0.09–0.40 = 0.31

0.31 corresponds to 0.78 μmols

∴ 0.1 mL of serum liberates 0.78 μmol

$$1 \text{ mL of serum liberates} = \frac{0.78 \times 1}{0.1} = 7.8 \ \mu\text{moL}$$

∴ 1000 mL of serum liberates = 7.8 × 1000 = 7800

So in 1 hour, 7800 μmoL of pyruvate is released from one liter.

$$\text{Therefore, in 1 min} = \frac{7800}{60} = 130 \text{ units/liter}$$

Lactate Dehydrogenase (LDH)

- LDH is present in almost all the tissues of the body.
- There are different forms of LDH, which are known as isoenzymes
- LDH is one of the best examples for isoenzymes.
- *Isoenzymes* are defined as *different forms* of *a single enzyme* and *exist in the same species*

which *have same catalytic activity* but *differ structurally, physically and chemically.*

- LDH has *five different forms.* Each consists of four subunits (polypeptide chains) in the following combinations:

Isoenzyme	*Subunits*	*Source*
LD_1	HHHH	Heart, RBC
LD_2	HHHM	RBC, heart
LD_3	HHMM	Liver, lungs, and spleen
LD_4	HMMM	Liver, lungs, and spleen
LD_5	MMMM	Skeletal muscle

- Since LDH is present in almost all the tissues, its increase in the serum is nonspecific.
- LDH level mainly increases in the following condition:
  - Myocardial infarction (LD_1 and LD_2 increased)
  - Skeletal muscle diseases (LD_5 increased)
  - Liver diseases (LD_3 and LD_4 increased)
  - Cancer of lung, liver and many other organ diseases (LD_3 and LD_4 increased)

Note: Hemolyzed serum samples should not be used because it affects the LDH level (it will be high, due to the release of LD_1 and LD_2 from the RBC).

Separation of LDH Isoenzymes in Serum

Electrophoresis

Serum LDH is separated into five distinct bands which represent five isoenzymes of LDH.

LDH_1 moves fast towards anode (+).

The LDH_5 is the slowest moving compared to other forms.

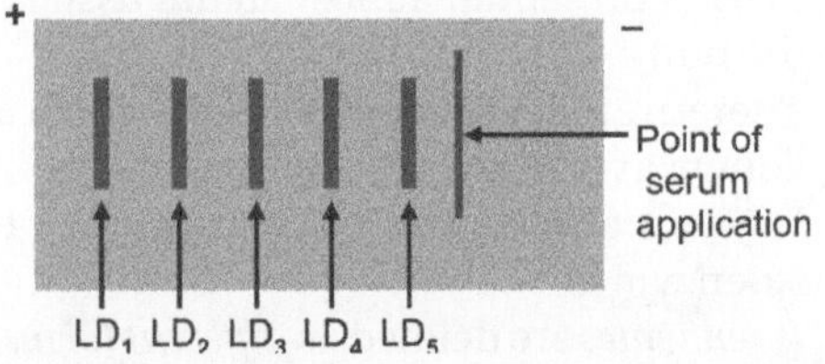

Chemical Method

- Various chemical compounds are found to inhibit the isoenzymes LD_2, LD_3, LD_4, and LD_5.
- LD_1 alone is stable to these compounds.
- When the serum sample is treated with any such compounds, the isoenzymes LD_2 to LD_5 are destroyed (except LD_1). The remaining LDH activity in the serum, which is due to LDH_1 only, is estimated.
- Urea solution at very high concentration is used for this purpose.

Selective Substrate Method

- In this method, L-ketobutyrate is used as a substrate, which is acted upon by LD_1 and LD_2 only.
- This method is used to estimate the level of LDH_1 in the serum.
- The test is also known as the L-hydroxybutyrate dehydrogenase reaction.

$$\text{L-ketobutyrate} + \text{NADH} \xleftrightarrow{\text{LHBDH}} \text{L-hydroxybutyrate} + \text{NAD}^+$$

Determination of Lactate Dehydrogenase in Serum

Methods available

1. *Spectrophotometric method:*
   a. Method of Wroblewski and LaDue (1955)
   b. Method of McQueen (1972)
   c. Method of Mactiners.
2. *Colorimetric methods:*
   a. Method of Amador et al. (1963)
   b. Method of Kind using dinitrophenylhydrazine with lactate
   c. Method using INT and PMS with lactate as substrate.

Wroblewski and LaDue Method

Principle

The pyruvate is converted to lactate in the presence of LDH.

During the reaction, the NADH is converted to NAD^+ and the decrease in the absorbance of NADH is measured at 340 nm. This is used to calculate the LDH activity.

$$\text{Pyruvate} + \text{NADH}^{+} + \text{H} \xleftrightarrow{\text{LDH}} \text{Lactate} + \text{NAD}^{+}$$

The optimum pH with pyruvate as substrate is 6.8–7.5, but with lactate, the pH is appreciably higher and is 9.0–10.0. Optimum pH also varies with different isoenzymes. The equilibrium is such that the forward reaction above is more than twice as fast as the backward reaction.

In this method, pyruvate is used as the substrate.

Lactate has the advantage of being more stable than pyruvate and NAD^+ is cheaper than NADH. NADH has a absorbance peak at 340 nm but NAD^+ has less absorption. Hence, with pyruvate as substrate, the progress of accompanying oxidation of NADH substrate to NAD^+ is monitored continuously by measuring the rate of decrease in absorbance at 340 nm in a spectrophotometer.

Reagents

1. *Phosphate buffer pH* 7.4, 100 mmoL/lit (13.97 g of K_2HPO_4 + 2.69 g of KH_2PO_4 in liter) or K_2HPO_4 0.698 g and KH_2PO_4-0.134 g in 50 mL.
2. *Reduced nicotinamide adenine dinucleotide* 2.5 mg of NADH is mixed in 1 mL of phosphate buffer. It is prepared fresh. It can also be kept frozen for a few days.
3. *Sodium pyruvate* 2.5 mg/mL of buffer. It can be kept in a refrigerator for a few days or a few weeks frozen.

Specimen

Serum or plasma (heparinized) is used. However, serum or plasma should be separated from the clot as soon as possible.

Plasma containing other anticoagulants should not be used.

Hemolyzed plasma or serum must not be used, since erythrocyte contains 100–150 times as much LDH as the serum.

Specimen can be stored at room temperature at which no loss of activity takes place for 2–3 days. If the specimen has to be stored for longer time it should be kept at 4°C with NAD^+ (10 mg/mL) or glutathione (3.1 mg/mL). (It is added to decrease the rate of isoenzyme LDH_4 and LDH_5).

Procedure

About 2.4 mL of phosphate buffer, 0.1 mL serum, and 0.1 mL NADH solution is taken in a test tube and allowed to stand for 20 minutes at 25°C for any ketoacids in the serum to be reduced. 0.1 mL of sodium pyruvate solution is added to the above solution, mixed and the absorbance is noted in spectrophotometer (cuvette with 1 cm light path). The rate of change of extinction at 340 nm and at 25°C is monitored at 60 second intervals for 4 minutes.

Sl. No.		Absorbance
0	-	0.650
60	-	0.600
120	-	0.560
180	-	0.540
240	-	0.52

Serum LDH activity (U/L)

$$= \frac{\Delta \text{E } 340/\text{min} \times 1000 \times \text{Vol in cuvette (mL)}}{\text{Volume of serum} \times 6.3}$$

Δ E = is the mean difference between 3 successive values

6.3 = molar absorption of NADH

Calculation

If Δ E = 0.03/min

Serum lactate dehydrogenase activity

$$= \frac{0.03 \times 1000 \times 2.7}{0.1 \times 6.3}$$

$$= \frac{30 \times 2.7}{0.63} = \frac{81}{0.63} = 128.51 \text{ U/L}$$

Normal values in serum: 60–200 U/L.

Creatine Kinase (CK) (Creatine Phosphokinase) (CPK)

- Creatine kinase catalyzes the reaction in the body as shown below:

$$\text{Creatine} \xleftrightarrow{\text{CK}} \text{Creatine phosphate}$$
ATP ADP

- Creatine (P) is a high-energy compound and acts as a ready source of energy in the muscles.
- CK has 3 isoenzyme forms, each having 2 subunits.

Isoenzyme	*Subunits*	*Source*
CK_1 (CKBB)	BB	Brain
CK_2 (CKMB)	MB	Heart muscle
CK_3 (CKMM)	MM	Heart and skeletal muscle

- Liver and RBC do not contain CK
- Creatine kinase increases in:
  - Muscular dystrophy
  - Injuries of the skeletal muscle. It is the CKMM form which increases due to destruction of the muscle cells
  - Myocardial infarction and other heart diseases (the isoenzyme CKMB will increase markedly)
  - Creatine kinase increases also in head injury and diseases of the brain. It is the CKBB form of CK that is increased.

Methods for the Estimation of CK

Kinetic Method

Principle

The reaction catalyzed by creatine kinase is coupled to hexokinase and glucose-6-phosphate-dehydrogenase (G-6-P-D) reaction. The NADPH formed in the reaction is measured at 340 nm.

1. $\text{Creatine (P)} + \text{ADP} \xleftrightarrow{\text{CK}} \text{Creatine} + \text{ATP}$
2. $\text{ATP} + \text{Glucose} \xleftrightarrow{\text{Hexokinase}} \text{Glucose 6 (P)} + \text{ADP}$
   G-6-PDH
3. $\text{Glucose 6 (P)} + \text{NADP} \longrightarrow$ 6-phosphoglucono-lactone + NADPH

Methods for the Separation of CK Isoenzymes

1. *Electrophoresis:* On electrophoresis CK_1 moves fastest, CK_3 is the slowest.

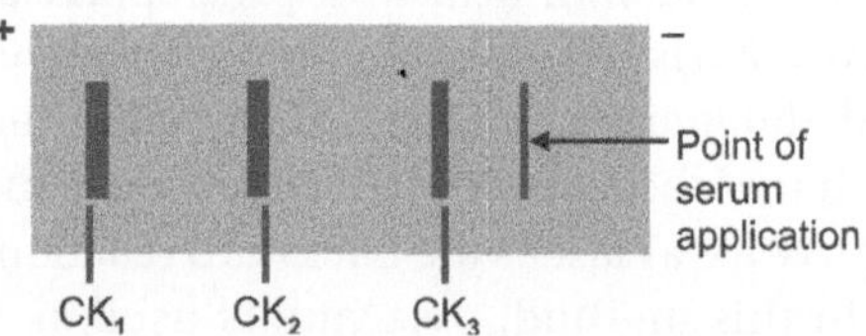

2. *Ion exchange chromatography:* Ion exchange chromatography is used to separate and analyze the different forms of CK but this method is laborious compared to other methods available.
3. *Immunological method:* In this method, antibody (Ab) to "M" subunits of CK are used. This Ab binds with "M" subunits and makes it inactive. The remaining activity is due to B subunits of CK and it is taken as CKMB activity. This method is used for the estimation of CKMB.

Cardiac Enzymes in Myocardial Infarction

The enzymes, such as CKMB, LDH, LDH_1 and AST are included under the cardiac enzyme panel. The estimation of above enzymes may help in the diagnosis, assessment and prognosis of the heart disease.

The increase or decrease in the levels of cardiac enzymes follows a particular pattern in myocardial infraction (MI). It is as follows:

CK and CKMB

Following myocardial infarction, the 1st enzyme to increase is CKMB. Immediately after the heart attack the CKMB level in serum, starts increasing. It goes on increasing and reaches a maximum level by the end of the 1st day. After reaching the peak level CKMB decreases and reaches the normal level by 3rd day. Total CK also follows the same pattern. Normally, CKMB is about 6% of the total CK value. In MI, CKMB may go up to 10–30% of total CK.

AST

The AST level in plasma increases after 6–8 hours of chest pain and it reaches the peak value by 2nd day, but comes to normal by the 4th or 5th day.

LDH1 and LDH

Total LDH and LDH_1 begin to increase 8 to 12 hours after the chest pain. They go on increasing and reach the maximum value by the 3rd day and slowly come to normal by about the 7th day.

The level of these enzymes in serum is related to the severe damage to heart muscle. Therefore, in severe MI the level of these enzymes are more.

The CKMB and LD_1 are the most sensitive and specific markers for the diagnosis of MI.

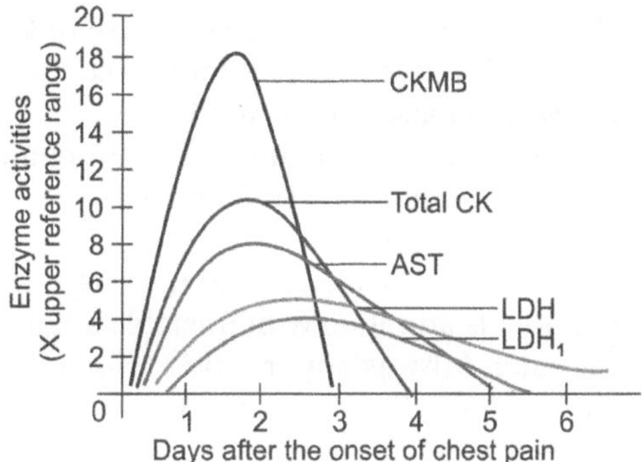

Pattern of change in serum enzyme activities following an uncomplicated myocardial infarction

Clinical Importance of Troponin and Myoglobin Estimation

Troponin

- There is a developing global epidemic of cardiovascular disease.
- Troponins and myoglobin have been investigated as markers of acute cardiac ischemia.
- Troponins are protein components of striated muscle.
- Troponin-T is the myofibrillar protein of the striated muscle, which is the building block of the contractile apparatus.
- Troponin is a protein complex consisting of 3 subunits with different structure and function, namely:
  1. Troponin T (TnT): Tropomyosin binding element
  2. Troponin I (TnI): Actinomycin ATPase inhibitory element.
  3. Troponin C (TnC): Calcium binding.

Troponin-T

It is normally measured because a small pool of it is not compartmentalized in the contractile apparatus and may be a precursor for synthesis of the troponin complex.

- The troponin fractions from different sources, such as skeletal and heart muscle are genetically and structurally different.
- The heart specific Troponin-T can be measured in the plasma by differential immunological method (ELISA or RIA) and provides a more specific tool for the diagnosis of myocardial infarction.
- It is released into the blood within about 4 hours after the onset of symptoms, peaks at 12–16 hours and remains, elevated for 5-9 days post-infarction.
- Therefore, cardiac troponin (CTT) is very useful as a marker at any time interval after the heart attack, which is its great advantage.
- A level > 1.5 μg/L is indicative of myocardial damage.
- Troponin-T is the specific and sensitive test for the diagnosis of myocardial infarction as compared to CPK and LDH enzymes.
- Troponin-T is a very useful indicator of myocardial ischemia in these cases.
- Cardiac troponin-T exhibits serum concentration changes depending upon the reperfusion of the infarct.
- Successful recanalization shows high serum peak levels on the first day whereas persistent release of Troponin-T detectable up to 10 days shows protracted release from infarcted area indicating irreversible myocardial necrosis.

- On the 4th day after onset of pain, a second peak of troponin-T occurs.
- The 14–32 hours ratio of troponin-T is a reliable indicator of the success of thrombolysis therapy and recanalization.
- A ratio of > 1 is a reliable indicator of early recanalization.
- Thus, this test is a noninvasive biochemical angiography.

Indications of Troponin-T

1. Acute myocardial infarction
2. Subacute myocardial infarction
3. Microinfarction
4. Size of infarction
5. Monitoring the outcome of thrombolysis therapy.

Advantages of Troponin-T

- Highly sensitive for detecting myocardial ischemia
- Levels may help to stratify risk afterward
- The 14/32 hour ratio of troponin is a reliable indicator of success and thrombolysis.

Disadvantages of Troponin-T

- Less specific than troponin I
- Increase in unstable angina
- Increase in chronic renal failure.

Troponin I elevation is useful for predicting in-hospital risk for unstable angina patients admitted to a community hospital.

The association of ECG changes and high troponin I identifies a population at very high-risk; however, the absence of both variables in patients with a diagnosis of unstable angina does not preclude the development of events.

Advantages of Troponin-I

- More specific than troponin T
- Is not increased in chronic renal failure.

Interpretation

- A level >1.2 suggests myocardial infarction
- Negative values predict low likelihood of coronary event—obtain two negative troponin values 4 hours apart
- Troponin T (cTnT) and troponin I (cTnI) are released only following cardiac damage
- CK and CKMB are found in skeletal muscle as well as cardiac muscle—therefore if there is damage to skeletal muscle; elevations of CK and CKMB will occur and can make the diagnosis of myocardial infarction difficult. In such a situation, levels of cTnT or cTnI will not rise unless myocardial infarction has occurred
- Troponin T and I are present for remain elevated for a long time
- cTnI is detectable in the blood for up to 5 days and cTnT for 7–10 days following MI. This allows an MI to be detected if the patient presents late. For example, if a patient comes to the surgery with a history of chest pain 2–3 days ago, measurement of cTnT or cTnI will allow the diagnosis or exclusion of MI as a cause of the chest pain.

Troponin T and I are Very Sensitive

- There is always a low level release of CK and CK-MB from skeletal muscle so there is always a background value.
- This is not the case for the cardiac structural proteins, such as cTnT and cTnI, and therefore, they are very sensitive.
- Studies have revealed that about one-third of patients admitted with unstable angina, in which MI was apparently excluded by CK and CK-MB measurement, have raised levels of cTnT and cTnI.
- Follow-up studies have revealed that these patients are at significantly greater risk of death, subsequent MI or readmission with unstable angina than patients who did not have detectable levels of cTnT or cTnI.

General Disadvantages

- Elevation of cTnT or TnI is indicative of cardiac damage, but this can occur because of causes other than MI, e.g., myocarditis, coronary artery spasm from cocaine, severe cardiac failure, cardiac trauma from surgery or a road traffic accident, and a pulmonary embolus can cause cardiac damage with an accompanying elevation of cardiac troponin(s).
- Both cTnT and cTnI may be elevated in patients with chronic renal failure and

indicate a higher long-term risk of death. They can be distinguished from changes due to myocardial infarction by repeating the tests. Myocardial infarction causes a rise and fall in cTnT or cTnI, but in renal failure the elevated levels are sustained reference ranges, which may vary between laboratories and are dependent on methods of measurement used.

Myoglobin

- Serum myoglobin determinations hold promise in early screening for myocardial infarction.
- It has structure similar to hemoglobin and mainly found in the muscle.
- Myoglobin is a protein found in skeletal and cardiac muscle.
- It is an oxygen binding protein, which serves as a reserve for oxygen and facilitates movement of oxygen within the muscle cells.
- Myoglobin released from skeletal and cardiac muscle tissue is indistinguishable.
- Myoglobin released from necrotic tissues into the serum returns to normal within 24 hours because it is quickly filtered through the glomerulus.

Myoglobinemia

- This is the increased myoglobin in the blood. Elevated myoglobin levels in serum have been used to screen patients for myocardial infarction because myoglobin is released from damaged cardiac muscle within 2 hours after the onset of symptoms. However, specificity may be limited because myoglobin can be elevated in serum from noncardiac related conditions.

Myoglobinuria

- This is the presence of myoglobin in the urine. This occurs after severe physical exercise or in trauma where muscle fiber necrosis has occurred.
- Myoglobinuria should be suspected when the urine test is positive for hemoglobin but the microscopic analysis of the sediment does not show red blood cells.

Phosphatases

These are enzymes, which catalyze the removal of PO_4^{2-} group from organic monophosphoric esters. Two types of phosphatases exist normally, *alkaline phosphatase,* which has maximum activity at pH 10, and *acid phosphatase* with maximum activity at acidic pH 5.0.

Alkaline Phosphatase (ALP)

- The alkaline phosphatase is present in all tissues of the body and its level is high in liver, bone, intestine, kidney and placenta.
- Each of the above mentioned organs contains a specific isoenzyme of alkaline phosphatase.
- There are totally 5 isoenzyme forms of ALP.
- Normal adult serum contains ALP, which is mainly from liver and bile duct.
- Whereas, in children the source of serum ALP is mainly from bone.
- Placental ALP is found in pregnancy only.
- The functions of ALP in the body are the transport of phosphate across the cell membranes and addition of phosphates during mineralization of the bone.

Determination of Alkaline Phosphatase by King and King Method

$$\text{Disodium phenyl phosphate} \xrightarrow{\text{ALP}} \text{Phenol + phosphate}$$

$$\text{Phenol + 4-aminoantipyrine} \xrightarrow{\text{Pot-Ferricyanide}} \text{Orange-red colored product measured colorimetrically}$$

The alkaline oxidizing agent, 4-amino-antipyrine gives a red or purple color with compounds containing a phenolic group. This reaction has been used to determine phenol produced by the reaction of alkaline phosphatase on disodium phenyl phosphate. The color developed is read at 510 nm.

Then the serum is incubated with phenyl phosphate buffered at pH 10 for 15 minutes at 37°C. The hydrolytic product is condensed with 4-aminoantipyrine and then oxidized with alkaline ferricyanide to give a red colored complex, which is measured photometrically at 510 nm.

Reagents

1. *Buffer (pH 10.14 at 20°C):* Dissolve 3.18 g of anhydrous sodium carbonate and 1.68 g of sodium bicarbonate in water and make up to 500 mL. Store at 4°C.
2. *Substrate (0.01 M):* Dissolve 1.09 g of disodium phenyl phosphate, in 500 mL boiled and cooled distilled water and 2 mL chloroform as a preservative.
3. *Sodium hydroxide 0.5 N:*
4. *Sodium bicarbonate 0.5 N:* 42.0 g of anhydrous sodium bicarbonate/L.
5. *4-Aminoantipyrine:* 6 g/liter, filter and store in a brown bottle.
6. *Potassium ferricyanide:* 24 g/liter. Store in a brown bottle. If slight green tinge appears, prepare fresh reagent.
7. *Standard phenol 1 mg/mL:* 100 mg of pure phenol in 100 mL of 0.1 N HCl. Keep at 4°C in a brown bottle. It lasts at least for one month.
8. *Working standard (0.05 mg/mL):* Dilute 5 mL of stock phenol standard to 100 mL with distilled water, preserve with a few drops of chloroform and keep at 4°C in a brown bottle. Stable for one week. Standardization of phenol must be done.

Procedure

Reagents	*Blank*	*Test*	*Standard*	*Control*
Buffer (mL)	2.0	0.9	1.5	0.9
Substrate	–	1.0	–	1.0
Serum (mL)	–	0.1	–	–
Standard (mL)	–	–	0.5	–
Incubate for 15 minutes at 37°C				
0.5 5 N NaOH	1.0	1.0	1.0	1.0
Serum (mL)	–	–	–	0.1
0.5 N sodium bicarbonate	1.0	1.0	1.0	1.0
4-amino-antipyrine (mL)	1.0	1.0	1.0	1.0
Potassium ferricyanide	1.0	1.0	1.0	1.0
Read the absorbance at 510 nm				

Note: Mix thoroughly after addition of reagents in each step otherwise irregular results may be obtained because the reaction is pH dependent.

Read the absorbance of reddish brown color immediately at green filter (510 nm) avoiding, exposure to strong sunlight. The amount of phenol present in the standard tube is 25 micrograms.

Calculation

$$0.1 \text{ serum liberates} = \frac{T-C}{S-B} \times 25\ \mu g$$

Hence, 100 mL serum would liberate,

$$\frac{T-C}{S-B} \times 25 \text{ mg of phenol}$$

Since one King Armstrong Unit is the production of 1 mg of phenol in 15 minutes under the conditions of the test.

$$= \frac{T-C}{S-B} \times 25 \text{ mg}$$

Advantages of the Method

1. Simple and popular.
2. Gives reproducible results.
3. Does not require deproteinization of serum.

Colorimetric Method

$$\text{P-nitrophenyl phosphate} \xrightarrow{ALP} \text{p-nitrophenol+ Phosphate}$$

In this method, p-nitrophenyl phosphate (PNPP or 4-NPP) is used as substrate. ALP acts on PNPP and liberates p-nitrophenol. As p-nitrophenol is yellow in color it can be measured directly at 405 nm. This method is being widely used. Results are expressed in U/L.

Separation of ALP Isoenzyme

The isoenzyme forms of ALP can be separated by using the following different techniques

1. Electrophoresis
2. Use of chemical inhibitors: Ethylenediaminetetraacetate (EDTA)

inactivates all the isoenzymes of ALP except placental ALP (chelating the Mg^{2+})

3. *Heat stability*: The placental ALP is stable to heat whereas, all the other enzymes are inactivated by heat at 56°C for 10 minutes.
4. *Urea*: Bone enzyme is more susceptible to urea treatment.

Liver enzyme has intermediate resistance and placental enzymes are most resistant.

Specimen: Serum or plasma is collected with heparin as an anticoagulant.

Normal range: 3–13 KA units/dL (35–140 U/L)

Serum ALP increases in:

1. Serum ALP level is high during growth period.
   Due to the active bone growth in children, the ALP level is about 2 times higher than the normal adult level.
   In pregnancy, serum ALP is higher due to the release of ALP from the placenta.
2. Disorders of liver and bile duct: Obstruction of the bile duct (obstructive jaundice) and liver cirrhosis.
3. Bone disorders, such as rickets, osteomalacia, bone tumors, etc.
   - ALP always increases in obstructive jaundice.
   - Therefore, it is considered as a marker for the diagnosis of obstructive jaundice.
   - Marked increase in serum ALP and direct bilirubin and moderate increase in AST and ALT (may be normal) level is a clear indication of obstructive jaundice.
   - In hepatitis, ALP level increase moderately and AST and ALT increase markedly.
   - Thus, ALP estimation is one of the indexes to differentiate hepatic and post-hepatic jaundice.
   - The decrease in ALP is also reported in severe anemia, in scurvy, and in Kwashiorkor.

Acid Phosphatase (ACP)

The prostate gland is the richest source for ACP.

Other sources are red blood cells, platelets, bone, etc.

Estimation of Acid Phosphatase

The 4-Aminoantipyrine Method

The reagents used for ALP can be used for the estimation of ACP, substituting a citrate buffer of pH 5.0.

Principle: At a pH of 4.9 and temperature of 37°C, the enzyme acid phosphatase present in the given serum sample liberates phenol and disodium phenol phosphate. The phenol liberated from it forms a red or purple colored complex which is measured photometrically at 520 nm.

Reagents

1. *Citric acid:* Sodium citrate buffer—dissolve 21 g of crystalline citric acid in water , add 18.8 mL of (1 mol/L) NaOH and make to 500 mL with distilled water. Adjust to pH 4.9, if necessary by adding drop by drop NaOH or HCl or alternatively dissolve 58.82 g of sodium dihydrate in 200 mol/L HCl and make to a liter with the acid. Check the pH and adjust if necessary.
2. Disodium phenyl phosphate
3. Buffer substrate (100 mL disodium phenyl phosphate + 100 mL sodium citrate-citric acid buffer).
4. 0.5 N NaOH
5. 0.5 N $NaHCO_3$
6. 0.6% 4-aminoantipyrine
7. 2.4% $K_3[Fe(CN)_6]$
8. *Phenol standards:* 1 mg/mL.
   100 mg of pure phenol in 100 mL of 0.1 N HCl. Keep at 4°C in a brown bottle. It is stable for one month.

Working standard: 0.05 mg/mL—dilute 5 mL stock phenol standard to 100 mL with deionized water, preserve with drops of chloroform, store at 4°C in a brown bottle. Stable for one week.

Reagents	Blank	Test	Standard	Control
Buffer (mL)	2.0	0.9	1.5	0.9
Substrate	–	1.0	–	1.0
Incubate for 3 mintues at 37°C				
Serum (mL)	–	0.1	–	–
Standard (mL)	–	–	0.5	–
Incubate for 60 minutes at 37°C				
0.5 N NaOH	1.0	1.0	1.0	1.0
Serum (mL)	–	–	–	0.1
0. 5 N sodium bicarbonate	1.0	1.0	1.0	1.0
4-amino-antipyrine (mL)	1.0	1.0	1.0	1.0
Potassium ferricyanide	1.0	1.0	1.0	1.0
Read the absorbance at 510 nm				

0.1 serum liberates = $\frac{T-C}{S-B} \times 25\ \mu g$

Hence, 100 mL serum would liberate,

$\frac{T-C}{S-B} \times 25$ mg of phenol

Since 1 King Armstrong unit is the production of 1 mg of phenol in 15 minutes under the conditions of the test.

Serum acid phosphate = $\frac{T-C}{S-B} \times 25$
in KA > Units/100 mL

Note:

1. Blood should be collected without any anticoagulants.
2. ACP is highly unstable at room temperature. Hence, ACP should be estimated without much delay.
3. If the estimation is not possible immediately acidify the serum by adding one drop of 5N acetic acid and store at 0–4° C stable for 3 days.
4. Hemolyzed samples are not suitable for ACP estimation.

Standard Graph

Excepting the buffer substrate and the standard, the other reagents are the same as used for the BST method.

Buffer substrate: 100 mL disodium phenyl phosphate + 100 mL sodium citrate-citric acid buffers.

Standard: 100 mg phenol in 100 mL 0.1 N HCl.

Working standard: 2.5 mL of stock phenol standard diluted to 100 mL with water.

Calculation

From the graph 0.08 OD corresponds to 4 μg i.e., 0.1 mL serum releases 4 μg of phenol

∴ 100 mL serum releases 4000 μg of phenol

∴ Specific activity of ACP in given sample = 4 KA units.

Interpretation

Normal value = 11 U/L

1. Serum ACP increased in:
   a. Carcinoma of the prostate gland
   b. May be in prostate gland enlargement
   c. Bone disease.

Determination of acid phosphatase with Thymolphthalein in monophosphate (substrate) (Roy and Colleagues modified by Ewen and Spitzer):

Principle

Thymolphthalein monophosphate is hydrolyzed by prostatic ACP at pH 5.4 and 37°C.

The reaction is stopped after 30 minutes by addition of NaOH and Na_2CO_3 solution.

This develops the alkaline color of the liberated thymolphthalein, which is measured at 595 nm.

Reagents

1. *Acetic acid 5 mol/L:* Transfer 28.87 mL of glacial acetic acid into a 100 mL volumetric flask and make up the volume with water and mix.

Procedure

Contents	*B*	S_1	S_2	S_3	S_4	S_5	S_6	S_7	C_1	T_1
Phenol	–	0.2	0.4	0.6	0.8	1.0	1.2	1.4	–	–
Conc (µg/tube)	–	5	10	15	20	25	30	35	–	–
Citric acid: Na citrate (mL)	2	1.8	1.6	1.4	1.2	1.0	0.8	0.6	–	–
Buffer substrate (mL)	–	–	–	–	–	–	–	–	2	2
Serum (mL)	–	–	–	–	–	–	–	–	–	0.1
Incubate at 37°C for 1 hour (C and T only)										
0.5 N NaOH (mL)	←--------				1.0 mL					--------→
Serum (mL)	–	–	–	–	–	–	–	–	0.1	–
0.5 N $NaHCO_3$ (mL)	←--------				1.0 mL					--------→
4-aminoantipyrine	←--------				1.0 mL					--------→
$K_3[Fe(CN)_6]$	←--------				1.0 mL					--------→
OD at 520 nm	.06⊠0	0.11	0.23	0.32	0.42	0.52	0.63	0.74	0.00	0.08

2. Sodium acetate 5 mol/L. Dissolve 68.0 g $CH_3COONa.3H_2O$ in water in a 100 mL volumetric flask and mix.
3. Acetate buffer 5 mol/L, pH 5.4 at 25°C. Add sufficient reagent 2 to acetic acid 5 mol/L (reagent 1) to adjust to pH 5.4 at 25°C.
4. Acetate buffer, 0.25 mol/L, pH 5.4 at 25°C. Pipette 5 mL of reagent 3 into a 100 mL volumetric flask. Dilute to volume with water.
5. *Buffered substrate:* Dilute a solution of Brij-35, 300 g/L, to a concentration of 3.24 g/L. Dissolve 82.8 mg disodium thymolphthalein monophosphate in 11 mL H_2O and make up to 100 mL. If a substrate preparation with a different water of crystallization is used, adjust the weight of salt appropriately. Add 1.92 g of sodium acetate (trihydrate) to the solution, mix to dissolve, adjust the pH of the solution to 5.4 with HCl, 0.1 mol/L and adjust volume to 100 mL with water. Store in a refrigerator. The solution is stable for up to 1 month.
6. Alkaline reagent, sodium carbonate (Na_2CO_3), 0.1 mol/L, in NaOH, 0.1 mol/L. Dissolve 10.6 g of anhydrous Na_2CO_3 and 4.0 g of NaOH in distilled water. Dilute to 1000 mL and mix. The reagent is stable at room temperature.
7. Thymolphthalein stock calibration solution, 3 mmol/L. Dissolve 129.3 mg of thymolphthalein in n-propanol—water (70:30, v/v) and make up to 100 mL. Mix well. Store at 4°C.

Procedure

1. For each specimen, pipette 0.55 mL buffered substrate (reagent 5) into a labeled test tube and place in a water bath at 37°C to reach temperature equilibrium.
2. At zero time, add 50 µL serum, mix well, and return tube rapidly to water bath.
3. While incubation is proceeding, prepare a "blank" tube for each specimen, containing 1.0 mL of alkaline reagent (6) Add 0.55 mL buffered substrate (5). Followed by 50 µL of the serum specimen to the appropriate

blank tube. Mix (ACP cannot act at the high pH of the alkaline reagent; the blank tube thus compensates for endogenous color of both specimen and reagent).

4. After exactly 30 minutes, add 1.0 mL of alkaline reagent (6) to each "test". Mix well to stop the reaction and develop the color.
5. Read absorbances of test and blank tubes for each specimen at 595 nm, with water as a reference. Substract the blank reading from the test to give the absorbance change, A, in 30 minutes due to ACP activity.
6. If a well-calibrated narrow-band pass spectrophotometer is used for measurement, the molar absorptivity of thymolphthalein (39.20×10^{-3} L × mmol-1 × cm^{-1}) can be used to calculate the catalytic activity concentration of the specimen from the following formula:

$$\text{Acid phosphatase} = \frac{A \times 1 \times 1.6}{30 \times 39.2 \times 10^{-3} \times 0.05}$$

$$= A \times 27.2 = U/L$$

Because, the final 1.6 mL reaction mixture contains 0.05 mL of the serum sample.

7. Alternatively, a calibration curve can be prepared from the stock calibration solution (7) by diluting 1.0, 2.0, 3.0, 4.0, 5.0 and 6.0 mL, volumes of the calibrator to 10 mL with n-propanol: water. Working calibrators consist of 50 µL of each of the respective standard dilutions, plus 0.55 mL buffered substrate (5), plus 1 mL alkaline reagent (6). The absorbance of these solutions at 595 nm corresponds to those produced by 10, 20, 30, 40 and 50 U/L of ACP.

Kit Method

Principle

Commonly 1-Naphthyl phosphate is used as a substrate. In acidic pH ACP hydrolyses 1-Naphthyl phosphate to PO_4 and 1-Naphthol. 1- Naphthol reacts with fast red salt to form a colored complex, which is measured at 405 nm. The rate of increase in absorbance is directly proportional to the rate of ACP activity.

$$\text{1-Naphthyl Phosphate} \xrightarrow{ACP} \text{1-Naphthol} + PO_4$$

$$\text{1-Naphthol} + \text{Fast red salt} \longrightarrow \text{Colored complex (405 nm)}$$

ACP in the plasma is broadly divided into 2 categories:

a. Prostatic ACP (PAP)
b. Non-prostatic ACP.

Estimation of Prostatic ACP (PAP)

Estimation of PAP is useful in diagnosis and monitoring of prostate cancer. PAP is cleared by tartaric acid. Other forms are stable to tartrate. This property is utilized in the estimation of prostatic ACP.

The following steps can be adopted to determine the prostatic ACP:

1. Estimate the total ACP in the serum sample
2. Add tartarate solution to the serum sample
3. Estimate ACP in the tartarate treated serum
4. Difference between two ACP values is the value of PAP.

   PAP = Total ACP – ACP in the tartarate treated serum.

Gamma Glutamyl Transferase (GGT)

Source

Liver and bile duct are the main sources of plasma GGT.

Pancreas, prostate gland and kidneys also contain this enzyme.

Estimation of GGT

Principle

GGT γ-glutamyl-P-nitroanilide + Glycyl glycine → γ-glutamyl-glycyl-glycine + P – nitroaniline

The GGT catalyzes the transfer of the γ-glutamyl group from the substrate γ- glutamyl peptides to another peptide, such as glycyl glycine forming γ-glutamylglycyl glycine and P-nitroaniline. The p-nitroaniline has maximum absorbance at 405 nm.

Clinical Significance

Normal Value

10–50 U/L

GGT levels increases in:

1. Obstructive jaundice
2. Hepatitis
3. Alcoholic cirrhosis.

Plasma GGT level is a very sensitive indicator to diagnose alcoholic cirrhosis.

Amylase

- Amylase helps in the digestion of starch in the small intestine.
- Amylase breaks α-1, 4-glycoside linkages of starch into maltose.
- Serum amylase originates from pancreas and salivary gland.

Clinical Significance

Normal Range

80–240 U/L

Serum amylase level increases in

- Acute pancreatitis
- Pancreas injury
- Carcinoma of pancreas
- Tumors of lung
- Mumps
- Salivary lesions.

Determination of Serum Amylase (Colorimetric Method of Kaplan)

Principle

Iodine forms a blue colored complex with starch. Amylase is the enzyme, which breaks down starch. Serum is incubated with starch substrate at 37°C for 10 minutes. The enzyme reaction is stopped by the addition of Iodine-EDTA solution. The remaining starch forms a blue color with iodine from which the amylase activity is calculated.

Reagents

1. *Nitric acid 1 mol/L:* Dilute 61 mL of concentrated HNO_3 to one liter with water.
2. *Buffered starch solution:* Make a paste of 125 mg of starch with about 3 mL of water in a 250 mL beaker. Add about 100 mL of water. Add 2.435 g of tris (hydroxymethyl) amino methane and 2.875 g of sodium chloride (AR Grade). Boil while stirring. Cool to room temperature. Add 250 mg of sodium azide as preservative. Adjust the pH to 7.4 by the addition of 1 M HNO_3. Transfer to a 250 mL volumetric flask and make up to mark.
3. *Stock iodine: EDTA solution:* Dissolve 12 g of potassium iodide (KI) in 125 mL of water taken in a 500 mL volumetric flask. Add 185 mg of disodium EDTA and stir until dissolved. Add 5.2 g of iodine and stir until dissolved. Make up to 500 mL with water. Store in a brown bottle.
4. *Working iodine: EDTA*—dilute the stock solution 10 in 100 with water every day.

Procedure

Label three test tubes "Test (T)", "Control (C)" and "Blank (B)". Add 2 mL of buffered starch solution to T, C, and B. Incubate the three tubes at 37°C for 5 minutes. Pipette 0.05 mL of serum to test tube T only. Incubate for 10 minutes. Add 15 mL of Iodine-EDTA working solution to test tubes T, C and B. To test tube C add 0.05 mL of serum. To test tube B add 0.05 mL of water. Mix each tube thoroughly. Let stand for 3 minutes.

Reagents	T	C	B
Buffered starch solution	2 mL	2 mL	2 mL
Incubate at 37°C for 5 minutes			
Serum	0.05 mL	–	–
Incubate at 37°C for 10 minutes			
Working iodine-EDTA solution	15 mL	15 mL	15 mL
Serum	–	0.05 mL	–
Water	–	–	0.05 mL
Kept for 3 minutes and read the OD at 640 nm or red filter			

Calculation

Units of enzyme activity: One amylase unit for this method is amount of enzyme catalyzes hydrolysis of 10 mg of starch in 45 minutes to a stage at which no color is given by iodine. In this case,

$$= \frac{\text{Conc of starch in 2 mL of buffer} \times 45 \text{ min}}{10 \text{ mg of starch} \times 10 \text{ min}}$$

$$= \frac{1}{10} \times \frac{45}{10} = 0.45 \text{ units}$$

∴ under condition of this procedure complete hydrolysis of the substrate per mg represents 0.45 amylase units per 0.05 mL of serum sample

∴ for 100 mL of serum sample

$$= \frac{0.45 \times 100}{0.05} = 900 \text{ units / dL}$$

$$\text{Amylase activity} = \frac{\text{OD of C} - \text{OD of T}}{\text{OD of C}} \times 900$$

in units/100 mL

If the amylase activity is above 1000, 1 in 5 dilution of the sample can be done.

Amylase assay using 4-Nitrophenyl-Glycoside substrates.

Some commercial kits use 4-NP-G substrate and alpha-glucosidase. The mixture is preincubated for a few minutes at the assay temperature. 50 or 100 μL of specimen is added and after a further incubation of 2 or 3 minutes, A/min is determined at 405. The A/min is proportional to the amylase activity of the specimen.

$$\text{4-NP-(glucose)} \xrightarrow{\alpha\text{-Amylase}} \text{4-NP-(glucose)} + \text{(glucose)}$$

$$\text{4-NP (glucose)} \xrightarrow{\alpha\text{-Glucosidase}} \text{4-NP (glucose)} + \alpha\text{-glucose} + \text{NP}$$

Lipase

The enzyme present in the intestine which hydrolyzes triglycerides (FAT) of the diet and finally helps to digest the fat.

Bile salts are essential for the action of lipase.

Source

Pancreas is the major source for lipase in the serum.

Clinical Significance

Serum lipase is increased in chronic pancreatitis.

Serum amylase is increased in mumps, pancreatic diseases or due to some other cause, whereas lipase is increased only in pancreatitis. Therefore, the determination of both amylase and lipase together helps in the diagnosis of acute pancreatitis.

Estimation of Lipase

Principle

A solution of triglyceride in water has a milky appearance (Turbid) when serum is added to this solution; lipase in the serum hydrolyzes triglyceride, which results in decreased turbidity. As the reaction proceeds there is decrease in turbidity and hence decrease in the absorbance. The decrease in the absorbance is read at 340 nm.

Normal range: 40–200 U/L.

Cholinesterases

Two types have been distinguished:

1. *True cholinesterase* (acetylcholine hydrolase, acetylcholinesterase)
   - Present in nerve tissue and RBC
   - Responsible for the hydrolysis of acetylcholine at the synapses and neuromuscular junction
2. *Pseudocholinesterase* (acetylcholine acylhydrolase, cholinesterase)
   - Present in the liver, heart muscle, intestine and sera
   - Function of this enzyme is not known
   - Estimation of pseudocholinesterase in serum or plasma is clinically useful.

Clinical Significance

- *Normal levels:* 4000–12000 U/L.
- Serum cholinesterase level is an important indicator of insecticide poisoning.

- Its level markedly decreased in persons who have consumed insecticides, which are organophosphorus compounds, such as parathion and tetraethyl pyrophosphate.
- Its level also decreases in uremia, shock, anemia, tuberculosis, cancer and in malnutrition.

Glucose-6-PO_4 Dehydrogenase (G-6-PD)

Glucose-6-Phosphate dehydrogenase is present within the RBC. Deficiency of G-6-PD is inborn and it is prevalent throughout the world. The deficiency is of the mild type, in most people. Deficiency is also observed in some rare cases and it is observed in childhood itself. G-6-PD is the enzyme required in HMP (Hexosemonophosphate) pathway of carbohydrate metabolism. It catalyzes the reaction, with the production of NADPH. NADPH is essential for the stability of RBC membrane (NADPH is required to maintain reduced glutathione range which maintains the stability of RBCs). In case of G-6-PD deficiency NADPH production will be decreased leading to breakdown of RBC and anemia. In the case of mild deficiency, a person will be healthy when he is treated with certain drugs, such as primaquine, sulfonamides cause severe hemolysis. When these drugs are given the NADPH supply is not sufficient to maintain the stability of RBC. So hemolysis takes place that may lead to anemia and death.

G-6-PDH estimation in blood is required in the following conditions:

1. When the patient is suffering from severe hemolytic anemia.
2. While treating a patient with malarial drugs.

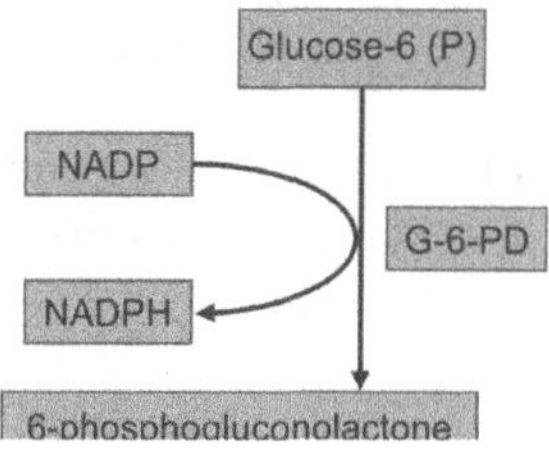

G-6-PD Estimation

Whole blood is collected with either heparin or EDTA.

Blood is centrifuged and plasma is discarded.

The RBCs are used for the estimation of G-6-PD.

RBC is lyzed and the hemolysate is taken for the estimation of G-6-PD.

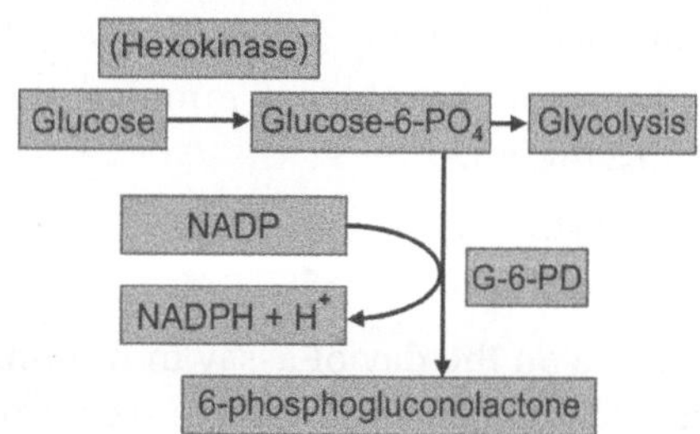

The glucose-6-Phosphate of dehydrogenase catalyzes the conversion glucose-6 phosphate to 6-phosphogluconolactone producing NADPH.

The absorbance of NADPH produced is measured at 640 nm.

Reagents

1. NaCl, 0.155 M (0.9%) - Keep at 4°C.
2. *Hemolyzing solution:* Place 10 mL of Na_2EDTA, 0.27 mol/L (1g/10 mL), (10%) pH 8.0 and 0.05 mL of 2-mercaptoethanol in a 1 L volumetric flask and make up the volume with distilled water. Store at 4°C.
3. Tris-HCl buffer, 1 M, pH 8.0. Place 121.14 g of tris (hydroxymethyl) in a 2 L beaker and add 800 mL distilled water. Adjust pH to 8.0 by adding drop by drop, 1 M HCl, while constantly stirring then transfer to a 1 L jar to make up the volume.
4. $MgCl_2$, 0.1 M, aqueous (2.0 g/dL).
5. NADP, 2 mmol, aqueous (Sigma) (1.53 mg/mL) freshly prepared.

$$\frac{(765.4 \times 2 \times 1)}{1000}$$

6. *Stock reagent mixture:* The reagents (3), (4) and (5) may be premixed in the following proportions:
   Tris-HCl buffer—5.0 mL
   $MgCl_2$—5.0 mL
   NADP solution—5.0 mL (8 mg NADP/5 mL H_2O).
   H_2O—29.0 mL
   The reagent mixture may be prepared in advance and stored frozen for 1 month.
7. Glucose-6-phosphate, 6 mmol, aqueous (1.82 mg/mL).

$$\frac{(6\times 304.1\times 1)}{1000}$$

Prepare on the day of assay in minimum volume of 0.3 mL for one assay and control.

Specimen: Whole blood, heparinized.

Procedure

Preparation of Hemolysate

1. Centrifuge 2 mL of whole blood at 1500 × g for 10 minutes. Remove and discard plasma and buffy coat (the topmost cream colored layer of cells).
2. Resuspend erythrocytes in 10 mL of cold NaCl (0.155 M), mix thoroughly.
3. Centrifuge at 1500 × g for 10 minutes at 4°C.
4. Discard supernatant and topmost layer of cells, including any residual buffy coat.
5. Repeat the suspension of cells in cold NaCl (0.155 M), centrifugation and discarding the supernatant and uppermost layer of cells, a total of three times.
6. Then resuspend the remaining cells in an equal volume of cold NaCl (0.155 M).
7. Add 0.2 mL of erythrocyte-NaCl suspension to 1.8 mL of hemolyzing solution in a glass tube. Keep in deep freezer till frozen.
8. If the hemolysate is turbid, centrifuge at 2250 × g for 30 minutes at 4°C.

Determination of G-6-PD Activity

1. Pipette the reagents into a glass tube in the following proportions:
   Stock reagent mixture—0.9 mL
   Hemolysate—20 mL
2. Cap with parafilm and invert twice to mix.
3. Incubate at 37°C for 10 minutes (pre-incubation).
4. Add 0.1 mL of glucose-6-phosphate solution to the above tube, invert to mix and immediately take the absorbance at 340 nm. Record the reading.
5. Incubate the tube in the water bath maintained at 37°C for 10 minutes.
6. Remove the tubes from the water bath, mix and measure the absorbance at 340 nm. Record the reading as 'TEST'.
7. $A\,340/\text{min} = \frac{T-B}{10}$
8. Add 0.1 mL of hemolysate to a tube containing 5.0 mL of Drabkin's solution (Hb reagent). Mix. Measure the absorbance at 540 nm (540). It is better to take a blank reading of the reagent alone first and then taking another reading with the hemolysate as above. Difference between the two will be A540.

Note: The dilution of Drabkin's solution is 1:50 instead of the usual 1:502. The factor calculating the hemolysate hemoglobin concentration is therefore proportionately smaller.

Calculation

$$\text{G-6-PD activity, U/g Hb} = \frac{14.67\times \Delta A340/\text{min}}{\Delta A540}$$

$$= \frac{804\times \Delta A340/\text{min}}{\Delta A540\times 5.48}$$

5.48 = factor for cyanmethemoglobin
(OD of the known concentration of Hb)
Reference: 8–18 U/g Hb.

SELF TEST

1. Explain the structure and composition of enzymes.
2. Write a note on apoenzymes and coenzymes. Give an example for each.
3. Classify enzymes. Give an example for each class.
4. Give examples of different classes of enzymes.
5. What are the factors affecting the enzyme activity?
6. Explain the effect of temperature on enzyme activity.
7. How pH will affect enzyme activity?
8. How do you differentiate functional enzymes from non-functional enzymes of plasma?
9. Expand the terms AST, ALT ALP, CKMB and CPK?
10. Define the enzyme unit.
11. Write a note on isoenzyme.
12. What are cardiac enzymes?
13. What are the isoenzyme forms of LDH. Write the normal level for it.
14. Explain the clinical significance of LDH estimation.
15. What are the isoenzymes of CK? Give the normal value for it.
16. Explain the clinical importance of CK.
17. How can you estimate CKMB?
18. In which diseases does the AST level increases?
19. Give the pattern of cardiac enzyme profile in myocardial infarction.
20. Write the principle of AST estimation. Write the clinical significance of AST.
21. Write a note on myoglobin.
22. How useful is myoglobin in the diagnosis of cardiac diseases?
23. Write the clinical significance of troponin T and troponin I.
24. Name the enzymes commonly estimated for liver diseases.
25. Write a note on ALT. In which disease do their levels increase more than normal in the blood?
26. State the isoenzymes of ALP. State the organ of origin for each.
27. Describe the clinical significance of ALP.
28. What is the importance of GGT estimation in liver diseases?
29. Name the enzymes estimated in suspected cholestatsis.
30. Write a note on prostatic acid phosphatase.
31. Explain the clinical significance of acid phosphatase.
32. How do you estimate acid phosphatase?
33. Write a note on amylase.
34. What is the clinical significance of amylase estimation?
35. How is lipase a better index than amylase in pancreatic diseases?
36. Write the clinical significance of lipase.
37. Write the clinical significance of choline esterase.

MULTIPLE CHOICE QUESTIONS

1. The enzyme amylase is secreted from:
   a. Liver
   b. Intestine
   c. Pancreas
   d. Bone

2. LDH has———-
   a. Two isoenzyme forms
   b. Only one form
   c. Four isoenzyme forms
   d. Five isoenzyme forms

3. The enzyme, which increases in obstructive jaundice is:
   a. LDH
   b. ACP
   c. ALP
   d. CK

4. The richest source of ACP is:
a. Kidney
b. Prostate gland
c. Adrenal gland
d. Platelets.

5. An important indicator of insecticide poisoning is:
a. Lipase
b. Phenobarbital
c. Cholinesterase
d. Glucose-6-phosphate dehydrogenase.

6. The optimum temperature for enzymes in our body is:
a. 30 °C
b. 32 °C
c. 37 °C
d. 27 °C.

7. G-6-PO_4 dehydrogenase deficiency leads to:
a. Increased production of NAD
b. Decreased production of NADPH
c. Increased production of NADPH
d. Decreased production of NADH.

15

UNIT

Liver Function Test

LEARNING OBJECTIVES

At the end of this unit, the learner should be able to understand:

- Different types of functions performed by liver.
- The various diagnostic tests performed to detect the functions of the liver.
- The different types of jaundice, causes and biochemical findings of it.
- The hepatitis markers test to detect the liver dysfunction.

INTRODUCTION

The human liver contains complex parenchymal cells that perform multiple functions, which are essential for life. The liver is one of the largest organs in the human body weighing 1.2 to 1.5 kg in the adult. The liver consists of two unequal lobes. The excretory apparatus of the liver consists of the common hepatic duct, the gallbladder, the cystic duct and the common bile duct **(Fig. 15.1)**.

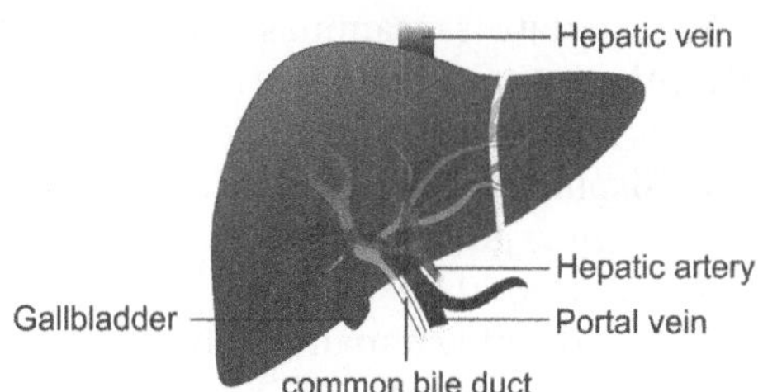

Fig. 15.1: Liver structure.

Liver function tests represent a wide range of normal functions performed by the liver. The diagnosis of liver disease depends upon a complete history, physical examination, and evaluation of liver function tests and further invasive and noninvasive tests. Many patients become confused regarding the meaning of a liver function test.

The hepatobiliary tree represents hepatic cells and biliary tract cells. Inflammation of the hepatic cells results in elevation in the alanine aminotransferase (ALT), aspartate amino-transferase (AST) and possibly the bilirubin. Inflammation of the biliary tract cells results predominantly in an elevation of the alkaline phosphatase. In liver disease, there are crossovers between purely biliary disease and hepatocellular disease. To interpret these, the physician will look at the entire picture of the hepatocellular disease and biliary tract disease to determine, which is the primary abnormality.

Functions of the Liver

1. The liver plays a major role in storing blood, i.e., it acts as a reservoir of blood.
2. Detoxification of blood.
3. The parenchymal cells of the liver are related to the breakdown of Hb to bilirubin and the removal of pigments, bacteria and other foreign materials by phagocytosis.

4. The parenchymal cells have a major role in maintaining homeostasis. They play a central role in the metabolism of carbohydrates (glycogenesis, glycogenolysis, gluconeogenesis and alcohol metabolism), proteins (transamination, oxidative deamination of amino acids, urea synthesis and protein synthesis), lipids, hormones, vitamins, bilirubin and bile acids.
5. Storing of vitamins, fat, cholesterol, and bile.
6. Metabolizing (processing) medications and nutrients.

Limitations of Liver Function Test

1. The liver does not easily demonstrate dysfunction at least in its metabolic activities. This is because of enormous reserve capacity and the marvelous regenerating power of the liver. Only a small portion of the liver is enough to perform all the functions. About 75 to 80% of the liver needs to be out of function for any of the tests to be positive.
2. The functions performed by the liver are numerous and varied. A large number of these functions are shared by other organs also.
3. There is no single test for measuring the liver function. Whole liver is not equally or simultaneously disturbed in hepatic disorders.

Indications of Liver Function Test

The results of LFT help in:

- The differential diagnosis of jaundice.
- Detection of liver diseases.
- Assessment of severity and prognosis of liver disease.
- Monitoring the treatment.
  Most of the LFT are performed on blood and urine.

Basic Processes in Liver Diseases

Liver Cell Damage

This may vary from areas of local damage to destruction of most of the liver cells leading to liver failure.

The main causes are:

a. *Acute hepatitis* may be mainly viral.
b. *Chronic hepatitis* is due to the continuing action of infective or toxic agents or that associated with autoimmune response.
c. Cirrhosis (destruction of hepatic cells).

Biliary Tract Involvement

The involvement of the biliary tract is associated with obstruction to bile flow (cholestasis) and may manifest as obstructive jaundice.

There are two types of obstruction:

1. *Intrahepatic cholestasis* mainly arises with liver cell destruction. The main causes are viral hepatitis, use of steroids (during pregnancy or in the case of women taking oral contraceptives).
2. *Extrahepatic cholestasis*

Causes: Gallstone in the common bile duct, carcinoma of the pancreas, cirrhosis of the bile duct.

The LFTs are considered in the following categories:

a. Tests indicating liver cell damage:
   1. Aspartate transaminase (AST)
   2. Alanine transaminase (ALT).
b. Tests indicating biliary tract involvement:
   1. Alkaline phosphatase (ALP)
   2. Gamma glutamyltransferase (GGT)
   3. 5' nucleotidase.
c. Tests indicating impaired function:
   1. Serum proteins
   2. Bilirubin.
d. Tests indicating etiology.

Tests Related to Protein Metabolism

- The liver plays a central role in protein metabolism.
- Extensive liver damage leads to reduced blood levels of these proteins.

- The level of serum immunoglobulins produced by plasma cells varies widely in liver disease and variation in their levels is a reflection of inflammation or immune response and role of hepatocyte dysfunction. The important tests related to protein metabolism are:
  - Serum total protein
  - Albumin
  - Globulins.

Total Protein, Albumin and Globulin

Albumin is the major protein present within the blood. Albumin and all globulins except γ-globulins are formed in the liver. As such, albumin represents a major synthetic protein and is a marker for the ability of the liver to synthesize proteins. It is only one of many proteins that are synthesized by the liver. However, since it is easy to measure, it represents a reliable and inexpensive laboratory test for physicians to assess the degree of liver damage present in any particular patient. When the liver has been chronically damaged, the albumin may be low. This would indicate that the synthetic function of the liver has been markedly diminished. Such findings suggest a diagnosis of cirrhosis. Malnutrition can also cause low albumin (hypoalbuminemia) with no associated liver disease.

Since albumin is catabolized slowly, even in complete cessation of albumin synthesis, the serum level falls by only 25% in 8 days. Hence, in acute liver disease (viral hepatitis) the albumin value may be normal.

The serum proteins are estimated by differential precipitation of albumin and globulin fractions and also by biuret method and dye binding method.

Normal range:

Total protein	-	6.0–8.0 g/dL
Albumin	-	3.5–5.0 g/dL
Globulin	-	2.5–3.0 g/dL
γ-globulin	-	0.5–1.5 g/dL.

By using an electrophoretic gel, major proteins can be separated. This results in four major types of proteins. These are (1) albumin, (2) alpha globulins, (3) beta globulins and (4) gamma globulins. This test is useful for evaluation of patients who have abnormal liver function tests since it allows a direct quantification of multiple serum proteins.

If the gamma globulin fraction is elevated, autoimmune hepatitis may be present.

In viral hepatitis α_1-globulin is decreased and β_1-globulin is increased.

In cirrhosis and inflammation, γ-globulin is elevated.

The average contents of the five main components of the serum proteins in percentages are:

Albumin	=	66%
α_1-globulin	=	3%
α_2-globulin	=	7%
β-globulin	=	9%
γ-globulin	=	12–15%

Prothrombin Time

Another measure of hepatic synthetic function is the prothrombin time (PT).

Liver synthesizes clotting factors, such as prothrombin, fibrinogen, factor V, factor VII and factor X.

Prothrombin time is affected by proteins synthesized by the liver. Particularly, these proteins are associated with the incorporation of vitamin K metabolites into clotting factors. This allows normal coagulation. Thus, in patients who have prolonged prothrombin times, liver disease may be present. Since a prolonged PT is not a specific test for liver disease, confirmation by other abnormal liver tests is essential. This may include reviewing other liver function tests or radiology studies of the liver. Diseases such as malnutrition, in which decreased vitamin K in gestion is present, may result in a prolonged PT time. An indirect test of hepatic synthetic function includes administration of vitamin K (10 mg) subcutaneously over 3 days.

Several days later, the prothrombin time may be measured. If the prothrombin time becomes normal, then hepatic synthetic function is intact. This test does not indicate that there is no liver disease, but is suggestive that malnutrition may coexist with (or without) liver disease.

Zinc Sulfate Turbidity Test

Serum is mixed with a buffered zinc sulfate solution and the resulting turbidity is read at 680 nm.

Reagent

Buffered zinc sulfate solution: Dissolve 24 mg zinc sulfate, ($ZnSO_4.7H_2O$), 280 mg barbitone and 210 mg sodium barbitone in carbon dioxide-free water and make up to a liter. The pH should be 7.5 ± 0.05.

Technique

Add 100 μL fresh serum to 6 mL zinc sulfate solution, incubate it for 30 minutes and read the turbidity at 680 nm.
Normal range: 0–10 units.

Tests Related to Conjugation and Excretion

These tests are based on the ability of the hepatocytes to clear certain substances from the blood by conjugation and excretion in the bile or urine. The tests, which are commonly performed, are:

- The tests related to bilirubin
- The tests related to hippuric acid synthesis
- BSP (Bromsulphalein) excretion test

Hippuric Acid Synthesis Test

The liver removes benzoic acid by conjugating it with glycine to form hippuric acid, which is excreted in the urine. This test depends on the ability of the liver to produce sufficient amount of glycine and to conjugate it with benzoic acid.

To carry out this test, the renal functions should be normal.

Procedure

Benzoic acid is given orally (5.0 g) or intravenously (IV = 1.8 g) in the form of sodium benzoate. The amount of hippuric acid excreted during a fixed period of time is determined.

In oral test, around 3.5 g of sodium benzoate should be excreted as hippuric acid in 4 hours urine sample in a normal person. Less than 3.5 g indicates hepatic dysfunction due to either decreased synthesis of glycine or decreased synthesis of the conjugating enzyme, during acute or chronic liver damage. Amounts lesser than 1 g may be excreted by patients with hepatitis.

In the intravenous test at least an equivalent of 0.9 g of sodium benzoate should be excreted as hippuric acid in the 1st hour and up to 1.3 g in 2 hours. If there is a defect in the intestinal absorption in a patient, an intravenous test can be performed in place of oral test.

Bromsulphthalein (BSP) Excretion Test

Bromsulphthalein (BSP) is a dye, which is taken up by the liver, conjugated and excreted in the bile. BSP shares several steps with bilirubin in this process, such as binding to albumin, hepatic uptake, intracellular transport, conjugation, and active secretion into the bile and enterohepatic circulation.

Procedure

1. Five mg dye/kg body weight is injected intravenously, and blood samples collected from the other arm at 4, 25 and 45 minutes after commencement of the infusion.
2. The serum is separated.

Estimation

Reagents

1. NaOH—0.1 N
2. HCl— 0.1 N
3. *Standard solution:* Dissolve 100 mg BSP in 100 mL H_2O.

Working Standard
One mL stock diluted to 10 mL with water.

Procedure

	B	S_1	S_2	S_3	S_4	S_5	T
BSP (mL)	–	0.2	0.4	0.6	0.8	1.0	–
Concentration (mg)	–	2.0	4.0	6.0	8.0	10.0	–
Sample (mL)	0.5	–	–	–	–	–	0.5
Water (mL)	2.5	2.8	2.6	2.4	2.2	2.0	2.5
HCl (mL)	3.0	–	–	–	–	–	–
NaOH (mL) 0.1 N	3.0	3.0	3.0	3.0	3.0	3.0	3.0

The development of purple color is read in a colorimeter and compared with the standard graph results, and is expressed as percentage of dye excreted.

Calculation

Ten mg dye/100 mL serum represents the maximum concentration reached. Twenty five and 45 minute readings are expressed as a percentage of the 4 minutes reading.

A retention of more than 10% of the dye after 30 minutes and more than 3% after 45 minutes indicates abnormality in liver function.

Normal value: 0–10% at 30 minutes
0–3% after 45 minutes.

Abnormal retention of the dye indicates:

1. Impaired hepatic uptake
2. Reduced ability of the parenchymal cells to take up the dye from blood
3. Faulty excretion into the bile.

Therefore, this test has little value in the differential diagnosis of jaundice.

This test has abundant complexities and occasional side effects, which may be fatal.

Tests Related to Bile Pigment Metabolism

Bilirubin

The bilirubin metabolism is altered when there is:

- Increased load of bilirubin to the liver
- Reduced hepatic uptake
- Reduced intracellular transport
- Reduced conjugation and excretion of bilirubin
- Obstruction to the flow of bile.

One or more of the above problems leads to elevated bilirubin, causing jaundice.

Jaundice

- Jaundice comes from the French word *jaune*, which means yellow.
- Normal serum bilirubin concentration is around 1.2 mg/100 mL.
- When the bilirubin level exceeds more than 2.0 mg%, it diffuses into the tissues. The skin and sclera of the eye turn yellow. The condition is called jaundice (icterus).
- The yellowish coloration is caused by an excess amount of bilirubin in the skin.
- Bilirubin is a yellowish-red pigment.
- Normally, small amounts of bilirubin are found in everyone's blood.
- When too much bilirubin is made, the excess is dumped into the bloodstream and is deposited in tissues for temporary storage.
- Jaundice in the infant appears first in the face and upper body and progresses downwards towards the toes.

Formation and Metabolism of Bilirubin

- Once bilirubin is formed, it binds to albumin and is transported to the liver.
- In the liver, it is separated from the albumin and the bilirubin is taken up by the liver cells.
- In the liver, the UDP glucuronyl transferase enzyme conjugates the bilirubin with two molecules of UDP glucuronic acid to form a conjugated bilirubin called bilirubin diglucuronide.
- Normally, the bilirubin is secreted into the bile through bile duct. The conjugated bilirubin reaches the intestine through the bile.
- The intestinal bacteria act on it and deconjugate the conjugated bilirubin.

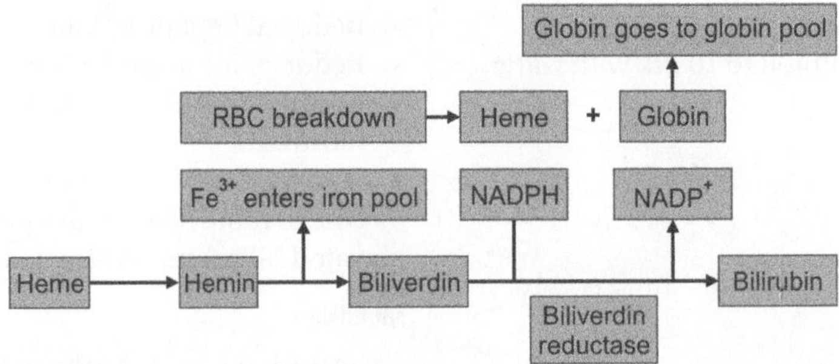

- The free bilirubin then gets reduced to colorless tetrapyrrole urobilinogen.
- Then 20% of this urobilinogen is reabsorbed from the intestine and returned to the liver by portal blood. The urobilinogen is again re-excreted.
- The urobilinogen is also excreted through blood, but it is negligible.
- The urobilinogen is further reduced to stercobilinogen and excreted through feces (around 200–300 mg/day).
- The urobilinogen and stercobilinogen are colorless compounds; but when they are exposed to atmospheric oxidation, they are converted to a colored urobilin and stercobilin respectively.
- The conjugated water-soluble bilirubin when treated with diazo reagent ($NaNO3^+$ sulfanilic acid) gives a red color immediately. This is called direct van den Bergh's test. The conjugated bilirubin reacts directly without adding methanol so it is also called direct bilirubin.
- The water insoluble unconjugated bilirubin gives a positive van den Bergh's test only if methanol is added to the serum. This is the indirect van den Bergh's test. This also called indirect bilirubin.
- The water-soluble free conjugated bilirubin can be filtered through the glomerular membrane and excreted in the urine when there is a increase in the blood levels of conjugated bilirubin.
- The water-insoluble unconjugated bilirubin is not filtered by the glomerular membrane as it is bound to albumin; hence, it does not appear in the urine, whenever the blood level of unconjugated bilirubin is increased.

There are three different types of jaundice.

Causes and Laboratory Findings of Different Types of Jaundice

Hemolytic Jaundice

This type of jaundice mainly arises due to excessive breakdown of red blood cells (RBCs).

This type of jaundice is common in newborn babies where bilirubin formed and released into the bloodstream when RBCs are broken down. Infants have too many RBCs. It is natural process for the baby's body to breakdown the excess red blood cells, forming a large amount of bilirubin. It is this bilirubin that causes the skin to take on a yellowish color. A newborn's liver is immature and cannot process bilirubin as quickly as it will be able to when it gets older. This slow processing of bilirubin has nothing to do with liver disease. It merely means that the baby's liver is not as fully developed, as it will be, and thus, there is some delay in eliminating the bilirubin.

Most babies with jaundice have physiologic jaundice.

Physiologic Jaundice

Occasionally, there are other factors that cause jaundice in an infant. Two of these are

Specimen	Prehepatic or hemolytic	Hepatic	Posthepatic or obstructive
Causes	Abnormal red cells; Antibodies; abnormal hemoglobin	Viral hepatitis; toxic hepatitis; intrahepatic cholestasis; drugs, and toxins	Extrahepatic cholestasis; gallstones; tumor of bile duct; carcinoma of pancreas
Blood			
Unconjugated bilirubin Conjugated bilirubin	Present (++) Normal	Present (++) Increases in early phase and later decreases	Normal Present (++)
Urine			
Bile salt (Hay's test)	Absent	Absent	Present
Conjugated bilirubin (Fouchet's test)	Absent	Present	Present
Urobilinogen (Ehrlich's test)	Present (+++)	Increases in early phase and later decreases	Absent
Feces			
Urobilins	Present (++)	In intrahepatic cholestasis decreases	Clay colored
Serum enzymes			
ALP	Normal	Moderately increased	Increased markedly
ALT	Normal	Increased markedly	Moderately increased
AST	Normal	Increased markedly	Moderately increased
GGT	Normal	Moderately increased	Increased

conditions known as ABO incompatibility and Rh incompatibility. Both of these conditions result in a very fast breakdown of RBCs. Also, jaundice may appear in infants with physical defects in the organs that work to eliminate bilirubin from the body and decrease conjugating enzymes.

Treatment for Neonatal Jaundice

If the level of bilirubin is high and needling treatment, it is usually treated with phototherapy. This means the undressed baby is placed under special lights. The lights may be white, blue or green. Or, the baby can be placed on a light producing blanket. The light helps to breakdown the bilirubin in the skin. It may cause the baby to have runny stools. It may not be good for babies to have bright light continuously shining in their eyes. The eyes are covered to protect them from so much light. If a baby has only the phototherapy blanket, the eyes do not need to be covered.

Biochemical Findings

Elevated total bilirubin (High Indirect Bilirubin).

Hepatic Jaundice

This type of jaundice mainly arises due to the damage of the parenchymal liver cells (refer table for details).

Biochemical findings: High total bilirubin (beginning direct bilirubin elevated then later it will be indirect bilirubin).

ALP increases moderately.

Very high AST and ALT.

Obstructive or Posthepatic Jaundice

Obstruction to the flow of bile causes the conjugated bilirubin to return to the blood.

Therefore, the serum contains increased amount of direct bilirubin.

Biochemical Findings

High total bilirubin (Direct bilirubin high).

Marked increase in serum ALP and direct bilirubin.

Moderate increase in AST, ALT (may be normal).

- Thus, ALP and bilirubin estimation can be used as one of the indices to differentiate hepatic jaundice and posthepatic jaundice.

Estimation of Serum Billirubin by Malloy and Evelyn Method

Principle

Bilirubin of serum reacts with diazo reagent to form a colored complex, which is measured at 540 nm photometrically. Conjugated bilirubin (direct bilirubin) undergoes color reaction directly, whereas unconjugated bilirubin (indirect bilirubin) forms color after the addition of alcohol. Total bilirubin is the sum of direct and indirect bilirubin. Indirect reaction gives the concentration of total bilirubin and direct reaction gives that of direct bilirubin. Concentration of indirect bilirubin is obtained by taking the difference between the total and direct bilirubin.

Reagents

1. Absolute methanol
2. *HCl 1.5%:* 4.2 mL concentration HCl diluted to 100 mL with distilled water.
3. *Diazo reagent:*
   - Solution A: 0.1 g of sulfanilic acid is dissolved in 1.5 mL concentrated HCl and made up to 100 mL with water.
   - Solution B: 0.5 g of sodium nitrite is dissolved in 100 mL of water.
   - Diazo reagent is prepared freshly by mixing 10 mL of solution A and 0.3 mL of solution B.
4. *Standard bilirubin:* 0.1 mg/mL: 5 mg of bilirubin is dissolved in 50 mL of chloroform stored in a brown bottle. Keep in dark place.

Procedure

Dilute 1 mL of serum to 20 mL with water in a conical flask and mix.

Total bilirubin: Label two tubes as Test (Tt) and Blank (Tb). Into Tb pipette 5 mL of methanol, 1 mL of 1.5% HCl and 4 mL of diluted serum (1 in 20).

Into Tt pipette 5 mL of methanol, 1 mL of diazo reagent and 4 mL of diluted serum. Mix both the tubes. Stand at room temperature for 30 minutes. After 30 minutes read the absorbance using green filter or at 540 nm.

Direct Bilirubin

Mark two test tubes as Test (Dt) and Blank (Db). Into Db, pipette 5 mL of water, 1 mL of 1.5% HCl and 4 mL of diluted serum. Into Dt pipette 5 mL of water, 1 mL of diazo reagent and 4 mL of diluted serum. Mix both the tubes. Let stand at room temperature for 30 minutes.

Standard

Label two test tubes as Standard (S) and Blank (Sb). Into S pipette 8.8 mL of methanol, 1 mL of diazo reagent and 0.2 mL of standard. Into Sb pipette 8.8 mL of methanol, 1 mL of 1.5% HCl and 0.2 mL serum. Mix and keep at room temperature for 30 minutes. Read absorbance at 540 nm or using green filter.

Reagents	*Tt*	*Tb*	*Dt*	*Db*	*S*	*Sb*
Methanol (mL)	5	5	–	–	8.8	8.8
Water (mL)	–	–	5	5	–	–
Diazo reagent	1 mL	–	1	–	1	–
1.5% HCl (mL)	–	1	–	1	–	1
Diluted serum	4	4	4	4	–	–
Standard bilirubin (mL)	–	–	–	–	0.2	0.2
Mixed and kept for 20–30 minutes						
Read the OD at 540 nm (Green)						

Calculation

$$\frac{\text{OD of Tt} - \text{OD of TB}}{\text{OD of S} - \text{0.0 of Sb}} \times 0.02 \times \frac{20}{4} \times 100$$

100 mL serum contains

$$= \frac{\text{OD of Tt} - \text{OD of TB}}{\text{OD of S} - \text{OD of Sb}} \times 0.02 \times \frac{100}{0.2}$$

$$= \frac{\text{OD of Dt} - \text{OD of Db}}{\text{OD of S} - \text{OD of Sb}} \times 10$$

Note: Bilirubin deteriorates in light. If the assay is delayed, store the serum in the dark and in refrigerator.

Estimation of Serum Bilirubin by Direct Spectral Method

Principle

The method is dependent on direct measurement of bilirubin natural yellow color by spectrophotometer (measurement of absorption at 450 and 575 nm). For this, a spectrophotometer is essential. The absorbance values are then applied to an equation of two unknown. The wavelength of minor Hb peak at 575 nm has been shown to be that at which Hb absorbance is almost equal to its contribution at a wavelength of normal bilirubin absorption.

Reagents

NaCl 0.9%: 0.9 g of NaCl in 100 mL H_2O.

Procedure

5 mL of 0.9% NaCl solution (normal saline) is taken in a test tube. To that 100 μL (0.1 mL) of serum is added, mixed and absorption is taken at 450 and 575 nm using spectrophotometer. At 450 nm bilirubin and Hb gives reading. At 575 nm only Hb answers.

Calculation

$$\text{Amount of bilirubin} = \frac{(a-b)\times 5000 - 0.44 \text{ mg/dL}}{\text{Vol. of serum}}$$

a = A × 1.28 = 0.084 × 1.28 = 0.1075
b = B × 1.43 = 0.017 × 1.43 = 0.0243
A = Absorbance at 450 nm
B = Absorbance at 575 nm

$$\text{Amount of bilirubin} = \frac{(0.1075 - 0.0243)\times 5000}{100} - 0.44$$

= 0.0832 × 50 - 0.44
= 4.16 - 0.44
= 3.72 mg/dL

1.28 and 1.43 are factors fixed for wavelengths 450 and 575 nm because there is no standard or control. Factors differ from instrument to instrument.

0.44 → is the correction factor for other pigments.

450 → maximum absorption including Hb (i.e., all the compounds containing porphyrin ring) 575 → at this nm Hb will give absorbance.

In the hemolyzed sample, at 450 nm, the value will be more because OD due to Hb will add to this increased value. At 575 nm, only Hb will give a value. So the difference between these will give the absorbance due to bilirubin.

Advantage

Less sample is required (convenient for neonatal cases).

Disadvantage

Only total bilirubin can be estimated.

Normal Values

Total bilirubin = 0.2–1 mg %
Direct bilirubin = 0–0.2 mg %
Indirect bilirubin = 0–0.8 mg %.

Estimation of Bilirubin by Capillary Method

Blood is collected in a capillary. Centrifuge the sample using a special centrifuge, which is meant for capillary tubes.

Take out the plasma from Hamilton syringe
Add 2.5 mL of normal saline (0.9% NaCl)
Read the absorbance at 450 nm and 575 nm separately in the spectrophotometer.

Calculation

$$\frac{\text{OD of 450 nm} \times \text{O.D of 575 nm} \times \text{volume of saline}}{\text{Sample volume}}$$

Final result - 0.44 = mg of bilirubin

At 450 nm both hemolyzed and nonhemolyzed bilirubin is measured.

At 575 nm only hemolyzed bilirubin is measured.

The bilirubin and bile salts in urine are detected by Fouchet's and Hay's test respectively.

Fouchet's Test

Add a few mL of barium chloride solution (100 g/L) and a pinch of magnesium sulfate to about 10 mL of urine in a test tube. Filter, dry the filtrate on a filter paper and add a drop of Fouchet's reagent [25 g TCA + 10 mL ferric chloride (100 g/L) + 100 mL water] on the filtrate. A greenish color, an oxidation product of bilirubin is obtained if bilirubin is present in the sample.

Hay's Test

Sprinkle the sulfur powder on the urine sample contained in a test tube. The sulfur powder sinks to the bottom of the tube if bile salts are present in the urine because bile salts have the property of lowering the surface tension.

In jaundice, with unconjugated hyperbilirubinemia, there is no excretion of bilirubin and bile salts in the urine and the urine is of a normal color. Jaundice with conjugated hyperbilirubinemia, there is an excretion of bilirubin and bile salts in urine, which results in deep yellow or dark color of urine. This will be seen usually in regurgitation jaundice, infective or toxic hepatitis.

Urobilinogen in Urine and Feces

The presence of urobilinogen in a test sample can be demonstrated by a test based on the production of red color when urobilinogen reacts with *Ehrlich's aldehyde reagent*.

The *excess bilirubin* formed in *hemolytic jaundice* enters the intestine through bile; there it will be converted to *urobilinogen*. Then it leads to excretion of *more urobilinogen* in the urine and feces.

In a patient with liver disease accompanied by hepatocellular damage, relatively less bilirubin is excreted in the intestine through the bile as compared to a normal person. However, during enterohepatic circulation the excretion of the urobilinogen by the hepatocytes is impaired, resulting in the release of higher proportion of urobilinogen, which subsequently appears in urine. Therefore, the amount of urobilinogen in urine is higher than normal in this condition. But in feces it is very low.

In patients with obstructive jaundice, the urobilinogen in urine and feces is reduced or absent. The stool in obstructive jaundice is clay colored. For several reasons, urine and feces urobilinogen determinations do not provide useful information for the evaluation of hepatobiliary disease.

Serum Enzymes in Liver Disease

The assay of serum enzymes is very useful for the differential diagnosis and monitoring of various hepatobiliary disorders.

There are three types of enzymes:

1. Enzymes, which are normally present inside the hepatocytes, released into the blood when there is hepatocellular damage → Markers for hepatocellular damage.
2. Enzymes, which are primarily membrane bound (plasma membrane or side of hepatocytes) → Markers for cholestasis.
3. Enzymes, which are synthesized in the hepatocyte → Indicates disturbances in the hepatocellular synthesis.

Evidence of Hepatocellular Damage

Serum Transaminases

- The aminotransferases catalyze chemical reactions in which an amino group from one amino acid (amino acids are building blocks of proteins) is transferred from a donor molecule to a recipient molecule. Hence, the names "aminotransferases". Another name for aminotransferase is transaminase.
- The enzyme aspartate aminotransferase (AST) is also known as serum glutamic oxaloacetic transaminase (SGOT).

- Alanine aminotransferase (ALT) is also known as serum glutamic pyruvic transaminase (SGPT).

Aspartate Transaminase (AST) and Alanine Transaminase (ALT)

- *Location:* AST present in cytosol and mitochondria.
- ALT located in cytosol of liver.
- In the liver, the concentration of ALT per unit weight of the tissue is more than AST.
- These enzymes are more important in assessing and monitoring the degree of liver cell inflammation and necrosis.
- The highest activities of ALT are found in hepatocytes and muscle cells.
- Again the hepatocytes has very high activity of ALT.
- Therefore, elevations in scrum ALT are considered to be relatively specific for liver disease.
- AST may be elevated in other forms of tissue damage, such as myocardial infarction, muscle necrosis and renal disorders.
- In liver disease, the ALT level is increased markedly compared to AST.
- In acute viral hepatitis, there is a 100–1000 times increase in both ALT and AST but ALT level is increased more than that of AST.
- A variety of medications can cause abnormal liver enzymes levels.
- Examples of some of the common medications with potential liver toxicity include: Aspirin, acetaminophen (Tylenol), ibuprofen (Advil, Motrin), naproxen (Naprosyn, Naprelan, Anaprox, Aleve), diclofenac (Voltaren, Cataflam, Voltaren-XR), phenylbutazone (Butazolidin), valproic acid (Depakote, Depakote ER, Depakene, Depacon), carbamazepine (Tegretol, Tegretol XR, Equetro), phenobarbital, tetracyclines, [for example, tetracycline (Achromycin)], sulfonamides, isoniazid (INH) (Nydrazid, Laniazid), sulfamethoxazole (Gantanol), trimethoprim cholesterol lowering drugs.

Estimation of AST and ALT: (Refer unit 14)

Evidence for Cholestasis

Alkaline Phosphate

- The serum alkaline phosphate (ALP) estimation is the most widely used biochemical test to put in evidence for cholestasis of intra-or extrahepatic origin.
- ALP is a phospho-monoesterase enzyme whose optimum pH is in the alkaline range.
- It is localized in the microvilli of biliary canaliculi, located in the plasma membrane.
- Besides liver, ALP is also located in other tissues, such as bone, kidney, placenta and the small intestine. There are five isoenzymes of ALP corresponding to five tissues of origin.
- The ALP from liver is the fastest moving isoenzyme in electrophoresis.
- Normal level = 4–13 KA units or 40–140 IU/L.
- Increase in serum level of alkaline phosphatase from liver is a very sensitive indicator of cholestasis.
- Elevated ALP in cholestasis may be due to two features:
  1. Regurgitation of ALP from bile to blood and
  2. Increased synthesis from the cells lining the biliary canaliculi.
- In obstructive jaundice the ALP level becomes very high (30 KA Units).
- The method for estimation is the *King and Armstrong* method.

In this method, the disodium phenyl phosphate is used as substrate. Action of ALP on this compound liberates phenol and phosphate. The phenol produced in the reaction is estimated by forming a colored product with 4-aminoantipyrine. The enzyme activity is expressed as King and Armstrong units (KA units).

Disodium phenyl phosphate $\xrightarrow{ALP}$ Phenol + phosphate

Phenol + 4-aminoantipyrine—red colored product → measured colorimetrically

For procedure refer unit 14.

Gamma Glutamyl Transferase (GGT)

This enzyme catalyzes the transfer of γ-glutamyl group from glutamyl peptides to another peptide or an amino acid.

Principle

γ-glutamyl-P-nitroanilide + Glycyl glycine $\xrightarrow{GGT}$

γ-glutamylglycyl glycine + P – nitroaniline

- GGT catalyzes the transfer of the γ-glutamyl group from the substrate γ-glutamyl peptides to another peptide, such as glycyl glycine forming γ-glutamylglycyl glycine and P-nitroaniline. P-nitroaniline has maximum absorbance at 405 nm.
- GGT is a marker of cholestasis.
- The GGT level is increased both in liver disease and in cholestasis but the level is very high in cholestasis.
- Both GGT and ALP are increased in liver disease.
- However, the GGT in blood is not affected in bone diseases (in children).
- Its activity is induced by alcohol and also drugs like phenytoin.
- The increased level of GGT is seen in cirrhosis of liver or chronic alcoholism as etiology.

Therefore, it is also considered as the marker enzyme for alcoholic cirrhosis.

Normal value: 10–50 U/L.

HEPATITIS MARKERS

- 'Hepatitis' the combination of 'hepatic'+ 'itis' means inflammation of the liver.
- The causes of hepatitis can be divided into infectious and noninfectious.
- The infectious causes include bacteria and more commonly viruses.
- Any attack by foreign organisms to the liver can kill hepatocytes and recruit inflammatory cells.
- Inflammatory diseases are long-term chronic conditions that must be managed medically. Among inflammatory disorders, infections are the most common.
- For correct diagnosis, it is important to understand the host immune response, the disease and clinical stage and the types of viral hepatitis.

The recognized types of viral hepatitis are:

- Hepatitis A—caused by hepatitis A virus (HAV)
- Hepatitis B—caused by hepatitis B virus (HBV)
- Hepatitis C—caused by hepatitis C virus (HCV)
- Hepatitis D—caused by hepatitis delta virus (HDV)
- Hepatitis E—caused by hepatitis E virus (HEV)

Of these, hepatitis A and E are spread through contaminated food and water, whereas hepatitis B, C and D are spread parenterally, sexually, through transfusion of infected blood, by use of infected needles.

Hepatitis A Viruses

- Hepatitis A virus (HAV) is an enterovirus.
- HAV does not cause chronic hepatitis or carrier state so fatality associated is only 0.1%.
- The hepatitis A antigen is a small unenveloped, single stranded RNA-containing virus and is the only hepatic virus, which has been grown in culture.
- It is spread by the ingestion of contaminated water and food and is shed in stool for 2–3 weeks before and 1 week after the onset of jaundice.
- Thus, close personal contact or fecal oral contamination during this period accounts for most cases.

- The prevalence of infection is measured by the presence of HAV Ag, HAV antibodies IgG and IgM.

HAV IgG

- It is used as a marker for past hepatitis infection.
- It peaks after the acute illness and remains detectable indefinitely, perhaps lifelong.
- The demonstration of HAV IgG indicates previous infections.
- It protects against subsequent infection with hepatitis A virus but is not protective against hepatitis B or other viruses.

HAV AB-M

- Determination of IgM antibody to hepatitis A virus (IgM anti-HAV) in serum or plasma aid in the diagnosis of acute or recent (usually present for up to 6 to 9 months) hepatitis A viral infection.
- Hepatitis A is a self-limiting disease and is often a subclinical disorder, particularly in children. Since symptomatic hepatitis A viral (HAV) infections can be clinically indistinguishable from infection with hepatitis B or C virus, serological testing is an important tool to achieve proper diagnosis.
- During the acute phase of HAV infection, IgM class antibody to HAV appears in the serum and is nearly always detectable at the onset of symptoms.
- In most cases, IgM anti-HAV response usually peaks within the first 6 months, declining to nondetectable levels within 12 months.
- IgM anti-HAV is not detected in normal subjects whether or nor they have the IgG antibody to the hepatitis A virus (IgG anti-HAV).

Hepatitis B Virus

- Hepatitis B virus (HBV) is a hepadnavirus.
- It is a small enveloped DNA virus containing 3.2 kb.
- The hepatitis B virus consists of a surface and a core.
- The core contains a DNA polymerase and the E antigen.
- The DNA structure is double stranded and circular.
- There are four major polypeptide reading frames (genes):
  1. The S (surface) gene codes for protein surface antigens (Hbs Ag) an envelope glycoprotein present on the outer surface.
  2. The C (core): The C gene is divided into two regions the precore and the core, and codes for two different proteins, the Core antigen (Hbc Ag) and the E antigen (Hbe Ag).
  3. The P (polymerase).
  4. The X (transcriptional transactivating).
- HBV is classically acquired through a blood transfusion.
- It is present in blood and all physiologic and pathologic body fluids.
- Thus, blood and body fluids are the primary vehicles of transmission.
- Virus may also be spread by contact with body secretions, such as saliva, sweat, semen, tears, breast milk and pathologic effusion.

HBs Ag

- It indicates the patient is infected with the HBV.
- It is a first serological marker to appear postinfection.
- Especially important for pretransfusion diagnosis.
- Persistence for more than 6 months indicates chronic state.

CORE-M

IgM antibody to HBV core antigen (IgM Anti-HBc).

- Determination of IgM antibody to HBV core antigen in human serum or plasma aid in the diagnosis of acute or recent (usually 6 months or less) hepatitis B viral infection.

- It is reliable marker for acute viral disease.
- Anti-HBc (both IgM and IgG antibodies) is detected in before or at the onset of symptoms; however, such reactivity can persist for years after illness, may even outlast anti-HBs and, occasionally, may be the only marker of either current or past infection.
- Several studies have demonstrated that IgM anti-HBc is the only specific marker for the diagnosis of acute infection with hepatitis B.

HBe Antigen

- HBe Ag determination can be used to monitor the progress of hepatitis B viral infection.
- HBe Ag is found in the early phase of hepatitis B infection after the appearance of hepatitis B surface antigen.
- The titers of both antigens rise rapidly during the period of viral replication.
- The presence of HBe Ag correlates with increased numbers of infectious viruses, the occurrence of core particles in the nucleus of the hepatocyte, and the presence of viral specific DNA polymerase in serum.
- During the HBe Ag positive stage, hepatitis B patients are at risk of transmitting the virus to their contacts.
- Persistence of HBe Ag in the HBV carrier is often associated with chronic active hepatitis.

Anti-HBe

- Detection of antibody to hepatitis Be antigen (Anti-HBe) in human serum or plasma aid in the diagnosis and monitoring of hepatitis B viral infection.
- Hepatitis Be antigen (HBe Ag) and its antibody, anti-HBe, are found only in association with hepatitis B viral infection.
- HBe Ag becomes undetectable after the peak of viral replication and onset of resolution of disease.
- A negative HBe Ag result alone may indicate—(a) early HBe antigenemia before the peak of viral infection or (b) early convalescence when HBe Ag has declined below detectable levels.
- The presence of anti-HBe serves to distinguish between these two periods.
- The appearance of anti-HBe indicates a reduced level of infectious virus due to a decrease in viral replication.

Hepatitis C Virus

- Hepatitis C Virus (HCV) is an envelope blood-borne virus closely associated with blood transfusion.
- Serological studies employing enzyme immunoassays for detection of antibodies to recombinant antigens of HCV (anti-HCV) have established HCV as the cause of most blood-borne as well as community, acquired non-A, non-B hepatitis.
- The presence of anti-HCV indicates that an individual may have been infected with HCV, may harbor infectious HCV and/or may be capable of transmitting HCV infection.
- Although the majority of infected individuals may be asymptomatic, HCV infection may develop into chronic hepatitis, cirrhosis or increased risk of hepatocellular carcinoma.
- The implementation of blood screening for anti-HCV before blood transfusion decreases the risk of transfusion-transmitted hepatitis.

Hepatitis D

- Hepatitis D virus (also called delta virus) is a small circular RNA virus.

- The hepatitis D virus is replication defective and therefore cannot propagate in the absence of another virus.
- In humans, the hepatitis D virus infection only occurs in the presence of hepatitis B infection.

Hepatitis E

- Hepatitis E virus is an important cause of enterically transmitted acute viral hepatitis in several developing countries and is transmitted by fecal-oral route.
- In disease endemic areas, individuals who have recovered from acute hepatitis E are unlikely to serve as a reservoir of HEV infection.

Importance of Various Hepatitis Markers (Complete Diagnosis of Hepatitis)

HAV IgG	Indicates past infection with HAV and immunity to HAV.
HAV IgM	Positive in acute hepatitis A infection. Peak at 3–4 weeks from onset of symptoms.
HAV Ab	Indicates acute infection when positive with HAV IgM. Remains positive during and after the resolving stage for a long time, falls slowly. HAV Ab is present post-vaccination.
HBs Ag (Hep B Surface Ag)	Indicates infection with the hepatitis B virus. First serological marker to appear postinfection. Especially important for pre-transfusion diagnosis. Persistence for >6 months indicates chronic state.
HBe Ag (Hep B Envelope Ag)	Indicates active viral replication. Patient is highly infectious. HBe Ag negative with HBV DNA positive indicates the person is infected with the precore mutant
HBc Ag	Extensively surrounded by HBs Ag Not freely detectable in the serum.
Anti-HBs	Marker of recovery and immunity Appears during convalescence A level > 10 IU following hepatitis B immunization is considered to be protective against HBV infection
Anti-HBe	Reduced viral replication. Inactive liver disease. Reduced infectious state.
Anti-HBc IgM	Differentiates between chronic and acute infection. Positive in acute infection.
Anti-HBc IgG	Indicates exposure to HBV. Always detected in HBV infection.
Anti-HCV	Indicates past or present HCV infection. All positive EIA results should be verified using supplemental assay (PCR/WB).
HCV RNA	Detects presence or absence of hepatitis C virus. Helps to differentiate between acute, chronic or past infection.
HDV IgM	With positive hepatitis B infection, HDV IgM reflects the presence of HDV Infection. High titers of HDV IgM are associated with superinfection. Positive with positive anti-HBc IgM is associated with hepatitis D coinfection.
HDV IgG	High titers during hepatitis D chronic superinfection.
HEV IgM	Acute HEV infection. Indicates recent exposure to HEV.

HEV IgG	Immunity/Old infection. Performed when HEV IgM is negative.

SELF TEST

1. List the tests under the LFT panel.
2. What are the indications of LFT?
3. What are the functions performed by the liver?
4. Name the tests related to protein metabolism.
5. Give the normal values for:
   a. Total protein
   b. Albumin
   c. Alanine transaminase
   d. Aspartate transaminase
   e. Total bilirubin
   f. Direct bilirubin.
6. Write the procedure of the hippuric acid test.
7. Draw a flowchart to show the formation of bilirubin from the RBC.
8. What are the steps involved during bilirubin excretion?
9. Mention the conditions in which bilirubin metabolism and excretion are disturbed.
10. Define jaundice.
11. What are the different types of jaundice?
12. Write the biochemical findings of any two types of jaundice.
13. State the method of bilirubin estimation.
14. What are direct and indirect van den Bergh's tests?
15. Which test is used to find the bilirubin in the urine and what is the procedure?
16. Why do bile salts sink to the bottom of the solution if it is present in the urine?
17. Which enzymes are considered as marker enzymes for hepatocellular damage?
18. State the enzymes, which are used as marker enzymes to detect the cholestasis.
19. How many isoenzyme forms of ALP exist?
20. Give the normal value of alkaline phosphatase.
21. Briefly discuss the following hepatitis markers:
    a. Hepatitis A
    b. Hepatitis B
    c. Hepatitis C.

MULTIPLE CHOICE QUESTIONS

1. ___________ increases in neonatal jaundice:
   a. Direct bilirubin
   b. Indirect bilirubin
   c. Direct and indirect bilirubin
   d. None of the above

2. The marker enzyme for alcoholic cirrhosis is:
   a. ALP
   b. AST
   c. GGT
   d. ALT

3. ___________ increases in obstructive jaundice.
   a. Direct bilirubin
   b. Indirect bilirubin
   c. Direct and indirect bilirubin
   d. None of the above

4. In the case of the direct van den Bergh's test:
   a. Only unconjugated bilirubin gives red color
   b. The conjugated bilirubin gives color without the addition of methanol
   c. Both conjugated and unconjugated bilirubin give red color
   d. The conjugated bilirubin gives color with the addition of methanol

5. The test used to detect bilirubin in blood is:
   a. Fouchet's test
   b. Malloy and Evelyn test
   c. Zak's method
   d. Ehrlich's test

6. **All the following are indications of LFT, *except:***
   a. Differential diagnosis of jaundice
   b. Detection of liver diseases
   c. Assessment of severity and prognosis of liver disease
   d. Detection of renal disease
7. **Which of the following is not a biochemical finding of hemolytic jaundice?**
   a. Elevated total bilirubin
   b. Reduced albumin
   c. Elevated indirect bilirubin
   d. Normal ALP
8. **The enzyme, which helps to differentiate between bone disease and jaundice is:**
   A.A a. ALP
   b. AST
   c. GGT
   d. ALT
9. **Which of the following helps in the differential diagnosis of jaundice?**
   a. Direct bilirubin
   b. AST
   c. Protein
   d. Prothrombin time

CASE STUDIES

1. Mr David, a 40-year-old man who travels lot and recently visited two countries. After a month of his return, he started getting the symptoms of dark urine, abdominal swelling, pruritus (itching), complaining loss of appetite, unexplained weight loss or gain, and abdominal pain. He rushed to the hospital and the physician after physical examination ordered for LFT and RFT. The requested laboratory tests revealed the following results:

Parameter	Result
Serum bilirubin	10.0 mg%
Direct bilirubin	5.2 mg%
Indirect bilirubin	4.8 mg%
AST	200 units/L
ALT	800 units/L
Alkaline phosphatase	170 units/L
HBS Ag	Positive
Urea	20 mg/dL
Creatinine	0.8 mg/dL
Blood sugar	80 mg/dL

   a. Which tubes were used for collecting blood for analyzing the above parameters?
   b. What diagnosis can be made using the above laboratory results?
   c. What could be the cause for his elevated bilirubin and enzymes?
   d. Explain with reasons for your diagnosis and symptoms mentioned.
2. Mr Jackman, a 40-year-old man who travels lot and recently visited two countries. After a month of his return he started getting the symptoms of dark urine, abdominal swelling, pruritus (itching), complaining loss of appetite, unexplained weight loss or gain, and abdominal pain. His wife took him doctor. The physician examined him and noticed swelling in liver below the ribs. He ordered for LFT test. The laboratory revealed the following results:

Parameter	Result
Serum bilirubin	10.0 mg%
Direct bilirubin	5.2 mg%
Indirect bilirubin	4.8 mg%
AST	200 units/L
ALT	800 units/L
Alkaline phosphatase	140 units/L
HBS Ag	Positive
Prothrombin time	Delayed

   a. What diagnosis made using the above laboratory results?
   b. Explain with reasons for your diagnosis and symptoms mentioned.
3. Mrs Lucy, admitted at gynecology ward, delivered a baby. The neonatologist examined the baby and noticed the yellowish skin and sclera of the eye and

decided to put the baby in phototherapy treatment.

Also he sent the blood sample for mini LFT from the laboratory. The laboratory results appear as follows:

Parameter	Result
Serum bilirubin	8.0 mg%
Direct bilirubin	0.2 mg%
Indirect bilirubin	4.8 mg%
AST	25 units/L
ALT	28 units/L

a. What type of jaundice the baby diagnosed with the available laboratory results?
b. Why phototherapy suggested?

4. Mr X, admitted to the adult emergency ward with a symptoms of anorexia and abdominal pain. The physician examined him and noticed yellowish discoloration of the skin and sclera of the eye. Then he requested for blood and urine test. The laboratory revealed the following results:

Parameter	Result
Serum bilirubin	12 mg%
Direct bilirubin	11.6 mg%
Indirect bilirubin	0.4 mg%
AST	55 units/L
ALT	60 units/L
Alkaline phosphatase	300 units/L
Urine bile pigments	++
Urine bile salts	++
Urobilinogen	Negative

a. What diagnosis would be made using the laboratory results?
b. Explain with reasons for the above mentioned symptoms.

5. Steve, a 35-year-old man was admitted to the hospital with the symptoms of anorexia (loss of appetite) vomiting, and diarrhea. He mentioned to the physician that his urine was dark in color and passed the light stools. Blood and urine analysis, which were requested revealed the following results:

Parameter	Result
Serum bilirubin	7.0 mg%
Direct bilirubin	4.2 mg%
Indirect bilirubin	2.8 mg%
AST	80 units/L
ALT	160 units/L
Alkaline phosphatase	80 units/L
Protein	7.5 g/dL
Albumin	4.5 g/dL
Urine bile salts	Absent
Urine bilirubin	Present
Urobilinogen	Present

a. What diagnosis can be made with the available laboratory results?
b. Give specific reasons for elevated bilirubin and transaminase enzymes?
c. Why the protein value remains normal?

6. A 36-year old man was admitted to a hospital following episodes of nausea, vomiting, and general malaise. His urine was darker than usual. Upon examination it was discovered that his liver was enlarged and tender to palpation. Liver function tests were abnormal; plasma ALT was 1500 IU/L; AST was 400 IU/L. During the next 24 hours, the man developed jaundice, and his plasma total bilirubin was 9.0 mg/dL (154 mmol/L). A diagnosis of hepatitis was made.
   a. What reactions are catalyzed by AST and ALT? What is the coenzyme?
   b. What conditions are important to maintain in performing the enzyme assays?
   c. Which other enzymes might have been elevated in the plasma?
   d. How does "total" bilirubin relate to "direct" and "indirect" bilirubin?
7. A 50-year-old woman complained to her physician of generalized severe itching during the previous 10 months. She had no other serious symptoms and she

mentioned that her alcohol consumption was 2–3 U/week. On clinical examination, she was slightly jaundiced with her eyes light yellow and bilirubin was detected both in blood and urine. The results of LFT were as follows:

Parameter	Result	Reference range
Total protein	7.0	5.0–8.0 g/dL
Albumin	3.9	3.5–5.0 g/dL
ALP	400	40–140 U/L
AST	200	5–40 U/L
ALT	450	5–40 U/L
Total bilirubin	6.0	0.2–1.0 mg/dL
Direct bilirubin	5.2	0–0.2 mg/dL
Indirect bilirubin	0.8	0–0.8 mg/dL

a. What is the most likely diagnosis?
b. How would you make a definite diagnosis?
c. Why ALT, ALP and direct bilirubin are high in this patient?
d. What is the cause for her itching?

16 UNIT

Factors Involved in Hemoglobin Synthesis

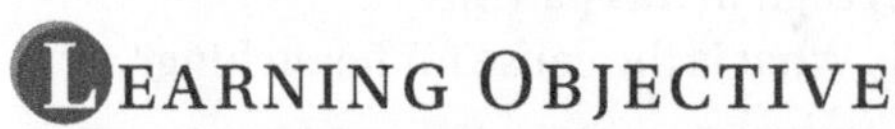

LEARNING OBJECTIVES

At the end of this unit, the learner should be able to understand:
- Structure and synthesis of hemoglobin.
- The role of iron, folic acid and vitamin B12 in the synthesis of hemoglobin.
- Importance of determination of iron, iron binding capacity and ferritin in determining anemia.
- Abnormal hemoglobin, sickle cell hemoglobin and thalassemia.

INTRODUCTION

- Hemoglobin is the iron-containing oxygen-transport conjugated metalloprotein in the red cells of the blood in mammals *and other animals.*
- Hemoglobin in vertebrates transports oxygen from the lungs to the rest of the body, such as to the muscles, where it releases the oxygen load.
- Hemoglobin synthesis takes place in the bone marrow.
- Its molecular weight is 68,000.
- Its blood level is 12–16 g/dL.
- The synthesis of hemoglobin depends on three important factors; they are iron, folic acid, and vitamin B_{12} along with amino acids.
- Deficiency of any of these factors decreases the ability of the bone marrow to synthesize RBC, thus causing anemia.
- Hemoglobin is the red pigment present in RBCs, which transports O_2 to the tissues.
- It consists of 4 heme molecules linked to the protein portion called "globin". Globin part consists of 4 polypeptide chains.
- Each heme molecule is located in a pocket formed by the folding of a polypeptide chain.
- The normal adult blood consists of two types of Hb, they are HbA_1 and HbA_2.
- HbA_1 comprises 96% and HbA_2 is about 3% of the total Hb.
- Less than 1% may be HbF.
- The blood of the newborn baby contains another type of Hb called fetal hemoglobin or HbF.
- The amount of HbF is up to 90% in the neonatal stage and falls gradually in about 4–5 months.

  The polypeptide chain compositions of the various hemoglobins are:

  HbA $\alpha_2\beta_2$ chains
  HbA_2 $\alpha_2\delta_2$ chains
  HbF $\alpha_2\gamma_2$ chains.

  The number of amino acids in the polypeptide chains is as follows:

α chain	141
β chain	146
δ chain	146
γ chain	146

STRUCTURE OF HEME (FIG. 16.1)

Heme consists of a porphyrin ring with one iron (Ferrous Fe^{2+}) at the center.

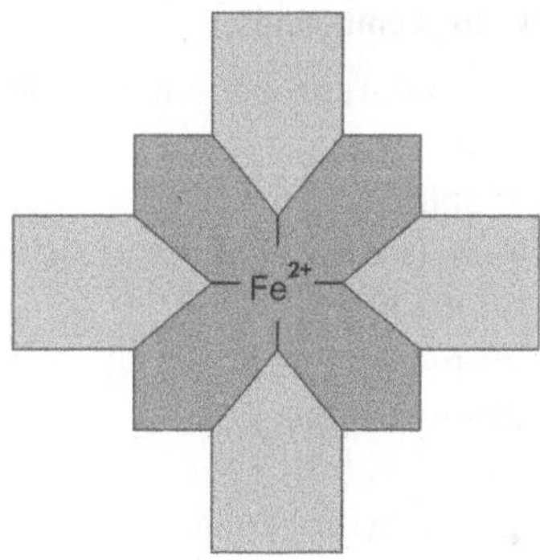

Fig. 16.1: Structure of heme.

The synthesis of normal hemoglobin is mainly dependent on the factors like iron, folic acid and vitamin B_{12}.

IRON

- Iron is a trace element.
- It is necessary for the *synthesis of hemoglobin.*
- It is present in the body in small amounts.
- It is required in the diet in very small amount.

Distribution of Iron in the Body

- Total body iron content is 3–4 g.
- Hemoglobin contains 70% (1.7–2.4 g) of iron.
- Reticuloendothelial system contains 25% (0.5–1.5 g).
- Muscle (myoglobin, enzymes) contains remaining 5%.
- Only 0.1%—circulates bound to transferrin (iron-binding protein).

Dietary Source

- Content and the amount of iron absorbed differ from food to food.
- Shell fish, meat, and liver have more iron than vegetables, eggs or milk foods.

Iron Absorption

It occurs mainly in the duodenum:

Factors favoring absorption	*Factors reducing absorption*
Ferrous form (Fe^{2+})	Ferric form (Fe^{3+})
Inorganic iron	Organic iron
Acids-HCl, vitamin C	Alkalis, antacids, pancreatic secretions
Iron deficiency	Iron excess
Increased erythropoiesis	Decreased erythropoiesis
Pregnancy	Infection

- Iron is absorbed in the small intestine.
- Heme iron is absorbed directly into the intestinal cells.
- Non-heme iron is absorbed in the ferrous form.
- Ferric form of iron present in the plant food is converted to ferrous form in the stomach in the presence of gastric HCl and ascorbic acid.
- In iron deficiency—more iron enters the cell and a greater proportion is transported into the portal blood.
- In iron overload state less iron enters the cell and a greater proportion of this is released back into the lumen.

Iron Transport and Transferrin

- Transferrin provides iron to the bone marrow for erythropoiesis.
- Iron is transported in blood bound to transferrin.
- Transferrin is synthesized in the liver and binds two atoms of iron per molecule.
- It is reutilized after it has given up its iron.

Storage

- Excess iron is stored in the cells of liver, spleen and bone marrow as ferritin.
- Ferritin is an iron protein complex, in which iron is present in the ferric (Fe^{3+}) form.

Excretion (Fig. 16.2)

- Dietary iron is absorbed in the small intestine.

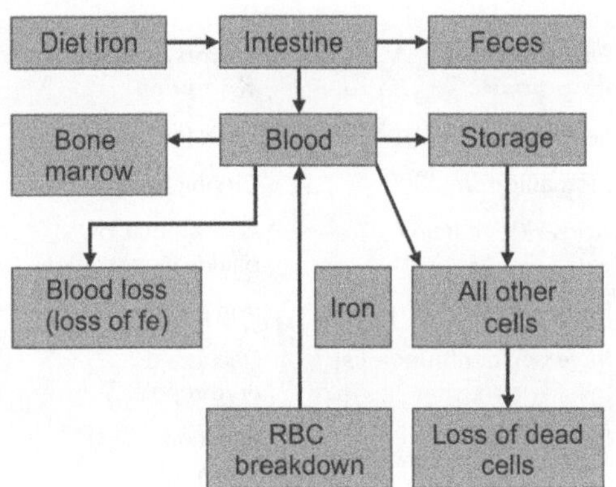

Fig. 16.2: Iron turnover in the body.

- The unabsorbed iron is excreted in the feces.
- From the intestine iron is transported to plasma.
- From plasma, iron is transported to bone marrow for RBC synthesis.
- If iron is in excess, it is transported to the liver or spleen, for storage as ferritin.
- Once the RBC breaks down, the hemoglobin is also broken down and iron is released.
- This iron returns to the plasma and is reutilized or stored as per the requirement.
- Iron is not excreted through urine.
- Thus, body iron is conserved very carefully.
- The iron level in the body is regulated at the level of intestinal absorption itself. This is a unique feature of iron metabolism.
- The only way iron lost from the body is through blood loss, or by the loss of dead cell of the epithelium of the intestine, urinary tract, skin, etc.

Iron Requirement

The amount of iron required each day to compensate for the loss depends on age and sex.

The requirement is higher in pregnancy and menstruating females.

Adult males	-	12 mg/day
Females	-	20 mg/day
Pregnancy and lactation	-	40 mg/day

Iron Containing Compounds

Iron is an essential component of the following compounds:
- Hemoglobin
- Myoglobin (stores O_2 in the muscles)
- Cytochrome b
- Cytochrome C
- Cytochrome oxidase
- Catalase
- Succinate dehydrogenase
- Xanthine oxidase.

In all these compounds, iron is present in the ferrous form, which is the functional form of iron.

Relationship between Serum Iron and Total Iron Binding Capacity

- Total iron binding capacity (TIBC) is typically measured along with serum iron to evaluate people suspected of having either iron deficiency or iron overload.
- The iron concentration divided by TIBC gives the transferrin saturation, which is a more useful indicator of iron status than iron or TIBC alone.
- In healthy people, about 20–50% of available sites in transferrin are used to transport iron.
- In iron deficiency, iron is low, but TIBC is increased, and transferrin saturation becomes very low.
- In iron overload states such as hemochromatosis, iron will be high and TIBC will be low or normal, causing the transferrin saturation to increase.
- Serum iron + Unsaturated iron-binding capacity (UIBC) = TIBC.
- Normal serum 2–4 g/L of transferrin.
- TIBC may be ordered along with serum iron when it appears that there is too much or too little iron in the body system.
- When the person has anemia, especially if the red cells are small and pale (microcytic and hypochromic), iron tests are usually performed.

- If a physician suspects that his patient has with too much iron, or has a family history of hemochromatosis, iron and TIBC may be used to see if further testing is needed.
- High TIBC or transferrin usually indicates iron deficiency, but it is also increased in pregnancy and with use of oral contraceptives.
- A low TIBC or transferrin may occur if the person has hemochromatosis, certain types of anemia in which iron accumulates, malnutrition, inflammation, liver disease, or nephrotic syndrome (a kidney disease that causes loss of protein in urine).

Iron Deficiency

Causes

1. Increased iron utilization during:
   - Growth
   - Pregnancy.
2. Blood loss during:
   - Menstruation
   - Gastrointestinal bleeding, gastric ulceration, colorectal cancer, peptic ulcer, gastric cancer
   - Hematuria.
3. Decreased iron intake:
   - Malabsorption—celiac disease, post-gastric resection

Laboratory findings of iron deficiency anemia:

- Low Hb percent
- Peripheral smear shows microcytic hypochromic RBCs
- Low serum iron
- Increased total iron-binding capacity (TIBC)
- Increased transferrin
- Decreased ferritin.

Iron Overload

- It is the condition in which excess iron is in the body.
- In this condition, iron has to be stored in the tissues because there is no method of excreting iron from the body. This results in iron overload.
- In this condition, iron is also stored as hemosiderin, which is another storage protein apart from ferritin. This condition is known as hemosiderosis.
- Hemochromatosis implies iron overload with injury to involved organs, as manifested by cellular degeneration and fibrosis.

Causes

1. *Hemolytic anemia*
   - Due to excessive breakdown of RBCs iron is released.
   - The utilization of this iron is low so it is stored in the tissues.
2. *Repeated blood transfusions.*

Laboratory Findings

1. Increased serum iron
2. Increased ferritin
3. TIBC, transferrin will be normal.
   - Measurements of serum iron concentration and total iron-binding capacity have been used as aids in the diagnosis of iron deficiency.

Biochemical Tests

Serum iron: Indicates the iron which is bound to serum transferrin.

It does not include the iron present in the Hb.

TIBC: The measurement of the maximum concentration of iron that is bound by transferrin. Normally, only 1/3rd of the binding sites of transferrin are occupied by iron.

UIBC: About 60–70% of the binding sites in transferrin are free and this is referred to as unsaturated iron-binding capacity (UIBC).

Assessing Iron and Iron Binding Capacity (Colorimetric Bathophenanthroline Method)

Iron

Principle: Serum iron bound to transferrin is released by reduction in acidic pH. Proteins and apoproteins are removed by precipitation. The ferric form of iron is reduced to the ferrous form by thioglycolic acid. The reduced iron forms a red colored complex with bathophenanthroline disulfonate, which is measured at 545 nm.

Total Iron-binding Capacity

Principle: Excess amount of iron (Fe^{3+}) is added to the serum to saturate all the iron-binding sites of transferrin. Excess of iron, which is unbound is removed by adding magnesium carbonate powder and then centrifuging. Iron content is estimated in the supernatant as per the serum iron estimation.

Reagents

1. *Precipitating reagent:* Take 16.6 mL of thioglycolic acid (mercaptoacetic acid), 49 g of trichloroacetic acid and 200 mL water in a 500 mL volumetric flask. Mix to dissolve slowly add 96 mL of concentrated HCl. Finally, make up the volume to 500 mL with water. Transfer the solution to a dark brown bottle. Store at room temperature. Stable for 3 months.
2. *Color reagent (25 mg/100 mL):* Dissolve 12.5 mg of bathophenanthroline disulfonic acid, sodium salt in 50 mL saturated sodium acetate solution. Transfer to 100 mL reagent bottle. Stable for one month.
3. *Iron standard (100 µg/mL):* Dissolve 70.2 mg of ferrous ammonium sulfate in about 25 mL of double distilled water in 100 mL volumetric flask. Add 0.1 mL of concentrated H_2SO_4. Make up the volume to 100 mL with water.
4. *Working standard (200 µg/dL):* To 2 mL of stock standard add 40 mL of double distilled water and mix well. Add 0.1 mL concentrated sulfuric acid. Make the volume to 100 mL. Transfer to 100 mL bottle and label (200 µg/dL). Stable for 10 months at room temperature.
5. *TIBC reagent (5 mg/mL):* Weigh 240 mg of ferric chloride and dissolve and make up to 100 mL with 0.5 M HCl.

Dissolve 5 mL of this solution in 500 mL of double distilled water. Transfer to 500 mL reagent bottle. Stable for several months at room temperature.

Note: Soak all the test tubes in 6N HCl overnight. Then wash the tubes with distilled water, dry in the oven and use.

Procedure

1. Iron

	Test	Std	Blank
Serum	0.6 mL	-	-
Iron std			
Reagent	-	0.6 mL	-
Water	-	-	0.6 mL
Precipitating reagent	0.6 mL	0.6 mL	0.6 mL
Mix well and keep for 30 minutes Centrifuge			
Supernatant	0.6 mL	0.6 mL	0.6 mL
Color reagent	0.6 mL	0.6 mL	0.6 mL
Mix well and measure the absorbance at 545 nm			

2. TIBC

To 0.6 mL serum, add 1.2 mL TIBC reagent. Mix well and keep for 10 minutes. Add one spatula (approximately 120 mg) of light magnesium carbonate. Mix and keep the tube for at least 30 minutes at room temperature. Mix vigorously 2 to 3 times in between. Centrifuge at 4000 rpm for 5 minutes. Pipette 0.6 mL of the supernatant to a labeled test tube and proceed as for the iron estimation.

Calculation

$$\text{Serum iron in µg/100 mL} = \frac{\text{OD of T} - \text{OD of B}}{\text{OD of S.} - \text{OD of B}} \times 200$$

$$\text{TIBC in µg/100 mL} = \frac{\text{OD of T} - \text{O.D of B}}{\text{OD of S} - \text{OD of B}} \times 600$$

UIBC = TIBC - Serum iron

$$\text{Transferrin saturation percent} = \frac{\text{Serum iron}}{\text{TIBC}} \times 100$$

Ferritin

In iron deficiency, the plasma ferritin is decreased. Measurement of serum ferritin level is a very good test to detect iron deficiency anemia.

Ferritin is estimated by any of the immunoassay methods like ELISA, FIA or RIA.

Normal Values

Iron → 65-170 μg /dL
TIBC → 200-450 μg/dL
Ferritin → 20-200 μg/L

Note: All the glassware used for the estimation one word of iron and TIBC should be free form iron contamination. This is achieved by soaking the glasswares in 6 N HCI for 24 hours followed by washing the tubes with deionized water thoroughly and drying. The dried tubes and glasswares are used for the estimation.

FOLIC ACID

- This is an organic compound, essential to animal growth and health and needed by bacteria as a growth factor.
- Part of the vitamin B complex, folic acid is necessary for synthesis of nucleic acids and formation of the heme component of hemoglobin in red blood cells.
- The coenzyme tetrahydrofolate is the active form of folic acid.
- The coenzyme of folic acid is a very important factor required for single carbon transfer through whom the purine and pyrimidine bases are synthesized; which are the major components of nucleic acids.

Sources: Fresh green vegetables, liver, whole grains, meat and legumes.

Requirement

Children	—	300 μg/day
Adults	—	400 μg/day
Pregnancy, lactation	—	800 μg/day

Function

- The coenzyme form of folic acid is tetrahydrofolic acid (FH_4).
- The FH_4 is the carrier of one carbon and it is involved in one carbon transfer reactions.
- Folate is required for the synthesis of purine and pyrimidine nucleotides, which are the components of nucleic acids. So FH_4 is directly involved in DNA synthesis (UMP TMP).
- This means that cell multiplication depends on folic acid.

Deficiency

Folic-acid deficiency anemia (megaloblastic anemia):

- It is a type of anemia that is a result of a deficient intake of folic acid.
- This B vitamin is needed for the formation of heme, the pigmented, iron-containing portion of the hemoglobin in red blood cells.
- A deficient intake of folic acid impairs the maturation of young red blood cells, which results in anemia.
- The disease is characterized by deficiency of red blood cells (anemia) and often white cells.

Causes:

- Most commonly caused by alcoholism (decreased intake, and impaired entero-hepatic circulation)
- Low dietary intake
- Intestinal malabsorption syndrome
- Pregnancy
- Due to drugs that inhibit dihydrofolate reductase (e.g., methotrexate)
- Due to drugs that interfere with absorption/storage of folate (e.g., some anticonvulsants)
- Deficiency of folic acid also results in growth failure.

Folate Antagonists

- Compounds, which resemble folate in structure.

- They cannot carry out the functions of folate.
- Instead, they inhibit the reactions in which folate is required.
- Hence, these compounds (folate antagonists) are used in the treatment of leukemias to prevent cell multiplication.
- Aminopterin and amethopterin (methotrexate) are the folate antagonists used in the treatment of cancer.
- Trimethoprim is also a folate antagonist, which is used to treat bacterial infections.

FIGLU Excretion Test

- In histidine metabolism, the formiminoglutamate is converted to further product with the help of an enzyme formiminotransferase, which needs FH_4.
- In the deficiency of FH_4, the formiminoglutamate (FIGLU) is not converted to the next metabolite. Therefore, the formiminoglutamate is accumulated and excreted in the urine.
- This helps to identify whether *megaloblastic anemia* is due to folic acid or vitamin B_{12} deficiency.

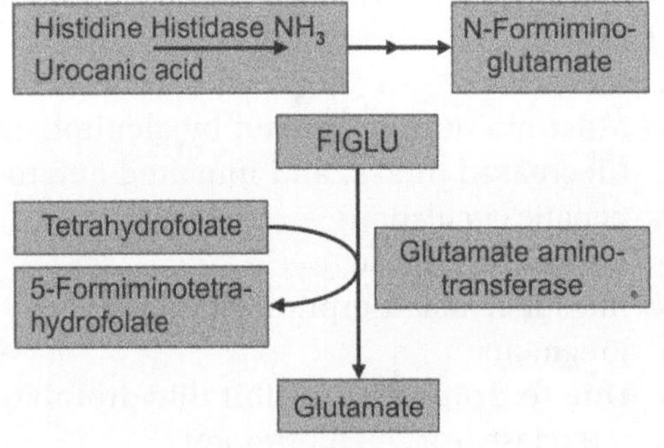

VITAMIN B_{12} (COBALAMIN)

Vitamin B_{12} is the largest and most complex of all the vitamins.

It is unique among vitamins in that it contains a metal ion, cobalt. For this reason, cobalamin is the term used to refer to compounds having B_{12} activity.

Methylcobalamin and 5-deoxyadenosylcobalamin are the forms of vitamin B_{12} used in the human body.

The form of cobalamin used in most supplements, cyanocobalamin, is readily converted to 5-deoxyadenosyl and methylcobalamin.

It is a water-soluble vitamin and it belongs to the B-complex group.

It consists of a corrin ring, which contains a cobalt atom in the center.

Dietary Source

Liver, meat, fish, eggs and milk.

Requirements

Children	: 2 μg/day
Adults	: 3 μg/day
Pregnancy and lactation	: 4 μg/day

Absorption

Absorption of vitamin B_{12} takes place in the small intestine and it requires an intrinsic factor, which is secreted by parietal cells of the stomach. A glycoprotein, castle's intrinsic factor and B_{12} is called extrinsic factor. Vitamin B_{12} of food binds to intrinsic factor in the stomach, this complex moves to the ileum and binds to specific receptors. Vitamin B_{12} is transported to mucosal cells and then to blood and carried by vitamin B_{12} binding proteins.

Storage

Vitamin B_{12} is unique among the other B-complex vitamins in that it can be stored in the liver and can be used whenever required.

Function

1. Vitamin B_{12} is required for the regeneration of tetrahydrofolate (FH_4) and synthesis of methionine.
   - Methylcobalamin is required for the function of the folate-dependent enzyme, methionine synthase.

- This enzyme is required for the synthesis of the amino acid, methionine, from homocysteine. Methionine is required for the synthesis of S-adenosyl-methionine, a methyl group donor used in many biological methylation reactions, including the methylation of a number of sites within DNA and RNA.
- Methylation of DNA may be important in cancer prevention.
- Inadequate function of methionine synthase can lead to an accumulation of homocysteine.

  Methyl FH_4 + Vit B_{12} + Homocysteine

  ↓

  Methyl B_{12} + FH_4 + Methionine

2. Vitamin B_{12} along with folic acid is required for the development of RBCs beyond the megaloblastic stage.
3. It acts as coenzyme for the mutase enzyme, which converts methyl malonyl CoA to succinyl CoA.
4. It is involved in the conversion of ribonucleotides to deoxyribonucleotides.

Deficiency

Cause: Intestinal malabsorption and poor dietary intake.

Symptoms

- Megaloblastic anemia
- Glossitis and inflammation of mouth
- Mucosal lining of mouth, tongue and intestine also show large fragile cells
- Methyl malonic aciduria.

Estimation of Vitamin B_{12} and Folic Acid

Various methods are available, they are:

1. Microbiological assay
2. Competitive protein-binding method
3. Immunometric assays.

Specimen

Fasting serum sample is preferred. Heparin should not be used during the collection of blood as it will interfere with the estimation of vitamin B_{12} and folate.

Normal serum levels

Vit B_{12}—200–1100 ng/L

Folate—2–9 μg/L

Relationship between Folate, Vitamin B_{12} and RBC Synthesis

Diminished activity of methionine synthase in vitamin B_{12} deficiency inhibits the regeneration of tetrahydrofolate (THF) and traps folate in a form that is not usable by the body, resulting in symptoms of folate deficiency even in the presence of adequate folate levels. Thus, in both folate and vitamin B_{12} deficiency, folate is unavailable to participate in DNA synthesis. This impairment of DNA synthesis affects the rapidly dividing cells of the bone marrow earlier than other cells, resulting in the production of large, immature, hemoglobin-poor red blood cells. The resulting anemia is known as megaloblastic anemia.

Vitamin B_{12} is not directly involved in RBC synthesis; its relationship is indirect through folate. Vitamin B_{12} is required for the regeneration of FH_4 (tetrahydrofolate, a form of folate) as follows:

Methyl FH_4 + Vit B_{12} → FH_4 + Methyl B_{12}

In case of severe B_{12} deficiency, folate is not regenerated and hence not available for DNA synthesis, leading to megaloblastic anemia. Hence in case of anemia, both folate and vitamin B_{12} are estimated in serum.

Role of Hemoglobin in Disease

- Decreased levels of hemoglobin, with or without an absolute decrease of red blood cells, leads to symptoms of anemia.
- Anemia has many different causes.
- Absence of iron decreases heme synthesis, red blood cells in iron deficiency anemia are *hypochromic* (lacking the red hemoglobin pigment) and *microcytic* (smaller than normal). Other anemias are rare.
- In hemolysis (accelerated breakdown of red blood cells), associated jaundice is caused

by the hemoglobin metabolite bilirubin, and the circulating hemoglobin can cause renal failure.
- Mutations in the globin chain are associated with the hemoglobinopathies, such as sickle cell disease and thalassemia.

ABNORMAL HEMOGLOBIN

The abnormal hemoglobin of sickle cell anemia was first demonstrated by Linus Pauling in 1949. Structurally, each globin chain has its own genetic locus. The individual chain of hemoglobin is under genetic control. Based on the genetics of the globin chain production structural abnormalities can be divided into four groups:

1. Amino acid substitutions: HbS, HbC, HbD and HbE.
2. Amino acid deletion (deletion of three nucleotides in DNA): Hb Gun Hill.
3. Elongated globin chains (result from chain terminations, shift mutations or other mutations).
4. Fused or hybrid chains (results from non-homologous crossing over): Hb Lepore.

Most of the hemoglobin variants arise by a single amino acid substitution which is called "point mutations".

Deletion of one or two nucleotide bases can shift the reading frame of all code words, which follow. Such an event observed in microorganisms is called a "Frameshift mutation".

Abnormal hemoglobins are inherited as autosomal codominants. Thus, subjects who inherit one normal and one abnormal gene are heterozygous and those who have two identical abnormal genes are homozygous.

Thalassemia

The name is derived from the Greek word, *thalassa*, which means "sea". Greeks inherited this disease present around Mediterranean sea. Absence or diminished synthesis of one of the polypeptide chains of human hemoglobin is characterized as "thalassemia". The reduction in the α-chain synthesis is called α-thalassemia and decreased synthesis of β-chain is called β-thalassemia. The β-thalassemia is more common.

Classification of Thalassemia

Thalassemia includes disorders affecting the alpha hemoglobin chain genes and the beta hemoglobin chain genes.

Alpha Thalassemia

Alpha thalassemia occurs when one or more of the four alpha chain genes fails to function.

Alpha chain protein production, for practical purposes, is evenly divided among the four genes.

a. The loss of one gene diminishes the production of the alpha protein only slightly. This condition is so close to normal that it can be detected only by specialized laboratory techniques that, until recently, were confined to research laboratories. A person with this condition is called a "silent carrier" because of the difficulty in detection.
b. The loss of two genes (two-gene deletion alpha thalassemia) produces a condition with small RBCs, and at most a mild anemia.
   An individual with this condition looks normal.
   The condition can be detected by routine blood testing.
c. The loss of three alpha genes produces a serious hematological problem (three-gene deletion alpha thalassemia). Patients with this condition have a severe anemia, and often require blood transfusions to survive. The severe imbalance between the alpha chain production and beta chain production causes an accumulation of beta chains inside the RBCs. Normally, beta chains pair only with alpha chains. With three-gene deletion, alpha thalassemia,

beta chains begin to associate in groups of four, producing abnormal hemoglobin, called "hemoglobin H". The condition is called "hemoglobin H disease".

d. The loss of all four alpha genes produces a condition that is incompatible with life. The gamma chains produced during fetal life associate in groups of four to form abnormal hemoglobin called "hemoglobin Barts".

Beta Thalassemia

The fact that there are only two genes for the beta chain of hemoglobin makes beta thalassemia a bit simpler to understand than alpha thalassemia. Unlike alpha thalassemia, beta thalassemia rarely arises from the complete loss of a beta globin gene. The beta globin gene is present, but produces little beta globin protein. The degree of suppression varies. Many causes of suppressed beta globin gene expression have been found.

a. One-gene beta thalassemia has one normal beta globin gene, and a second, affected gene with a variably reduced production of beta globin. The degree of imbalance with the alpha globin depends on the residual production capacity of the defective beta globin gene.
b. Two-gene beta thalassemia produces a severe anemia and a potentially life-threatening condition.

   There are two types of β-thalassemias:

   1. *β-thalassemia major:* This is the homozygous state for the β-thalassemia gene. It is a severe disease. Splenomegaly and skin pigmentation are the clinical symptoms. Blood picture show anemia and erythrocyte shows marked anisocytosis. The MCV and MCH decreases and MCHC increases. Both HbA and HbF are present (HbF 10–98%)
   2. *β-thalassemia minor:* This is the heterozygous state for the β-thalassemia gene both HbA and HbF are present.

      Less symptoms occur.

Hemoglobinopathy

Presence of abnormal hemoglobin in blood is called hemoglobinopathy.

It is a genetic disorder due to an alteration in the structure of hemoglobin molecule.

The examples are sickle cell anemia and sickle cell trait.

Sickle Cell Hemoglobin (HbS)

- The sickle cell hemoglobinopathies are hereditary disorders in which the red cells contain HbS.
- They include **heterozygous** (sickle cell trait: HbA and HbS present) and **homozygous** (sickle cell anemia: only HbS is present with the complete absence of HbA) for HbS.
- The presence of HbS causes a condition called sickle cell anemia.
- The HbS differs from HbA in the substitution of **valine** for **glutamic** acid in the **6th** position from the N-terminal end of the β-**chain**.
- HbA-Val-His-Leu-Thr-Pro-**Glu**-Glu-Lys.
- HbS-Val-His-Leu-Thr-Pro-**Val**-Glu-Lys.
- The side chain of valine is distinctly non-polar, whereas that of glutamate is highly polar.
- So, this alteration in polarity markedly reduces the solubility of deoxygenated HbS.
- HbS being less soluble aggregates together and distorts the red cells into sickle shaped (crescent-shaped) cells. Hence, this condition is known as sickle cell anemia.
- The change in the shape of the cell causes hemolysis leading to anemia.

Clinical Symptoms

1. Chronic hemolytic anemia
2. Hypoxia (breathlessness) due to low blood supply to the tissues and decreased oxygen
3. Pain and swelling in the joints.

Detection of Abnormal Hb

Electrophoresis: Different types of hemoglobins can be separated from each other by electrophoresis. The Hb variants move with different speed in an electrical field, and appear as separate bands. These differences in the migration are the result of different electrical charges of each Hb variant brought about by various amino acids in the polypeptide chains of Hb molecules. The support medium used for Hb electrophoresis is a cellulose acetate membrane strip.

Reagents

1. Barbitone buffer, pH 8.6, ionic strength 0.05 (for electrophoresis).
   Dissolve 350 mg disodium EDTA disodium and 10.3 g of sodium barbitone in water and make up to one liter. Adjust the pH with 2 M HCl.
2. *Strip soaking buffer:* Tris EDTA Borate buffer (stock).
   Dissolve 3.22 g Tris base and 0.31 g EDTA (disodium) in 40 mL water. Adjust the pH to 8.8 with saturated boric acid and make up to 50 mL.
   For use: Dilute 1:10 with water.
3. *Staining solution*: Freshly prepare by mixing the following solutions:
   - Benzidine, 0.2% in ethanol—5 mL
   - Acetic acid, 3% in water—10 mL
   - Sodium nitroprusside, 1% in water—1 mL
   - Hydrogen peroxide, 3% in water—1 mL.

Hemolysate Preparation

Centrifuge the specimen and remove the plasma. Cells are washed three times with normal saline. For each volume of packed cells, add one volume of distilled water and 0.5 volume of chloroform and shake vigorously for 2 minutes. Centrifuge at 3000 rpm for 20 minutes. Transfer the upper layer of hemolysate into another tube.

Determination of Hb in Hemolysate

Hb Reagent

Dissolve 220 mg potassium ferricyanide ($K_3Fe(CN)_6$), 50 mg KCN or sodium cyanide and 140 mg KH_2PO_4 in about 900 mL H_2O. Add 0.5 mL of sterox Se (Hartman-Leddon Co.) and mix quickly to dissolve. Adjust the pH to 7.2 ± 0.1 with 0.1 N H_2PO_4 or 0.1 N KOH. Make up the volume to 1 liter with H_2O. Stable for several months if stored in a dark bottle in refrigerator.

Procedure: Take 5 mL of Hb reagent + 20 µL of hemolysate. Mix and read at 540 nm.

Calculation

OD at 540 nm × MEC of Hb × DF = g of Hb%

$$\text{OD at 540 nm} \times \frac{1.47}{10} \times 251 \text{ g of Hb\%}$$

OD at 540 nm × 36.8 = g of Hb%

MEC of Hb is 1.47 for 1 liter. Here as we are calculating Hb%, i.e. for 100 mL

$$\text{MEC becomes} = \frac{1.47}{10} = 0.147$$

$$\text{DF} = \frac{5020}{20} = 251$$

OD at 540 nm × 36.8 = g of Hb%

Dilute the hemolysate to 5% with water and use for electrophoresis.

Procedure

Immerse the cello gel strip in buffer for at least 20 minutes. Excess buffer is removed from strips with the help of Whatman No. 1 filter paper. Care must be taken not to damage the gelatin coating. Fill the electrophoresis tank with buffer. The strips are stretched on the strip supporters and both ends are connected with the Whatman No. 1 filter paper into buffer. The 5% hemolysate is applied once with the macro-applicator and electrophoresis is carried out at a constant voltage of 150 for about 1 and ½ hours. Remove the strip and place it in the staining solution for about 3 to 5 minutes. Wash the solution with water **(Fig. 16.3)**.

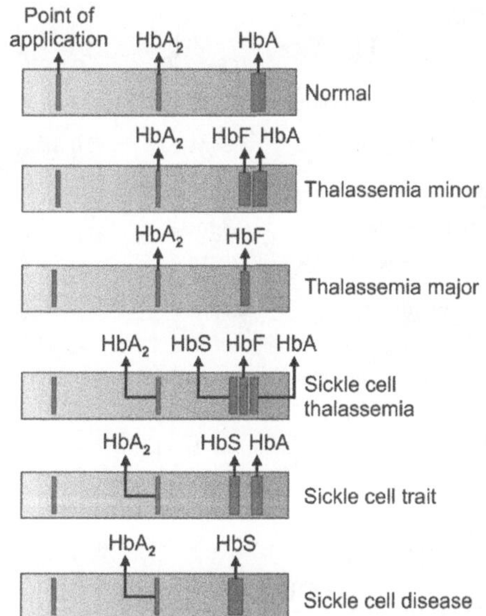

Fig. 16.3: Normal and abnormal hemoglobin patterns on cellulose acetate electrophoresis.

Detection of HbS

Sickling Test

Principle: Red cells containing HbS mixed with a freshly prepared solution of sodium metabisulphite (reducing agent) and observed under microscope. This test is simple and will detect both homozygous and heterozygous sickle gene. False results may be obtained if the patient had a recent transfusion of normal red cells or if the blood sample is contaminate.

Solubility Test

Principle: HbS is less soluble in a concentrated buffer solution at a pH of 6.5 whereas normal Hb is soluble. This principle is used in differentiating HbS from normal Hb. When Hb is added to a solution of sodium hydrosulfite, (a reducing agent) in phosphate buffer, the solubility decreases. The solution becomes turbid if HbS is present.

Reagents

1. Buffer reagent, pH 6.5, 2.24 M.
   Dissolve 25.1 g of dipotassium hydrogen orthophosphate and 14.2 g of potassium dihydrogen orthophosphate in about 60 mL of water and make up the volume to 100 mL. This is stable at 2–8°C for several weeks.
2. Sodium hydrosulfite (sodium dithionite). Ready to use.
   Store in desiccators at room temperature (dark place).
   Stable for several months.
3. Saline reagent—0.9% NaCl: Dissolve 0.9 g of sodium chloride in about 60 mL of water and make up to 100 mL. Stable for at least several weeks.
4. Chloroform.
   Specimen: Heparinized or oxalated blood. Preserve the RBC for hemolysate preparation.

Procedure

	Test	*Control*
Hemolysate	200 μL	10 μL
Phosphate buffer	1.8 mL	–
Water	–	15 mL
Sodium hydrosulfite	25 mg	–
Stand for 15 minutes and filter		
Take 30 μL test filtrate and add 4.5 mL of phosphate buffer. Mix and read at 415 nm		

Calculation

$$\text{HbF in \%} = \frac{\text{OD test}}{\text{OD control}} \times 100$$

Reference range:

	Percentage solubility
Normal	90–95%
HbAs	25–35%
HbSs	3–10%

If the value is less than 80% it indicates the presence of HbS.

Detection of HbF by Alkali Denaturation Test

Principle: Hemoglobin F is resistant to alkali treatment compared to other hemoglobins.

All hemoglobins are converted to cyanmethemoglobin and denatured hemoglobin is precipitated by ammonium sulfate and the alkali resistant HbF in the filtrate is measured.

Reagents

1. *Cyanide reagent:* Dissolve 0.1 g of potassium cyanide and 0.2 g of potassium ferricyanide in distilled water and dilute to 500 mL. Stable at room temperature for several months.
2. *Ammonium sulfate reagent:* Add 75 g of ammonium sulfate to 100 mL of distilled water. Warm and agitate to dissolve. Stable at room temperature for several weeks.
3. Alkali reagent.
   Dissolve 4.8 g of sodium hydroxide in distilled water and dilute to 100 mL.
4. *Saline reagent:* Dissolve 4.5 g of sodium chloride in about 300 mL of distilled water and make up to 500 mL. Stable at room temperature for several weeks.
5. *Chloroform:* Ready to use.
   Specimen: Heparinized or oxalated blood. Stable for at least one week at 4°C if hemolysate is prepared.

Preparation of Hemolysate

Centrifuge the specimen and remove the plasma. Wash the cells three times with saline reagent. For each volume of packed cells, add one volume of distilled water and 0.5 volume of chloroform and shake vigorously for 2 minutes. Centrifuge at 3000 rpm for 20 minutes. Pipette off the upper layer of hemoglobin. Filter, if necessary.

Procedure

	Test	Control
Hemolysate hemoglobin	0.2 mL	0.1 mL
Cyanide reagent	3.8 mL	2.0 mL
Water	–	10.5 mL
Alkali reagent	0.3 mL	–
Mix and stand for exactly 2 minutes		
Ammonium sulfate reagent	2.0 mL	
Mix, after 5 minutes filter through Whatman's filter paper		
Read OD of filtrate at 540 nm		

Calculation

$$\text{HbF in \%} = \frac{\text{OD test}}{\text{OD control}} \times 25$$

Reference Range

HbF% (Alkali denaturation test).

Normal	0.5–2
Thalassemia major	10–100
Thalassemia minor	0.5–8.0
Sickle cell β-thalassemia	5–20
Normal newborn	60–90

Precaution: This method is suitable when HbF is less than 5%. Do not pipette cyanide reagent by mouth.

Osmotic Fragility

The osmotic fragility test is employed to diagnose different types of anemia, where the physical properties of the red blood cell alteration. The main causative factor, is in turn dependent upon the column, surface area and functional state of the red blood cell plasma membrane. An increased osmotic fragility is found in hemolytic anemia, hereditary spherocytosis and whenever spherocytes are found. Decreased osmotic fragility occurs following splenectomy, in liver disease, sickle cell anemia, iron deficiency anemia, thalassemia and polycythemia vera.

Specimen

Heparinized venous blood or defibrinated whole blood (10 to 20 mL).

Principle

If RBCs are placed in an isotonic solution (0.85% sodium chloride), water will neither enter nor leave the red cell. However, if red cells are placed in a 0.25% solution of sodium chloride, water enters the red cells, the cell swells up and eventually hemolyzes or ruptures. A spherocyte, which is almost round, swells up in 0.25% sodium chloride and ruptures more than red cells, or more quickly than cells that have a large surface area per volume, such as target cells or sickle cells. The fragility of the red cell is increased when the rate of hemolysis increases. When the rate of hemolysis is decreased, the fragility of the red cells is considered to be decreased. In the osmotic fragility test, whole blood is added to varying concentrations of buffered sodium chloride solution and allowed to incubate at room temperature. The extent of hemolysis is then determined by reading the supernatants on a spectrophotometer. Normal blood (a control) runs at the same time.

Reagents

1. Buffered sodium chloride (NaCl) stock solution, pH 7.4. Dissolve 25 g of NaCl, 4.3 g of $Na_2H_2PO_4 . 2H_2O$ and 1.5 g $NaH_2PO_4 . 2H_2O$ in 250 mL water. Stable for several months at room temperature.
2. Buffered NaCl solution, 1%. Dilute 2 mL of stock solution to 20 mL with water.

Procedure

Prepare the following dilutions of buffered sodium chloride and place in the appropriately labeled tubes in duplicates.

Tube No.	mL 1% NaCl	Distilled water	Concentration of buffered NaCl
1	5.00	0.00	1.00
2	4.25	0.75	0.85
3	3.75	1.25	0.75
4	3.25	1.75	0.65
5	3.00	2.00	0.60
6	2.75	2.25	0.55
7	2.50	2.50	0.50
8	2.25	2.75	0.45
9	2.00	3.00	0.40
10	1.75	3.25	0.35
11	1.50	3.50	0.30
12	1.00	4.00	0.20
13	0.50	4.50	0.10
14	-	5.00	0.00

Mix well using parafilm, one set of dilutions will be used for the normal control blood.

If defibrinated blood is to be used, proceed as follows:

a. Place 15 to 20 mL of whole blood into an Erlenmeyer flask containing 15 glass beads.
b. Gently rotate the flask until the noise of the beads on the glass can no longer be heard (about 10 minutes).
   1. Add 0.03 mL of the patient's heparinized or defibrinated sample to each of the 14 tubes. Repeat the addition of normal control blood to the set of 14 control tubes. Mix each tube immediately by gentle inversion.
   2. Allow tubes to stand at room temperature for 30 minutes.
   3. Remix the tubes gently and centrifuge at 2000 rpm for 5 minutes.
   4. Carefully transfer the supernatants to cuvettes and read on a spectrophotometer at a wavelength of 550 nm. Set the optical density at 0, using the supernatant in tube

no. 1, which represents the blank, with 0% hemolysis. Tube No. 14, represents 100% hemolysis.

5. Calculate the percent hemolysis for each supernatant as follows:

$$\% \text{ of hemolysis} = \frac{\text{OD of supernatant}}{\text{OD of supernatant in tube No 14}} \times 100$$

6. The results of the test should then be graphed, with the percent hemolysis plotted on the ordinate or vertical axis and the sodium chloride concentration on the abscissa or horizontal axis.

Normal Range

Tube No.	*NaCl*	*Hemolysis %*
1	1.00	0
2	0.85	0
3	0.75	0
4	0.65	0
5	0.60	0
6	0.55	0
7	0.50	0–50
8	0.45	0–45
9	0.40	50–90
10	0.35	90–99
11	0.30	97–100
12	0.20	100
13	0.10	100
14	0.00	100

Note:

1. Instead of determining the amount of hemolysis on the spectrophotometer, the test may be read visually. By this method, the first tube (the highest concentration of sodium chloride) shows a trace of hemolysis in the supernatant.
2. The pH of the blood—saline mixture is important and should be 7.4.
3. There are many possible sources of technical error in this procedure. It is, therefore, important to report the control results and interpret the patient's test values.
4. Oxalated blood is not recommended for use in this test. The salts present in the anticoagulant may alter the pH of the blood saline mixture.

Reference

1. Dacie JV, Lewis SM. Practical Hematology, 5th edn. New York: Churchill Livingstone, 1975.

Determination of HbA_2

HbA_2 can be quantitatively estimated by ion-exchange chromatography, using DEAE cellulose, followed by spectrophotometry.
Normal value: 1–3%.

In β-thalassemia, minor HbA_2 may go up to 5–6%.

Abnormal Hb, which does not separate in alkaline pH, is separated by electrophoresis under acidic pH and here, the support medium used is agar gel plates. Abnormal Hbs like HbD, HbE can be separated by this method.

Derived Hemoglobin Compounds

Hemoglobin derivatives are formed by the joining of different groups with the heme part or by a change in the oxidation state of iron.

1. *Oxyhemoglobin (Hb-0)*
   - It is the form of Hb present in the RBC, of human body.
   - Oxygen is combined with Hb through Fe^{2+} (Ferrous).
   - It is dark red in color and the λ maximum is 577 nm.
2. *Reduced Hb or deoxyhemoglobin (Hb)*
   - This Hb is without oxygen.
   - This is purple red in color.
3. *Carboxy Hb (Hb-CO)*
   - Carboxy Hb is formed by the binding of carbon monoxide (CO) with Hb.
   - The CO-binds with the iron atom in the same way as oxygen binds.

- The CO has a higher affinity towards Hb, than O_2, hence even small quantity of CO present will bind to the Hb, λ maximum of Hb-CO is 572 mm.
- Exposure to CO occurs in the following conditions:
  - In the mines (also deep wells)
  - Heavy cigarette smoking
  - Incomplete burning of petrol.

4. *Methemoglobin (Met-Hb)*
   - A substitution of tyrosine for the histidine at either the proximal or distal histidine residues of either the α or β chains locks the heme iron into a trivalent state (Fe^{3+}) or the action of oxidizing agents on ferrous form of Hb converts the Fe^{2+} to the Fe^{3+} state. Fe^{3+} cannot bind oxygen and hence oxygen transport is not possible.
   - Increased Met-Hb in the blood is known as methemoglobinemia.
   - *Causes of methemoglobinemia*
     - Congenital Met-Hb reductase deficiency.
     - Ingestion of nitrites, nitrates, sulfa drugs, or certain dyes (aniline dyes)..
     - Exposure to household substances like shoe polishes (nitrobenzene).
   - When Met-Hb in the blood increases up to 15% of the total pigment, cyanosis occurs (bluish color of the skin).
   - Normally, a small amount of Met-Hb is produced in the blood.
   - The enzyme Met-Hb reductase present in the RBC converts the Fe^{3+} to the Fe^{2+} form thus converting the Met-Hb to normal Hb.

Signs and Symptoms

- If the Met-Hb concentration increases more than 55% acidosis, hypoxia and coma may result, if it exceeds more than 70%, death may occur.

Complications

Hyperkalemia and renal failure.

Thus under normal conditions Met-Hb concentration is less than 1% of the total Hb.

λmax of Met-Hb = 630 nm

There are again two types of methemoglobinemia:

- Hereditary methemoglobinemia associated with cytochrome b_5 reductase deficiency. This is an autosomal recessive trait and affected subjects are persistently cyanotic.
- Hereditary methemoglobinemia associated with HbM: This is associated with cyanosis. This disorder is transmitted as an autosomal dominant trait.

Determination of Methemoglobin

Principle: The absorbance spectrum of methemoglobin exhibits a small, characteristic peak at 630–635 nm. Addition of cyanide eliminates this peak converting methemoglobin to cyanmethemoglobin. The decrease in absorbance is proportional to the methemoglobin concentration.

$HbFe(II) + FeIII(CN)_6^{3-} \rightarrow HbFe(III) + Fe(II)(CN)_6^{4-}$

(Hb monomer) (meth Hb monomer)

$HbFe(III) + CN^- \rightarrow HbFe(III)CN$ (Monomer of cyanmethemoglobin)

The normal absorbance spectrum of oxyhemoglobin shows very little absorbance above 600 nm. However, if sulfhemoglobin is present in a hemolysate, there is a broad increase in the absorption curve in the range of 600–620 nm. This sulfhemoglobin plateau is not affected by treatment with cyanide.

Specimen: Fresh blood anticoagulated with heparin, EDTA or ACD (acid citrate-dextrose) solution. No fluid or food restriction is needed.

Reagents

1. *Potassium ferricyanide:* Dissolve 2.0 g of potassium ferricyanide in distilled water and dilute to 10 mL. If stored in a brown bottle at 4°C, stable for at least one year.

2. *Potassium cyanide solution (Caution: Lethal poison):* Dissolve 500 mg of KCN in distilled water and dilute to 10 mL.
3. *Potassium phosphate buffer, 0.15 mol/L, pH 6.6 (20°C):* Dissolve 17.1 g of $K_2HPO_4 \cdot 3H_2O$ (or 13.2 anhydrous) in 500 mL of distilled water. Transfer the KH_2PO_4 solution to a 2 L beaker and add an equal volume of K_2HPO_4 solution. Place a pH electrode in the beaker. Then slowly add more of the K_2HPO_4 solution, with constant stirring, until the mixture has a pH of 6.6. Store at 4°C. Discard whenever the solution appears turbid. New buffer should be prepared at least once in every 3 months.

Procedure

Preparation of hemolysate:
1. Pipette 0.1 mL of whole blood into a test tube containing 3.9 mL of distilled water; mix.
2. Add 4 mL of potassium phosphate buffer and mix thoroughly.

	C_1	C_2	C_3
Water	1.5 mL	–	–
Phosphate buffer	1.5 mL	–	–
Hemolysate	–	3.0 mL	3.0 mL
Potassium ferricyanide	–	–	0.1 mL
Mix and measure the absorbance of C_2 and C_3 at 630 nm after 2 minutes using C_1 as blank Record as A_2a and A_3a			
Potassium cyanide	0.1 mL	0.1 mL	0.1 mL
Mix by inverting 3 times and allow to stand for 5 minutes			
Measure absorbance C_2 and C_3 with C_1 as blank			
Record as A_2b and A_3b			

Calculations

Methemoglobin (% of total pigment)

$$= \frac{A_2a - A_2b}{A_3a - A_3b} \times 100$$

Reference range = 0–1%.

Laboratory Findings

Arterial Blood Gas (ABG)

- Normal arterial pO_2
- Decreased oxygen saturation curve.

Venous Blood

- Chocolate brown appearance of blood
- No changes on exposure to O_2
- Color fades with exposure to 10% potassium cyanide.

Sulfhemoglobin (HbS)

- This is an abnormal sulfur containing Hb (attached to the porphyrin ring).
- It does not act as an oxygen carrier and it is not present in the normal RBCs.
- It is formed by the toxic action of drugs and chemical agents that contain sulfur.
- It results in cyanosis.

Cyanmethemoglobin

- Hb is converted to cyan-MetHb by Drabkin's reagent (potassium ferricyanide + potassium cyanide).
- It is a complex formed by MetHb with cyanide and it is a stable compound having λmax at 540 nm.
- This provides an accurate method for the estimation of Hb in the blood.

Carbonyl Hb (Hb-CO_2)

- This is the form of Hb transporting CO_2 from tissues to the lungs.

SELF TEST

1. Write briefly on the structure of normal hemoglobin.
2. What is sickle cell hemoglobin?
3. What is thalassemia and what are its types?
4. Name the tests used to detect abnormal hemoglobin.
5. Explain the significance of the alkali denaturation test.
6. What are the different types of hemoglobin derivatives?
7. Write short notes on methemoglobin.
8. Name the factors which are important for hemoglobin synthesis.
9. Give the laboratory findings of iron deficiency anemia.
10. Briefly discuss the function of folate.
11. Name the storage and transport forms of iron.
12. Write a note on the role of vitamin B_{12} during hemoglobin synthesis.

MULTIPLE CHOICE QUESTIONS

1. The storage form of iron is:
a. Transferrin
b. TIBC
c. Ferritin
d. Hemoglobin

2. The iron requirement for a pregnant woman is:
a. 20 mg/day
b. 40 mg/day
c. 80 mg/day
d. 120 mg/day

3. All the following are iron-containing compounds, *except:*
a. Hemoglobin
b. Ceruloplasmin
c. Cytochrome C
d. Catalase

4. Megaloblastic anemia is due to the deficiency of:
a. Iron
b. Vitamin B_{12}
c. Iron overload
d. None of the above

5. The following are the biochemical findings of iron deficiency anemia, *except:*
a. Decreased ferritin
b. Increased TIBC
c. Increased ferritin
d. Increased transferrin

6. The polypeptide chain composition of the HbF is:
a. α_2 and β_2
b. α_2 and λ_2
c. α_2 and γ_2
d. α_2 and ε_2

7. Sickle cell hemoglobin is due to the substitution of Valine for:
a. Glutamic acid
b. Glycine
c. Alanine
d. Tyrosine

8. Alkali resistant hemoglobin is:
a. HbS
b. HbA
c. HbC
d. HbF

9. All the following are the symptoms of Vitamin B_{12} deficiency, *except:*
a. Megaloblastic anemia
b. Glossitis and inflammation of mouth,
c. Scurvy
d. Methyl malonic aciduria

10. Which of the following is not a laboratory finding of iron overload?
a. Increased serum iron
b. Increased ferritin
c. TIBC
d. Elevated transferrin

17

UNIT

Renal Function Tests

LEARNING OBJECTIVES

At the end of this unit, the learner should be able to understand:

- Various functions performed by kidney.
- The diagnostic tests performed to determine the functioning status of the kidney.
- Diagnostic tests to determine the concentrating and diluting mechanism of the kidney.
- Different metabolic inborn errors and the tests to determine them.
- Pathological conditions of the kidney.

INTRODUCTION

Kidney performs many important functions to regulate the internal environment of the body. It is the main regulator of all the substances of body fluids and is responsible for maintaining homeostasis. Kidney has cortex and medulla **(Fig. 17.1)**. The functional unit of kidney is nephron **(Fig. 17.2)**. It has glomerulus, proximal convoluted tubule, distal convoluted tubule, desending limb, loop of Henle, ascending limb and collecting duct. Bowmans capsule is a part of the nephron that forms a cup like sack surrounding the glomerulus **(Fig. 17.3)**.

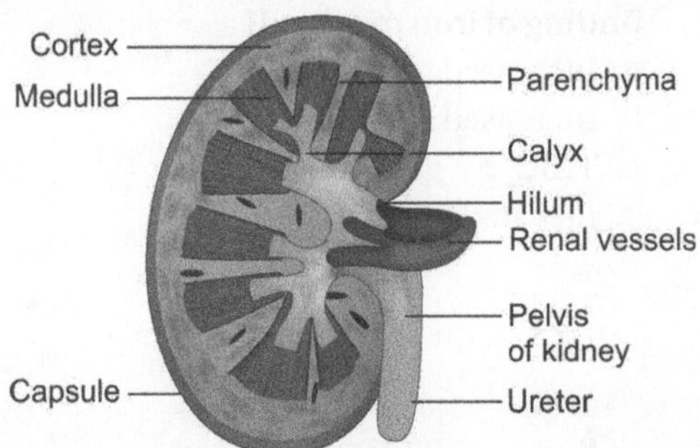

Fig. 17.1: Kidney.

FUNCTIONS OF KIDNEY

Kidney has five functions:

1. Urine formation
2. Regulation of fluid and electrolyte balance
3. Regulation of acid-base balance
4. Hormonal function
5. Excretion of nonprotein nitrogenous (NPN) substances.

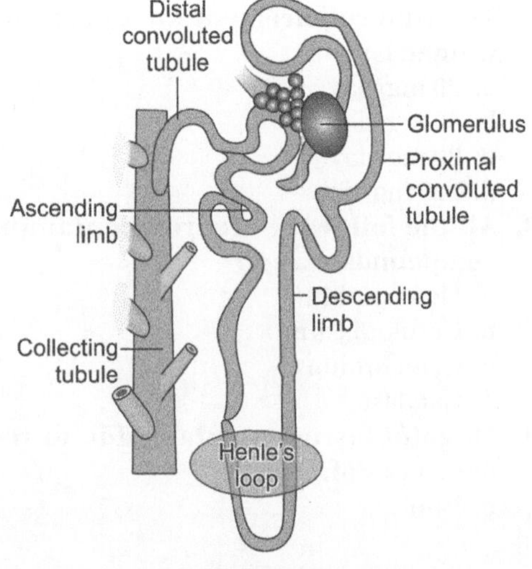

Fig. 17.2: Nephron.

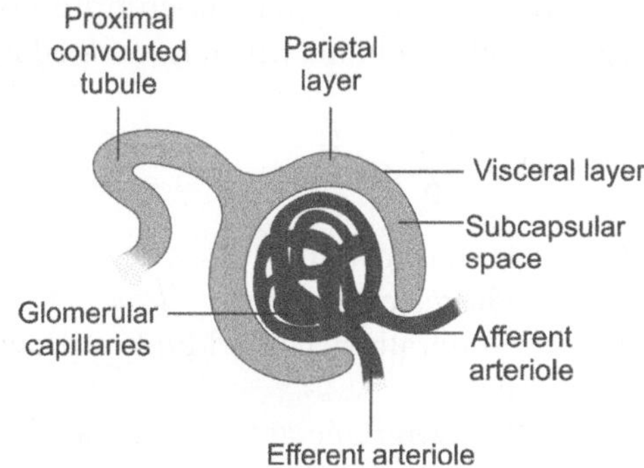

Fig. 17.3: Bowman's capsule.

Urine Formation

Removal of waste products from blood and preservation of essential solutes are accomplished through the formation of urine. This process involves:

1. *Ultrafiltration*: This occurs in the glomerulus, which allows water and electrolytes to pass through but not larger molecules like plasma proteins. The substances are filtered from the glomerulus into the Bowman's capsule at a rate of 125 mL/min. This is called the glomerular filtration rate (GFR).
2. *Selective reabsorption:* This takes place in the tubular system, which is divided into *proximal convoluted tubules* (PCT)—here the reabsorption of glucose and other carbohydrates takes place.
   Loop of Henle: Sodium and water absorption takes place.
   Distal convoluted tubules (DCT): Water reabsorption takes place
3. Secretion.

Regulation of Fluid and Electrolyte Balance

The water content of the body is 60% of the body weight so water balance is achieved through the concentrating and diluting mechanism of the kidney, which occurs in loop of Henle. A concentrating mechanism becomes effective when human body needs water. The urine osmolality increases during this mechanism.

Diluting mechanism takes place when there is excess water in the body. Therefore, osmolality decreases.

Acid-base Balance

Kidney is the one of the organs among the three systems that controls acid-base balance. (Discussed in the Acid-base Balance Chapter)

Hormonal Action

Kidney acts as a target organ for many hormones, such as ADH and aldosterone.

It acts directly as an endocrine organ secreting hormones, such as:

a. 1, 25 dihydroxycholecalciferol
b. Renin
c. Prostaglandins
d. Erythropoietin.

Excretion of NPN Products of Metabolism

Urea, creatinine, and uric acid are the substances eliminated by kidney.

Kidney functions are affected by the following:

- Prerenal causes
- Renal causes
- Postrenal causes.

Prerenal Causes

Dehydration (diarrhea, shock, and cardiac failure).

Renal Causes

The diseases affecting GFR and tubular function.

Any changes of the renal tubular system, which decreases the blood flow.

Postrenal Causes

Obstruction to urine flow (prostate enlargement, constriction).

Depending on the comments on the causes for decreased renal function and renal physiology, the renal function tests are divided into two groups.

Tests Measuring GFR

1. *Clearance tests:*
   a. Inulin clearance test
   b. Urea clearance test
   c. Creatinine clearance test.
2. *Study of elimination of NPN substances. Tests measuring the retention of NPN substances in serum:*
   a. Urea
   b. Uric acid
   c. Creatinine
   d. Amino acids
   e. Ammonia.

Clearance Test

The clearance tests are an extremely useful, effective and sensitive way of measuring the actual excretory capacity of the kidney.

Clearance is defined as the volume of plasma completely cleared off a substance, which is excreted in the urine.

Clearance can be calculated by:

$$\frac{UV}{P}$$

where U = Concentration of substance in the urine

P = Concentration of substance in plasma

V = Volume of urine

In order to determine GFR, the substance should be selected in such a way that it is:

1. Freely filtered by the glomerulus
2. Not reabsorbed or secreted
3. Not metabolized by the kidney
4. Not toxic.
   Urea is not preferred because:
   - This is produced within the body
   - It undergoes reabsorption
   - So it does not fulfill all the requirements of an ideal substance.

Creatinine Clearance Test

- It is the preferred clearance test used to find out the glomerular filtration rate.
- It is the volume of plasma completely cleared off creatinine, which is excreted in the urine.
- Formula = $\frac{UV}{P}$ or $\frac{U \times V \times 1.73/A}{P}$

U = Urine creatinine

P = Plasma creatinine

1.73 = Generally accepted body surface urea

A = Body surface area of the patient, under investigation

- The creatinine clearance is very convenient to measure GFR
- Because it fulfills all the requirements of a substance which is ideal for measuring GFR
- In addition to this, the amount of creatinine produced is relatively constant and it is not affected by the dietary intake.

Procedure

1. A minimum of 600 mL water is given to the patient. The first urine sample is discarded.
2. Then start the collection of urine for 24 hours with a preservative. Starting and ending times of collection are recorded.
3. During this time, a specimen of blood is also collected.
4. Creatinine concentration is determined in the urine and also in the blood.
   The GFR is influenced by—(a) renal blood flow, and (b) plasma colloidal osmotic pressure.

Determination of Urine Creatinine and Calculation of Creatinine Clearance

- The urine creatinine is estimated using Jaffe's method.
- Urine creatinine level can be used as a screening test to evaluate kidney function, or as part of the creatinine clearance test.
- Normal values are highly dependent on the age and lean body mass of the person.
- Normal range value vary from laboratory to laboratory

- Urine creatinine (24-hour sample) values may therefore be quite variable and can range from 500 mg/day to 2000 mg/day.

Reagents

1. *Picric acid, 0.04 M:* Dry some picric acid crystals by putting over a pad of filter paper. Dissolve 9.16 g of dry picric acid in water and make up to one liter.
2. *Sodium hydroxide, 0.75 N:* Weigh about 7 g of sodium hydroxide and prepare 200 mL solution in water. Determine the normality by titrating against 0.667 N sulfuric acid (Reagent 1). Adjust the normality of sodium hydroxide to 0.75 N by proper dilution.
3. Stock standard creatinine solution, 1 mg per mL. Dissolve 100 mg of creatinine in 0.1 N HCl (1 mL concentrated HCl diluted 100 mL) and make up to 100 mL with acid. Store in refrigerator. Stable for one month.
4. *Working standard, 0.02 mg per mL:* Dilute 2 mL of stock standard to 100 mL with water. Urine sample 1 mL diluted to 50 mL in a conical flask.

Procedure

Contents	Blank	Standard	Test
Water (mL)	4.0	3.5	2.0
Standard	—	0.5	—
Diluted urine	—	—	2.0
Picric acid	1.0	1.0	1.0
NaOH	1.0	1.0	1.0
Kept at room temperature for 15 minutes and read the absorbance at 520 nm			

Calculation

$$= \frac{T-B}{S-B} \times 0.01 \times \frac{50}{2} \times 100$$

$$= \frac{T-B}{S-B} \times 25 \text{ mg of creatinine in 100 mL of urine}$$

Given that the urine creatinine is 52 mg%, volume of the urine is 1400 mL and plasma creatinine is 0.6 mg% then

Applying the formula that is $= \frac{U \times V}{P}$

U = Urine creatinine concentration
V = Volume of the urine
P = Plasma creatinine

$$\frac{52 \times 1400}{0.6 \times 24 \times 60} = \frac{72800}{864} = 84.2 \text{ mL/min}$$

$$\frac{52 \times 1400}{100} = 728 \text{ mg of creatinine/volume}$$

Normal values

Males	105 ± 20 mL/min.
Female	95 ± 20 mL/min.

Abnormal results are lower than normal GFR measurements, and they indicate.

- Acute tubular necrosis
- Congestive heart failure
- Dehydration
- Glomerulonephritis
- Shock
- Acute nephrotic syndrome
- Acute and chronic renal failure.

Study of Elimination of NPN Substances

The intermediates or the end products of protein metabolism include urea, creatinine, uric acid, amino acid and NH_3.

Urea

- Urea is the end product of protein metabolism.
- The ammonia formed during amino acid metabolism is toxic to the human body.
- So, it should be converted to a nontoxic substance (urea) and excreted normally **(Fig. 17.4)**.
- Urea constitutes about 45% of NPN substances.
- Study of their elimination by simultaneous study of blood and urine may help in understanding renal disturbances.

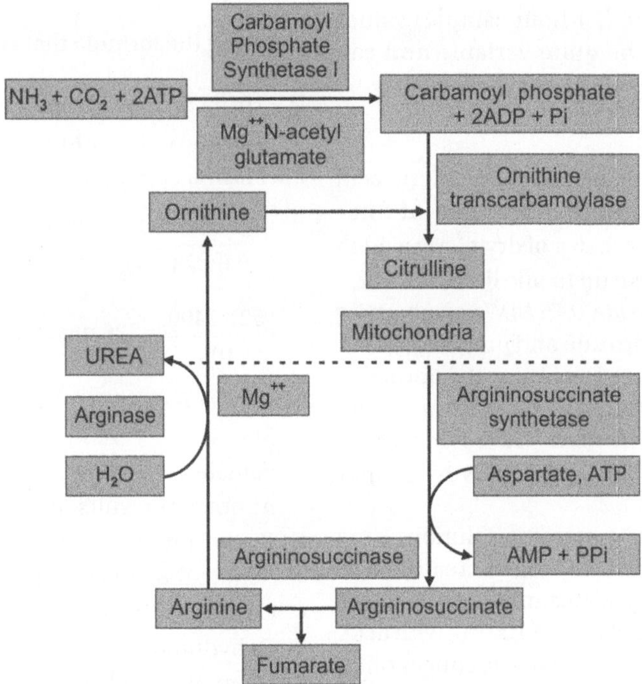

Fig. 17.4: Formation of urea

Chemical Method

Blood Urea Determination by Diacetyl Monoxime (DAM) Method

- The urea test is somewhat a routine test used primarily to evaluate renal (kidney) function.
- The test is often performed on patients with many different diseases.
- Urea is formed in the liver as the end product of protein metabolism.
- During digestion, protein is broken down to amino acids.
- Amino acids contain nitrogen, which is removed as NH_4^+ (ammonium ion), while the rest of the molecule is used to produce energy or other substances needed by the cell.
- The ammonia is combined with other intermediates to produce urea.
- The urea makes its way into the blood and it is ultimately eliminated in the urine by the kidneys.
- Most renal diseases affect urea excretion so that urea levels increase in the blood.
- Patients with dehydration or bleeding into the stomach and/or intestines may also have abnormal urea levels.
- Numerous drugs also affect urea by competing with it for elimination by the kidneys.

Principle

Urea reacts with diacetyl monoxime under strongly acidic conditions in presence of ferric ions and thiosemicarbazide to give a pink-colored complex.

$$\text{Diacetyl monoxime} + H_2O \xrightarrow{H^+} \text{Diacetyl} + \text{Hydroxylamine}$$

$$\text{Diacetyl} + \text{Urea} \xrightarrow{H^+} \text{Diazo derivative, read at 540 nm}$$

Specimen: Serum or plasma can be used.

Reagents

1. *Diacetyl monoxime:* Dissolve 1.56 g diacetyl monoxime in 250 mL water.

2. *Ferric chloride:* Dissolve 324 mg of ferric chloride in 10 mL of 56% orthophosphoric acid. Store in a brown bottle.
3. *Thiosemicarbazide*: Dissolve 41 mg of thiosemicarbazide in 50 mL of water.
4. *Sulfuric acid 20%*: Add 200 mL of concentrated sulfuric acid to 800 mL of water in a beaker slowly with stirring and cooling.
5. *Acid reagent:* Mix 1 liter of 20% sulfuric acid (Reagent 4) with 1 mL of ferric chloride reagent (Reagent 2).
6. *Trichloroacetic acid, 10%:* Dissolve 10 g of TCA in water and make up to 100 mL.
7. *Preservative diluent for standard*: Boil 250 mL water and add 40 mg of phenylmercuric acetate, mix to dissolve. Transfer to one liter graduated cylinder. Add 0.3 mL concentrated sulfuric acid and make up the volume to one liter and mix. The use of preservative diluent is optional.
8. *Stock standard urea:* 0.5 mg per mL. Dissolve 50 mg of urea (GR Grade) in 100 mL of preservative diluent (Reagent 7) or can be dissolved in deionized water it is stable for a week if it is refrigerated.
9. *Standard urea for use:* 0.01 mg per mL. Dilute 1 mL of stock standard (Reagent 8) solution to 50 mL with deionized water.

Procedure

Reagents	*Blank*	*Standard*	*Test*
Water	—	—	3.4 mL
Serum	—	—	0.1 mL
TCA, 10%	—	—	1.5 mL
Mix wait for 10 minutes centrifuge			
Supernatant	—	—	1.0 mL
Water (mL)	1.0	—	—
Standard urea for use	—	1.0 mL	—
Diacetyl monoxime	1.0 mL	1.0 mL	1.0 mL
Thiosemicarbazide	1.0 mL	1.0 mL	1.0 mL
Acid reagent	3.0 mL	3.0 mL	3.0 mL
Place in a boiling water bath exactly for 15 minutes and cool			
Read the absorbance at 540 nm or blue filter			

Calculation

Mg urea in 100 mL of blood $= \frac{T-B}{S-B} \times \frac{5}{1} \times 0.01 \times \frac{100}{0.1}$

$$= \frac{\text{OD of T} - \text{OD of B}}{\text{OD of S} - \text{OD of B}} \times 50$$

- Dilute the sample if optical density rises above 0.6 and perform the test again
- Dilution factor should be taken into consideration during calculation.

Determination of Urea Using (Standard Graph)

1. *TCA:* H_2O mixture (3:7): Dissolve 3 mL of 10% TCA in 7 mL of water.
2. *Stock standard urea:* 0.8 mg per mL. Dissolve 80 mg of urea (GR Grade) in 100 mL of water it is stable for a week if it is refrigerated.
3. *Working standard:* Transfer 2.5 mL of stock standard to 100 mL volumetric flask and make up to 100 mL with deionized water.

Other reagents are same as given for urea estimation by diacetyl monoxime method using single standard.

Procedure

Serum 0.1 mL + 0.9 mL of 10% TCA centrifuge for 10 minutes and use the supernatant for the estimation.

0.4 OD corresponds to 10.0 μg of urea

So 0.2 mL supernatant contains 10.0 μg of urea

1 mL supernatant contains:

$$\frac{1.0 \times 10}{0.2} = 50 \text{ μg of urea}$$

Therefore, 0.1 mL serum contains 50 μg urea 100 mL serum contains:

$$\frac{100 \times 50}{0.1} = 50{,}000 \text{ μg} = 50 \text{ mg\% of urea}$$

Direct Nesslerization Method for Urea Estimation

Principle

The urease enzyme hydrolyzes urea to ammonium carbonate, which on treatment with

Reagents	Blank	S_1	S_2	S_3	S_4	S_5	S_6	S_7	T
Standard (mL)	–	0.1	0.2	0.3	0.4	0.5	0.6	0.7	
Concentration (μg)	–	2	4	6	8	10	12	14	
Supernatant (mL)									0.2
TCA:H_2O (mL)	1	0.9	0.8	0.7	0.6	0.5	0.4	0.3	0.8
DAM (mL)	1.0	1.0	1.0	1.0	1.0	1.0	1.0	1.0	1.0
Thiosemicarbazide	1.0	1.0	1.0	1.0	1.0	1.0	1.0	1.0	1.0 mL
Acid reagent (mL)	3.0	3.0	3.0	3.0	3.0	3.0	3.0	3.0	3.0
Place in a boiling water bath exactly for 15 minutes and cool									
OD at 540 nm-------→ or blue filter	0.03>0	0.08	0.16	0.24	0.32	0.41	0.48	0.55	0.40

Nessler's reagent produces yellowish orange color. The absorbance of the color produced is measured photometrically using green filter or at 540 nm.

Specimen: Venous blood is collected with potassium oxalate as anticoagulant.

Reagents

1. *Sodium tungstate, 10%:* Dissolve 100 g sodium tungstate in water and make up to one liter.
2. *Sulfuric acid 0.667:* Dissolve 10 mL of concentrated sulfuric acid in 500 mL water. Determine the normality by titrating against 0.667 N sodium carbonate. Adjust the normality to 0.667 N by dilution.
3. *Urease suspension:* Grind 1 g horse gram powder with 10 mL water and 500 mg of potassium chloride. Use supernatant. Keep in refrigerator. Stable at least a week.
4. *Nessler's reagent:* Into a 500 mL volumetric flask, add 50 g mercuric iodide, 35 g potassium iodide and 200 mL distilled water. Mix to dissolve. In a beaker, dissolve 50 g sodium hydroxide in 250 mL water. Add this solution to volumetric flask with stirring and make up to 500 mL with water. Use only the clear supernatant. The reagent is stable if stored in polythene bottles.
5. *Standard urea solution:* 60 mg per 100 mL. Dissolve exactly 60 mg urea, AR grade in water and make up to 100 mL. Store in refrigerator. Prepare fresh every week.

Procedure

Reagents	B	S	T
Water	–	3 mL	3 mL
Blood	–	–	0.5 mL
Standard urea	–	0.5 mL	–
Urease suspension	–	0.5 mL	0.5 mL
Incubate at 55°C for 15 minutes			
Sulfuric acid 0.667 N	–	0.5 mL	0.5 mL
Mix, stand for 3 minutes			
Sodium tungstate 10%	–	0.5 mL	0.5 mL
Mix, centrifuge for 5 minutes			
Supernatant	–	2 mL	2 mL
Water	7 mL	5 mL	5 mL
Nessler's reagent	1 mL	1 mL	1 mL
OD at 540 nm or green filter			

Calculation

$$\text{Mg urea per 100 mL} = \frac{T-B}{S-B} \times \frac{0.12}{0.2} \times 100$$

$$= \frac{T-B}{S-B} \times 60$$

Note:
- Ammonium oxalate should not be used as an anticoagulant
- Do not mix after adding Nessler's reagent. It may form turbidity
- To avoid turbid formation, add one drop of saturated sodium-potassium-tartrate solution
- If turbidity occurs due to a high content of urea, repeat the color development step (Nessler's reagent addition) taking 1 mL supernatant. Apply dilution factor in calculation.
- Sulfuric acid was added to T and S to stop the enzyme action.

Enzymatic Method

Estimation of Urea by Glutamate Dehydrogenase (GLDH)/kinetic Method

Reagents
1. Urease, glutamate dehydrogenase and NADH.
2. *Standard:* Urea 50 mg/dL. Ready to use.

Specimen: Serum is preferred.

Procedure

Reaction temperature: 30°C.

Contents	Standard (S)	Test (T)
Working	1.0 mL	1.0 mL
Standard	0.005 mL	—
Sample	—	0.005 mL

Mix and record the change in absorbance of the test (ΔA_T) and standard (ΔA_S) between 20 seconds and 80 seconds at 340 nm wavelength.

Calculation

$$\text{Urea concentration (mg/dL)} = \frac{\Delta A_T}{\Delta A_S} \times 50$$

- Blood urea nitrogen (BUN) concentration (mg/dL) = 0.467 × urea concentration (mg/dL).
- To convert urea concentration (mg/dL) to mmol/L, use equation mmol/L = 0.167 × urea concentration (mg/dL)
- The method is linear up to 300 mg/dL of urea
- For sample values higher than 300 mg/dL, dilute the sample with 0.9% saline and repeat the assay. Apply proper dilution factor to calculate the final result.

Clinical Significance

Normal values

Serum/plasma urea: 8.0–40 mg/dL
2.49–7.47 mmol/L
BUN: 7–21 mg/dL

Greater-than-normal levels may indicate:

a. *Prerenal causes:*
   - Congestive heart failure
   - Myocardial infarction
   - Hypovolemia due to burns, shock or dehydration
   - Excessive protein catabolism
   - Gastrointestinal bleeding.

b. *Renal causes:*
   - Acute glomerulonephritis
   - Chronic nephritis
   - Pyelonephritis
   - Nephrotic syndrome
   - Acute tubular necrosis.

c. *Postrenal causes:* Urinary tract obstruction to urine flow (stone, tumor, enlarged prostate).

   Lower-than-normal levels may indicate:
   - Liver failure
   - Low protein diet
   - Malnutrition
   - Overhydration.

Creatinine

- Creatinine is a breakdown product of creatine, which is an important part of muscle
- The most important source of energy inside cells is the ATP molecule, with its high-energy phosphate bonds

- When one of these bonds is broken, energy is released, and ATP becomes ADP
- Creatine phosphate represents a backup energy source for ATP because it can quickly reconvert ADP back to ATP
- Over time, the creatine molecule gradually degrades to creatinine
- Creatinine is a waste product, that is, it cannot be used by cells for any constructive purpose
- The daily production of creatine, and subsequently creatinine, depends on muscle mass, which fluctuates little in most normal people over long periods.
- Creatinine is excreted from the body entirely by the kidneys.
- With normal kidney function, the serum creatinine level should remain constant and normal.
- A measurement of the serum creatinine level is used to evaluate kidney function.
- Urine creatinine levels can be used as a screening test to evaluate kidney function, or as part of the creatinine clearance test.

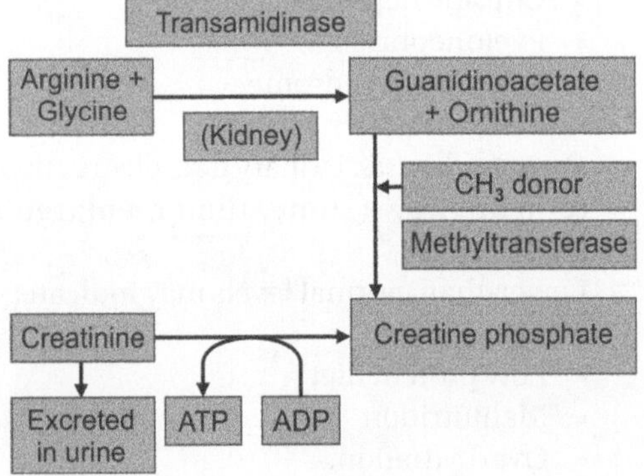

Determination of Serum Creatinine

The test is performed to evaluate kidney function. If kidney function is abnormal, creatinine levels will increase in the blood, due to decreased excretion of creatinine in the urine. Creatinine levels also vary according to a person's size and muscle mass.

Jaffe's Method (Bonsnes and Tausky)

1. The serum creatinine does not increase until renal function is below 50% of normal.
2. Simultaneous urea N_2 and creatinine N_2 determination have more clinical significance.

Principle

Creatinine in alkaline conditions reacts with picric acid to form alkaline creatinine picrate. The reddish yellow color so formed is measured colorimetrically at 520 nm and creatinine is determined.

Reagents

1. *Sulfuric acid, 0.667 N:* Dilute 10 mL of concentrated sulfuric acid to 500 mL water. Determine the normality by titrating against 0.667 N sodium carbonate. Adjust the normality to 0.667 N by dilution.
2. *Sodium tungstate, 5%:* Dissolve 5 g of sodium tungstate in water and make up to 100 mL.
3. *Picric acid, 0.04 M:* Dry some picric acid crystals by putting over a pad of filter paper. Dissolve 9.16 g of dry picric acid in water and make up to one liter.
4. *Sodium hydroxide, 0.75 N:* Weigh 7 g of sodium hydroxide and prepare 200 mL solution in water. Determine the normality by titrating against 0.667 N sulfuric acid (Reagent 1). Adjust the normality of sodium hydroxide to 0.75 N by proper dilution.
5. *Stock standard creatinine solution, 1 mg per mL:* Dissolve 100 mg of creatinine in 0.1 N HCl (1 mL concentrated HCl diluted 100 mL) and make up to 100 mL with acid. Store in refrigerator. Stable for one month.
6. *Working standard, 0.04 mg per mL:* Dilute 4 mL of stock standard to 100 mL with water.

Procedure

Reagents	B	S	T
Water	4 mL	2 mL	2 mL
Serum	–	–	2 mL
Standard for use solution	–	2 mL	–
Sulfuric acid, 0.667 N	2 mL	2 mL	2 mL
Sodium tungstate, 5%	2 mL	2 mL	2 mL
Mix Stand for 10 minutes. Centrifuge			
Take supernatant in 3 different test tubes	3 mL	3 mL	3 mL
Picric acid 0.04 M	1 mL	1 mL	1 mL
Sodium hydroxide, 0.75 N	1 mL	1 mL	1 mL
Mix and incubate at room temperature for 15 minutes			
Read the optical density at 520 nm or green filter			

Calculation

$$\text{Mg creatinine/100 mL serum} = \frac{\text{OD of T} - \text{OD of B}}{\text{OD of S} - \text{OD of B}} \times 0.03 \, \frac{100}{0.75}$$

$$= \frac{T-B}{S-B} \times 4$$

Determination of Creatinine (Standard Graph)

The reagents are same as used for BST procedure.

Stock standard: 100 mg of creatinine is dissolved in 100 mL of 0.1 N HCl.

Working standard: 4 mL of stock diluted to 100 mL with 0.1 N HCl.

Mix 3 mL of working standard, 3 mL 5% sodium tungstate , 3 mL water and 3 mL 0.667 N H_2SO_4 in a test tube. The concentration of standard at this dilution will be 10.0 mg/ml. From this, range of standard from 0.5–3.0 mL is taken.

In another centrifuge tube take 0.5 mL of serum, 0.5 mL water, 0.5 mL 5% sodium tungstate and 0.5 mL, 0.667 N H_2SO_4 (add H_2SO_4 dropwise). Keep the contents for 10 minutes and centrifuge. Use the supernatant for the assay.

Calculation

OD of 0.10 corresponds to 4.6 µg
1 mL supernatant contains 4.6 µg
Therefore, 2 mL contains 9.2 µg
0.5 mL serum contains = 9.2 µg

Procedure

Contents	B	S_1	S_2	S_3	S_4	S_5	S_6	T
Volume of standard (mL)	—	0.5	1.0	1.5	2.0	2.5	3.0	—
Concentration (mg)	—	5	10	15	20	25	30	—
Supernatant (mL)								1.0
Water (mL)	3.0	2.5	2.0	1.5	1.0	0.5	0.0	2.0
Picric acid (mL)	1.0	1.0	1.0	1.0	1.0	1.0	1.0	1.0
NaOH (mL)	1.0	1.0	1.0	1.0	1.0	1.0	1.0	1.0
Read the absorbance at 520 nm after 15 minutes of incubation at room temperature								
	0.07	0.09	0.17	0.27	0.36	0.45	0.53	0.10
	↓							
	adjusted to 0.00							

$$1 \text{ mL serum contains} = \frac{9.2 \times 1}{0.5} = 18.4\,\mu g$$

$$100 \text{ mL serum contains} = \frac{100 \times 18.4}{1} = 1.8 \text{ mg\%}$$ of creatinine

Interpretation

Normal value: 0.8 to 1.4 mg/dL.

Normal value ranges may vary slightly among different laboratories.

Higher-than-normal levels may indicate:
- Nephrotic syndrome
- Chronic glomerulonephritis
- Acute tubular necrosis
- Dehydration
- Diabetic nephropathy
- Reduced renal blood flow
- Pyelonephritis
- Renal failure
- Urinary tract obstruction.

Lower-than-normal levels may indicate:
- Muscular dystrophy (late stage)
- Myasthenia gravis.

ESTIMATED GLOMERULAR FILTRATION RATE

Various different diseases, conditions, and drugs can affect the function of the kidneys. The estimated glomerular filtration rate (eGFR) does not diagnose any kidney disease but is a test to assess how well your kidneys are working.

The estimated glomerular filtration rate (eGFR) is a test that is used to assess how well the kidneys are working. The test estimates the volume of blood that is filtered by your kidneys over a given period. The test is called the estimated glomerular filtration rate because the glomeruli are the tiny filters in the kidneys. If these filters do not do their job properly then the kidney is said to have reduced or impaired kidney function.

The eGFR test involves a blood test, which measures creatinine. Creatinine is normally cleared from the blood by the kidneys. If kidneys are not working properly, the level of creatinine in the blood goes up. The eGFR is then calculated from the age, sex and blood creatinine level. An adjustment to the calculation is needed for people with African-Caribbean origin.

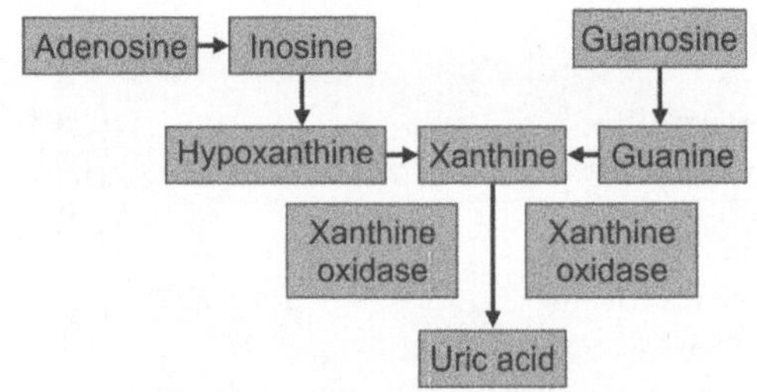

Fig. 17.5: Purine metabolism.

Uric Acid

It is the end product of purine metabolism **(Fig. 17.5)**.

Determination of Uric Acid (Henry et al. Method)

Principle

Uric acid oxidized to allantoin and CO_2 by a phosphotungstic acid reagent in alkaline solution. Phosphotungstic acid is reduced to tungsten blue, which is measured at 710 nm.

The uric acid concentration in serum is affected by renal as well as extrarenal factors.
1. The uric acid determination is helpful in the diagnosis of gout.
2. When there is severe impairment in the renal function the uric acid level will be varied.

Specimen: Serum or plasma.

Reagents

1. *Sulfuric acid 0.667 N:* Dilute 10 mL concentrated sulfuric acid to 500 mL. Determine the normality using 0.667 N sodium carbonate standard solution. Adjust the normality of acid to 0.667 N by dilution.
2. *Sodium tungstate 10% (w/v):* Dissolve 10 g of sodium tungstate in water and make up to 100 mL.

3. *Sodium carbonate 14%:* Dissolve 14 g of sodium carbonate in about 80 mL of water and make up to 100 mL.
4. *Phosphotungstic acid reagent:* Dissolve 40 g of sodium tungstate in 300 mL water in a liter round bottom flask. Add 32 mL of syrupy phosphoric acid (85%) and several glass beads or porcelain bits. Attach a reflux condenser and boil gently for 2 hours. Cool to room temperature. Add 32 g of lithium sulfate and dissolve. Dilute to one liter. Store in brown colored bottle.
5. *Stock standard uric acid, 1 mg per mL:* Dissolve 60 mg of lithium carbonate in 20 mL of water. Heat the solution to about 60°C and add exactly 100 mg of uric acid. Stir until dissolved. Cool, transfer to a 100 mL volumetric flask with rinsing. Add 2 mL of formalin (40%) and 1 mL of 10% acetic acid solution. Make up to 100 mL mark with water. Keep in a well stoppered bottle in the dark or in a refrigerator. The solution is stable for one month.
   Working standard: 0.01 mg/mL—Dilute 1 mL of the stock solution to 100 mL with water.

Procedure

Reagents	*B*	*S*	*T*
Water	—	—	8.0 mL
Serum or plasma	—	—	1.0 mL
Sulfuric acid, 0.667	—	—	0.5 mL
Sodium tungstate, 10%	—	—	0.5 mL
Mix, centrifuge for 10 minutes			
Supernatant	—	—	3.0 mL
Water	3.0 mL	—	—
Working standard	—	3.0 mL	—
Phosphotungstic acid	1.0 mL	1.0 mL	1.0 mL
Sodium carbonate, 14%	1.0 mL	1.0 mL	1.0 mL
Kept at room temperature for 15 minutes			
Read the absorbance at 710 nm or red filter			

Calculation

$$\text{Mg of uric acid per 100 mL serum} = \frac{\text{OD of T} - \text{OD of B}}{\text{OD of S} - \text{OD of B}} \times 0.03 \, \frac{100}{0.3}$$

$$= \frac{\text{T} - \text{B}}{\text{S} - \text{B}} \times 10$$

Interpretation

Normal value: 2.5–7 mg%

Higher-than-normal levels may indicate:
- Renal failure
- Acute gout
- Pneumonia
- Sepsis
- Leukemia
- Polycythemia
- Anemia.

Lower-than-normal levels may indicate: Acromegaly.

Aminoaciduria

- The presence of amino acids in the urine.
- Small amounts of amino acids are also present in normal urine
- The aminoaciduria test screens for increased levels of amino acid excretion in the urine that indicates possible inborn errors of metabolism caused by a specific enzyme deficiency
- Aminoacidurias may be primary or secondary
- Primary aminoaciduria is due to an inherited enzyme deficiency, this is also called an inborn error of metabolism
- The defect is located in the pathway by which amino acid is metabolized or the renal tubular system by which the amino acid is absorbed
- Secondary aminoaciduria may be due to disease of the liver or renal tubular dysfunction or protein-energy malnutrition
- In both the conditions, metabolites of amino acids accumulated in the blood are excreted in the urine.

There are several tests to detect these amino acids and their metabolites in the urine.

Determination of Amino Acids

Amino acids are a part of NPN.

Their determination is helpful only in some congenital renal disorders.

If there is defect in reabsorption, more amino acid may appear in urine, this condition is called aminoaciduria. For example, cystinuria, homocystinuria.

Principle

In a more recent colorimetric method, the reaction of 2,3-dinitrofluorobenzene (DNFB) with the amino group in alkaline solution is used, a reaction introduced by Sanger (1945) to estimate free amino groups in insulin and subsequently applied to blood by Dublin (1960), who extracted the dinitrophenyl compounds formed in acidified dioxane before reading at 420 nm.

Reagents

1. Stock DNFB—Dilute 0.65 mL of 2,4-dinitro-fluorobenzene in 50 mL acetone.
   Stable for 32 months at 4°C.
2. Sodium tetraborate, 132 mmol/L—Dissolve 50.35 g in one liter water. Stand overnight before use (Borax).
3. Working DFNB solution—Prepare freshly by diluting 1 mL of stock DFNB with 9 mL of sodium tetraborate.
4. Acidified dioxane—Dilute 1 mL of concentration HCl with 50 mL of dioxane.
5. HCl, 110 mmol/L.
6. Sodium tungstate—Dissolve 13.3 g sodium tungstate, 2 H_2O in water and make up to 100 mL.
7. Protein precipitant—Mix 1 mL of sodium tungstate and 9 mL of HCl solution. Prepare freshly.
8. Stock standard, 20 mmol/L—Dissolve 147 mg glutamic acid and 75.1 mg glycine in about 10 mL water. Add 200 mg sodium benzoate and 70 mL in HCl. Dilute to 100 mL with water.
9. Working standard—Dilute 0.1, 0.2 and 0.4 mL of stock standard to 1.0 mL with water. These contain 2.0, 4.0 and 8.0 mmol/l or 28.56 and 112 μg amino acid N/mL.

Procedure for Serum

	Blank	Std	Test
Water	0.5	0.3	—
Standard	—	0.2	—
Serum	—	—	0.5
Protein precipitant	4.0	4.0	4.0
Mix well, centrifuge			
Clear supernatant	1.0	1.0	1.0
Working DNFB	1.0	1.0	1.0
Incubate at 70°C for 15 minutes			
Kept for 10 minutes at room temperature			
Acidified dioxane	5.0	5.0	5.0
Mix and read at 420 nm			

Calculation: mg amino acid/100 mL serum

$$= \frac{(T-B)}{(S-B)} \times \frac{5.6}{0.1} \times \frac{100}{1000} \text{ or } \frac{(T-B)}{(S-B)} \times 5.6$$

Procedure for Urine

- Mix 1.0 mL urine with 10 mL water.
- Add 2 to 4 drops of phenolphthalein indicator and 0.2 N NaOH until the mixture turns pink.
- Boil gently for 15 minutes.
- Add further alkali dropwise to retain the pink color.
- Cool, dilute to 20 mL.
- Mix 1.0 mL of above titrated solution with 1.0 mL of DNFB and then follows the procedure of serum.

Calculation: mg amino acid/24 hours volume =

$$\frac{(T-B) \times 5.6 \times 20 \times \text{volume}}{(S-B) \times 1000} = \frac{(T-B) \times 0.112 \times \text{volume}}{(S-B)}$$

Note: Urine should be kept frozen (below 0°C) before analysis or fresh urine should be immediately processed.

Increased total urine amino acids may indicate any of the following:

- Alkaptonuria
- Phenylketonuria
- Cystinosis
- Cystathioninuria
- Hartnup disease
- Homocystinuria
- Hyperammonemia
- Hyperparathyroidism
- Maple syrup urine disease
- Methylmalonic acidemia
- Multiple myeloma
- Ornithine transcarbamylase deficiency
- Osteomalacia
- Propionic acidemia
- Rickets
- Tyrosinemia type 1
- Tyrosinemia type 2
- Viral hepatitis.

Alkaptonuria

- Alkaptonuria is a rare disease that is *inherited.*
- The disease results from a deficiency of the enzyme homogentisic acid oxidase.
- This enzyme deficiency leads to a buildup of homogentisic acid in tissues of the body.
- It is a classic recessive condition. The gene for it is autosomal chromosome.
- Parents of a person with alkaptonuria each have one alkaptonuric gene and a normal gene paired with it.
- Ochronosis is the darkening of the tissues of the body that is caused by pigment composed of the excess homogentisic acid in patients with alkaptonuria. The pigment accumulates in the cartilage of the joints and ears, skin, and whites (sclerae) of the eyes. Bluish discoloration of the nails is also characteristic.
- Alkaptonuria leads to premature progressive degeneration of the cartilage of the joints due to the accumulation of homogentisic acid in the cartilage.
- This results in osteoarthritis of joints throughout the body at an unusually early age.
- Typical joints affected include the spine, knees, hips, and shoulders. Joint symptoms include stiffness, pain, swelling, and limited motion.
- Homogentisic acid accumulated in the urine will cause it to turn black.
- The urine from a person with alkaptonuria turns dark on standing if it is alkaline.

Phenylketonuria (PKU)

It is an inherited disorder that increases the amount of the amino acid phenylalanine to harmful levels in the blood, due to the defect of phenylalanine hydroxylase.

If PKU is not treated, excess phenylalanine can cause mental retardation and other serious health problems.

Identification of Amino Acids

Paper Chromatography

When the test shows increased levels of amino acids in the urine, a 24-hour quantitative urine chromatography is necessary to accurately measure the elevated levels of the specific amino acids. (The detailed procedure is discussed in Unit 6).

Metabolic Screening

The inborn errors of metabolism (hereditary) results in mental retardation

Several qualitative tests are done on the urine samples to detect excess excretion of accumulated metabolites.

Specimen : random urine.

Ferric chloride test for phenylketonuria (PKU)

Due to the defect of phenylalanine hydroxylase the phenylalanine and its metabolites (phenylacetate, phenylactate and p-hydroxy-phenyl-acetate) are accumulated in the blood and are excreted in the urine. So, the disease is called phenylketonuria. The common test for the qualitative detection of the above metabolite in urine is ferric chloride test.

Reagents

10% $FeCl_3.6H_2O$

Procedure

Take 2 mL urine + 0.5 mL 10 percent ferric chloride. If the color changes to blue or green, it indicates the presence of phenylalanine and its metabolites in the urine.

Dinitrophenylhydrazine (DNPH) test for PKU and Alpha Keto acid Catabolites

Reagents

0.5% Dinitrophenylhydrazine

0.5 N NaOH.

Procedure

1 mL urine + 1 mL dinitrophenylhydrazine. If yellow precipitate is formed, then add 0.5 mL of 0.5 N NaOH. If more precipitate forms on adding NaOH, then the test is considered as positive.

Nitroprusside test for Homocystinuria

Reagents

1. Sodium chloride: Solid
2. Ammonia: 3 mL concentrated ammonia is diluted to 10 mL with water.
3. Silver nitrate solution $AgNO_3$ (1%), freshly prepared: Dissolve 100 mg silver nitrate in 10 mL water.
4. Sodium nitroprusside solution (1%): Dissolve 100 mg in 10 mL water (prepared freshly).
5. Sodium cyanide (0.7%): 70 mg in 10 mL water.

Procedure

Saturate 5 mL urine with sodium chloride and filter or centrifuge.

Control	*Test*	
Filtered urine	2.0 mL	2.0 mL
Ammonia	0.2 mL	–
$AgNO_3$ 1%	–	0.2 mL
Mix and keep for 1 minute		
Nitroprusside	0.2 mL	0.2 mL
Mix well		
Na cyanide	0.2 mL	0.2 mL
Mix and observe		

Observe the color as the reagent reaches the solution. Immediate development of pink color indicates a positive test. Appearance of pink color in the control shows the presence of cysteine. Pink color in the test shows the presence of homocysteine.

Note: If sodium cyanide is added in excess, it will give a false-positive result.

Silver Nitrate Test for Alkaptonuria

Reagents

- *Silver nitrate 3%:* Dissolve 3 g of silver nitrate in 100 mL water
- *Ammonia 4%:* Dissolve 4 mL of concentrated ammonia in 100 mL water.

Procedure

Add 5 mL silver nitrate solution to 0.5 mL urine and add drops of diluted ammonia slowly. If dark black color appears, it indicates that urine contains homogentisic acid and test is positive. Development of black color afterwards is not considered.

Nitrosonaphthol test for tyrosine and its P-OH catabolites

Tyrosine and its metabolites react with 1-nitroso-2-naphthol in the presence of sodium nitrite in a weak acid solution to give an orange-red color.

Procedure

To 1 mL 2.63 N nitric acid, add a drop of sodium nitrite, mix and add 0.2 mL of 0.1% nitrosonaphthol (prepared in ethanol). Mix the contents again and add 0.15 mL urine. Observe the color within 5 minutes. The orange-red color indicates the presence of tyrosine and its catabolites in the urine.

TESTS MEASURING TUBULAR FUNCTION

a. *Excretory function test:* Phenolsulfonphthalein test (PSP test)
b. *Tests to measure the concentrating and diluting ability:*
   - Specific gravity determination
   - Osmolality determination.

Concentrating and Diluting Mechanism of Kidney

Twelve-hour Specific Gravity Test

Procedure

The diet is divided into 3, i.e., taken at 8 am, 12 noon and 5 pm. The bladder is emptied at 8 am immediately before breakfast. The urine is collected at 2 hours intervals from 8 am to 8 pm. The night urine is collected as a single specimen for the 12th hour period.

The specific gravity is determined with the help of urinometer **(Fig. 17.6)**. Urinometer consists of a thin stem graduated from 1000 to 1060 corresponding to specific gravities of 1.0 to 1.06. The bulb at the bottom is suitably weighted. Urinometer is calibrated at 60°F (15°C). Take sufficient amount of urine in a container. Allow the urinometer to float in urine without touching the sides. Observe the specific gravity reading corresponding to the meniscus of urine. Note the temperature of the urine.

Suppose the meniscus of the urine coincides with the reading 1012 and temperature of urine is 37°C. Since the urine is at a higher temperature than the temperature of calibration of urinometer, a temperature correction has to be applied.

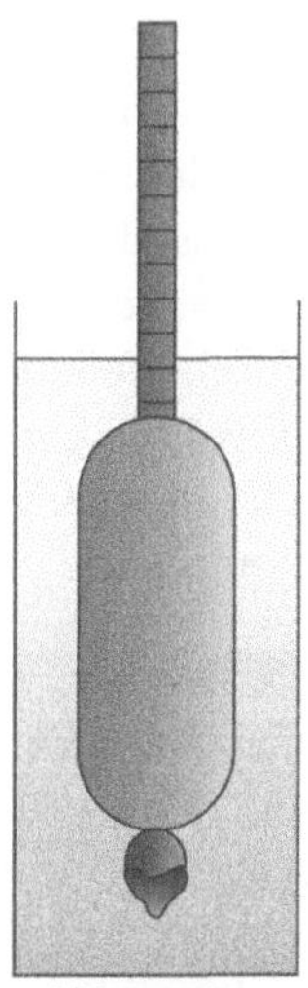

Fig. 17.6: Urinometer.

Correction is for every 3°C rise over the temperature of calibration, a correction factor of "one" is added to the observed reading. The difference between 37 and 15 is 22°C. This when divided by 3 gives 7.

Corrected specific gravity = 1012 + 7 = 1019

Applying the decimal point, the specific gravity of the given urine is close to 1.019.

In normal subjects, the specific gravity of urine is 1.016–1.022.

Determination of Osmolality of Urine and Serum

The urine osmolality measurement test will be the more accurate test to check the concentrating ability of renal tubules.

Osmolality is a measure of total concentration of dissolved particles in a solution.

Normal values

Serum = 275–295 mosmols/kg

Urine = 1400 mosmols/kg water.

Elimination of Water (Water Dilution Test)

If renal function is impaired, the quantity of eliminated urine will be very low. In this condition, increased specific gravity may be seen.

A urine test checks different components of urine, a waste product made by the kidneys. A regular urine test may be done to help find the cause of symptoms. The test can give information about your health and problems you may have.

Urinalysis

The kidneys take out waste material, minerals, fluids, and other substances from the blood to be passed in the urine. Urine has hundreds of different body wastes. More than 100 different tests can be done on urine. A regular urinalysis often includes the following tests:

Color

Many things affect urine color, including fluid balance, diet, medicines, and diseases. How dark or light the color is tells you how much water is in it. Vitamin B supplements can turn urine bright yellow. Some medicines, blackberries, beets, rhubarb, or blood in the urine can turn urine red-brown.

Clarity

Urine is normally clear. Bacteria, blood, sperm, crystals, or mucus can make urine look cloudy.

Odor

Urine does not smell very strong, but has a slightly "nutty" odor. Some diseases cause a change in the odor of urine. For example, an infection with *E. coli* bacteria can cause a bad odor, while diabetes or starvation can cause a sweet, fruity odor.

Specific Gravity

This checks the amount of substances in the urine. It also shows how well the kidneys balance the amount of water in urine. The higher the specific gravity, the more solid material is in the urine. When you drink a lot of fluid, your kidneys make urine with a high amount of water in it which has a low specific gravity. When you do not drink fluids, your kidneys make urine with a small amount of water in it which has a high specific gravity.

pH

The pH is a measure of how acidic or alkaline (basic) the urine is. A urine pH of 4 is strongly acidic, 7 is neutral (neither acidic nor alkaline), and 9 is strongly alkaline. Sometimes, the pH of urine is affected by certain treatments. For example, your doctor may instruct you how to keep your urine either acidic or alkaline to prevent some types of kidney stones from forming.

Protein

Protein is normally not found in the urine. Fever, hard exercise, pregnancy, and some diseases, especially kidney disease, may cause protein to be in the urine.

Glucose

Glucose is the type of sugar found in blood. Normally, there is very little or no glucose in urine. When the blood sugar level is very high, as in uncontrolled diabetes, the sugar spills over into the urine. Glucose can also be found in urine when the kidneys are damaged or diseased.

Dipsticks employing the glucose oxidase reaction for screening are specific for glucose but can miss other reducing sugars, such as galactose and fructose. For this reason, most newborn and infant urines are routinely screened for reducing sugars by methods other than glucose oxidase (such as the Clinitest, a modified Benedict's copper reduction test).

Nitrites

Bacteria that cause a urinary tract infection (UTI) make an enzyme that changes urinary nitrates to nitrites. Nitrites in urine show a UTI is present.

Leukocyte Esterase

Leukocyte esterase shows leukocytes [white blood cells (WBCs)] in the urine. WBCs in the urine may mean a UTI is present.

Ketones

When fat is broken down for energy, the body makes substances called ketones (or ketone bodies). These are passed in the urine. Large amounts of ketones in the urine may mean a very serious condition, diabetic ketoacidosis, is present. A diet low in sugars and starches (carbohydrates), starvation, or severe vomiting may also cause ketones to be in the urine.

Bilirubin and Urobilinogen

Unconjugated bilirubin is water insoluble and not normally present in the urine. Conjugated bilirubin only appears in urine in the presence of liver disease or obstruction of the bile ducts.

A small amount of urobilinogen is normally found in urine, but significant amounts suggest that further assessment for hemolytic and hepatocellular disease is indicated.

Urobilinogen levels can be increased in conditions associated with elevated nitrite levels (e.g., UTIs).

Microscopic Analysis

In this test, urine is spun in a special machine (centrifuge) so the solid materials (sediment) settle at the bottom. The sediment is spread on a slide and looked at under a microscope. Things that may be seen on the slide include the following:

Red or White Blood Cells

Blood cells are not found in urine normally. Inflammation, disease, or injury to the kidneys, ureters, bladder, or urethra can cause blood in urine. Strenuous exercise, such as running a marathon, can also cause blood in the urine. White blood cells may be a sign of infection or kidney disease.

Casts

Some types of kidney disease can cause plugs of material (called casts) to form in tiny tubes in the kidneys. The casts then get flushed out in the urine. Casts can be made of red or white blood cells, waxy or fatty substances, or protein. The type of cast in the urine can help show what type of kidney disease may be present.

Crystals

Healthy people often have only a few crystals in their urine. A large number of crystals, or certain types of crystals, may mean kidney stones are present or there is a problem with how the body is using food (metabolism).

Bacteria, Yeast Cells, or Parasites

There are no bacteria, yeast cells, or parasites in urine normally. If these are present, it can mean you have an infection.

Squamous Cells

The presence of squamous cells may mean that the sample is not as pure as it needs to be. These cells do not mean there is a medical problem, but your doctor may ask that you give another urine sample.

Urine Strip Test

Methods for Urine Collection

1. Random collection taken at any time of day.
2. Clean-catch, midstream urine specimen collected after cleansing the external urethral meatus.
3. A cotton sponge soaked with benzalkonium hydrochloride is useful and nonirritating for this purpose.
4. A midstream urine is one in which the first-half of the bladder urine is discarded and the collection vessel is introduced into the urinary stream to catch the last half.

Procedure

Immerse the dipstick completely in fresh urine **(Fig. 17.7)** and withdraw immediately, drawing edge along rim of container to remove excess. Hold dipstick horizontally before reading.

This strip consist of a ribbon made of plastic or paper of about 5 millimeter wide, plastic strips have pads impregnated with chemicals which react with the compounds present in urine producing a characteristic color.

On paper strips, the reactants are absorbed directly thereon. Paper strips are often specific to a single reaction, while the strips with pads allow several determinations simultaneously.

There are strips with different objectives, there are qualitative strips that only determine if the sample is positive or negative, and there are semiquantitative ones that in addition to providing a positive or negative reaction approaching a quantitative result, in the latter, color reactions are approximately proportional to the concentration of substance in the sample.

The reading of the results obtained by comparing the colors with a color scale provided by the manufacturer, no equipment needed.

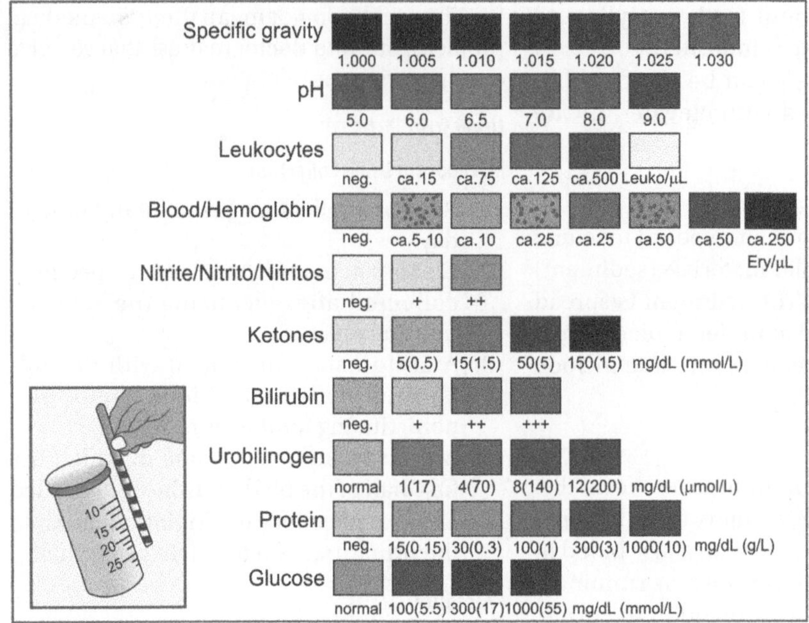

Fig. 17.7: Dipstick test and interpretation.

This type of analysis is very common in the control and monitoring of diabetic patients. The test can be read from a few minutes to 20 minutes after immersion of the strip in the urine.

Semiquantitative values can be reported, usually expressed as trace, 1+, 2+, 3+ and 4+. In the test areas also provides an estimate in milligrams per deciliter. Automated readers of test strips also provide units of the International System of Units.

They are used in the physicochemical stage of a urinalysis to determine glucose bilirubin, acetone, specific gravity, blood, pH, protein, urobilinogen, nitrite and leukocytes, or to reaffirm the suspicion of infection by different pathogens.

CONSEQUENCES OF CHRONIC RENAL FAILURE

Chronic kidney disease (CKD), also known as **chronic renal disease**, is a progressive loss in renal function over a period of months or years.

The symptoms of worsening kidney function are unspecific, and might include feeling generally unwell and experiencing a reduced appetite. Often, chronic kidney disease is diagnosed as a result of screening of people known to be at risk of kidney problems, such as those with high blood pressure or diabetes and those with a blood relative with chronic kidney disease. Chronic kidney disease may also be identified when it leads to one of its recognized complications, such as cardiovascular disease, anemia or pericarditis.

Chronic kidney disease is identified by a blood test for creatinine. Higher levels of creatinine indicate a lower glomerular filtration rate and as a result a decreased capability of the kidneys to excrete waste products. Creatinine levels may be normal in the early stages of CKD, and the condition is discovered if urinalysis (testing of a urine sample) shows that the kidney is allowing the loss of protein or red blood cells into the urine

The CKD is initially without specific symptoms and can only be detected as an increase in serum creatinine or protein in the urine. As the kidney function decreases:

- **Blood pressure** is increased due to fluid overload and production of vasoactive hormones created by the kidney via the RAS (renin-angiotensin system), increasing one's risk of developing hypertension and/ or suffering from congestive heart failure
- **Urea** accumulates, leading to azotemia and ultimately uremia (symptoms ranging from lethargy to pericarditis and encephalopathy). Urea is excreted by sweating and crystallizes on skin ("uremic frost").
- **Potassium** accumulates in the blood (known as hyperkalemia with a range of symptoms including malaise and potentially fatal cardiac arrhythmias).
- **Erythropoietin** synthesis is decreased (potentially leading to anemia, which causes fatigue).
- **Fluid volume overload** — impaired ability of the kidney to regulate water balance leads to fluid overload or fluid depletion very easily. Symptoms may range from mild edema to life-threatening pulmonary edema.
- **Hyperphosphatemia**—due to reduced phosphate excretion.
- **Hypocalcemia**—due to 1, 25 dihydroxy vitamin D_3 deficiency. The 1,25 dihydroxy vitamin D_3 deficiency is due to stimulation of fibroblast growth factor-23.
  - Later this progresses to secondary hyperparathyroidism, renal osteodystrophy and vascular calcification that further impair cardiac function.
- **Metabolic acidosis**, due to accumulation of sulfates, phosphates, uric acid, etc. This may cause altered enzyme activity by excess acid acting on enzymes and also increased excitability of cardiac and neuronal membranes by the promotion of hyperkalemia due to excess acid (acidemia). As chronic renal failure develops the ability of the kidneys to regenerate bicarbonate and excrete hydrogen ions in the urine become impaired. The retention of hydrogen causes metabolic acidosis.

People with chronic kidney disease suffer from accelerated atherosclerosis and are more likely to develop cardiovascular disease than the general population. Patients afflicted with chronic kidney disease and cardiovascular disease tend to have significantly worse prognoses than those suffering only from the latter.

- **Anion gap:** In normal serum there is balance between cations (Na^+, K^+, Ca^{2+}, Mg^{2+}) and anions, such as Cl^-, HCO_3^-, proteins, organic acids, sulfates and phosphates (*refer* Unit 13). This may be varied in renal failure.

PATHOLOGICAL CONDITIONS OF THE KIDNEY

Acute Glomerulonephritis (AGN)

It is an acute inflammation of the glomeruli. There are two types of glomerulonephritis—acute and chronic. The acute form develops suddenly and may appear after an infection in throat or on skin.

The early symptoms of the acute disease are:

- Puffiness of face in the morning
- Blood in urine (or brown urine)
- Urinating less than usual.

Acute GN is defined as the sudden onset of hematuria, proteinuria, and red blood cell (RBC) casts. This clinical picture is often accompanied by hypertension, edema, azotemia [i.e., decreased glomerular filtration rate (GFR)], and renal salt and water retention. Acute GN can be due to a primary renal disease or to a systemic disease.

Causes of Acute Glomerulonephritis (AGN)

In diffuse glomerulonephritis (GN), all of the glomeruli are aggressively attacked, leading to acute renal failure (ARF).

Disorders that attack several organs and cause diffuse GN are referred to as secondary causes. Secondary causes of diffuse GN include the following:

- Cryoglobulinemia

- Goodpasture's syndrome (membranous antiglomerular basement membrane disease)
- Lupus nephritis
- Vasculitis (e.g., Wegener's granulomatosis).

Primary diseases that solely affect the kidneys and cause AGN include the following:

- Immunoglobulin A nephropathy
- Membranoproliferative nephritis (kidney inflammation)
- Postinfectious GN.

Signs and Symptoms of Acute Glomerulonephritis (AGN)

Patients who have secondary causes of AGN often exhibit these symptoms:

- Cough with blood-tinged sputum
- Fever
- Joint or muscle pain
- Rash
- Oliguria
- Hematuria
- Proteinuria
- Anemia
- Increased blood urea and creatinine.

  The presence of RBCs in the urine is insufficient evidence for AGN, because the blood may arise from urinary tract too.

Tests that may be done are:

- Blood electrolytes
- Blood urea nitrogen (BUN)
- Creatinine—blood
- Creatinine clearance
- Potassium test
- Protein in the urine
- Urinalysis.

A kidney biopsy will show inflammation of the glomeruli, which may indicate the cause of the condition.

Tests to find the cause of acute nephritic syndrome may include:

- ANA titer (lupus)
- Antiglomerular basement membrane antibody
- Antineutrophil cytoplasmic antibody for vasculitis (ANCA)
- Blood culture
- Serum complement (C_3 and C_4).

The chronic form may develop silently (without symptoms) over several years. It often leads to complete kidney failure. Early signs and symptoms of the chronic form may include:

Blood or protein in the urine (hematuria, proteinuria)

- High blood pressure
- Swelling of ankles or face (edema)
- Frequent nighttime urination
- Very bubbly or foamy urine.

Symptoms of kidney failure include:

- Lack of appetite
- Nausea and vomiting
- Tiredness
- Difficulty sleeping
- Dry and itchy skin
- Nighttime muscle cramps.

Nephrotic Syndrome

Nephrotic syndrome (also called nephrosis) happens when kidneys start losing large amounts of protein in urine. As kidneys get worse, extra fluids and salt buildup in the body. This causes swelling (edema), high blood pressure and higher levels of cholesterol. Nephrotic syndrome may come from kidney diseases or from other illnesses, such as diabetes and lupus.

Increased membrane permeability leads to massive proteinuria (mainly albumin loss). There will be reduction in plasma osmotic pressure and the fluid movement from vascular to interstitial space that leads to edema.

It is characterized by:

- Massive proteinuria
- Edema
- Hypoalbuminemia
- Hyperlipidemia
- Lipiduria
- The syndrome has multiple causes.

Tubular Disease

Renal Tubular Disease

There are a variety of disorders of tubular function, both generalized and specific. These disorders may be isolated defects, generalized tubular defects as in Fanconi's syndrome, or associated with more generalized disease processes.

1. Fanconi's syndrome
2. Renal tubular acidosis
3. Glycosuria
4. Nephrogenic diabetes insipidus
5. Phosphate-handling disorders
6. Calcium-handling disorders
7. Aminoacidurias.

Fanconi's Syndrome

Fanconi's syndrome is a disturbance of renal tubular function resulting in:

- Generalized aminoaciduria
- Phosphaturia
- Glycosuria
- Rickets (children) or osteomalacia (adults)
- Renal tubular acidosis (RTA) type 2.

Causes

- *Inherited:*
  - Primary idiopathic: Sporadic or familial. Occurs in the absence of any identifiable cause, and most cases are sporadic. Some cases are inherited, but the mode of inheritance appears to be variable (autosomal dominant, autosomal recessive, X-linked).
  - Secondary: Cystinosis, tyrosinemia, Wilson's disease, Lowe's syndrome (oculocerebrorenal syndrome: bilateral congenital cataracts, glaucoma, general hypotonia, hyporeflexia, severe mental retardation and Fanconi's syndrome), galactosemia, glycogen storage disorders and mitochondrial cytopathies.
- *Acquired:*
  - Intrinsic renal disease: Acute tubular necrosis, interstitial nephritis, hypokalemic nephropathy, myeloma, amyloidosis, Sjögrens syndrome
  - Hyperparathyroidism
  - Kwashiorkor
  - Drugs: Cisplatin, ifosfamide, gentamicin, valproate
  - Toxins: Glue sniffing, heavy metals.

Renal Tubular Acidosis

Type 1 (Classic Distal) Renal Tubular Acidosis

- Inability to form acid urine in the distal tubule
- May be inherited as a primary disorder or associated with autoimmune disorders (e.g., Sjögren's syndrome, systemic lupus erythematosus (SLE)), hyperparathyroidism, analgesic nephropathy, renal transplant rejection, obstructive uropathy and chronic urinary tract infections
- Without treatment, leads to progressive renal failure
- *Findings:*
  - Hyperventilation, muscle weakness, cardiac arrhythmias (hypokalemia) and bone pain (due to rickets or osteomalacia).
  - Renal calculi, recurrent UTI, renal failure.
- *Investigations:*
  - Hypokalemia, hyperchloremic metabolic acidosis.
  - Urinary pH is above 6, hypercalciuria.
- *Treatment:*
  - Acute: Correct hypokalemia before acidosis.
  - Chronic: Oral bicarbonate; long-term potassium supplements are usually not required as alkali therapy prevents excessive urinary potassium loss.

Type 2 (Proximal) Renal Tubular Acidosis

- May occur in isolation but is more often associated with other tubular defects as part of the Fanconi's syndrome.

- Defective secretion of hydrogen ions and bicarbonate reabsorption in the proximal tubule leads to an excess of bicarbonate in the urine.
- *Findings:*
  - Polyuria, polydipsia, proximal myopathy
  - Osteomalacia or rickets.
- *Investigations:*
  - Hypokalemia
  - Hyperchloremic metabolic acidosis.
- *Treatment:* High doses of bicarbonate are required but the prognosis is good.

Type 4 (Hyperkalemia) Renal Tubular Acidosis

- *Occurs in diseases associated with reduced aldosterone activity;* causes include:
  - Addison's disease, inborn errors of steroid metabolism, diabetes mellitus, SLE, amyloidosis, chronic tubulointerstitial disease.
  - Drugs: ACE-inhibitors, beta-blockers, potassium-sparing diuretics, NSAIDs.
  - Mineralocorticoid deficiency: Reduced hydrogen secretion in the distal nephron causes reduced ammonium excretion.
- *Findings:*
  - Urinary pH
  - Hyperkalemia, hyperchloremic metabolic acidosis.
- *Treatment:* Fludrocortisone is required if there is acidosis or hyperkalemia.

Glycosuria

- Renal glycosuria occurs when there is failure of tubular mechanisms to reabsorb the entire filtered load of glucose under conditions of normoglycemia.
- The isolated form of renal glycosuria is familial with a mixed inheritance pattern.
- Many patients with chronic renal insufficiency of mild-to-moderate degree exhibit renal glycosuria, usually in combination with other disorders of tubular function.

Nephrogenic Diabetes Insipidus

- Caused by renal insensitivity to antidiuretic hormone
- It may be primary (familial, X-linked) or secondary to a number of causes:
  - Drugs, e.g., lithium, diuretics
  - Metabolic: Hypokalemia, hypercalcemia
  - Tubulointerstitial disease—partial obstruction, pyelonephritis, cystic diseases, granulomatous diseases, sickle-cell disease.
- *Presentation:*
  - Polyuria
  - Hypernatremia
  - Uremia.

Phosphate-handling Disorders

There are several types of phosphate transport defect causing hypophosphatemia and inappropriate phosphaturia. The most common forms include:

- Hereditary hypophosphatemic rickets (Vitamin D-resistant rickets)
- Hypophosphatemia with rickets or osteomalacia
- Presents with growth retardation and early bone deformity
- Does not respond to vitamin D but resistance to 1,25-dihydroxy vitamin D only occurs with functional defects of the vitamin D receptor
- Treatment is with 1,25-dihydroxy vitamin D plus amiloride and thiazide to reduce calcium reabsorption.
- X-linked hypophosphatemic rickets.
- Presentation is with poor growth and rickets in early childhood.
- There is a defect in proximal tubular phosphate transport that results in persistent hypophosphatemia and inappropriate phosphaturia.
- Large doses of oral phosphate supplements are required, together with 1,25-dihydroxy vitamin D.

- Hypoparathyroidism and pseudohypoparathyroidism (renal resistance to parathyroid hormone) causing reduced renal phosphate excretion.

Calcium-handling Disorders

Relatively common disorders causing hypercalciuria and, less commonly, hypocalciuria.

- *Idiopathic hypercalciuria:*
  - High risk of calcium stone formation with hypercalciuria but normal blood calcium.
  - Usually results from calcium hyperabsorption in the intestine with hypercalciuria being of overspill type.
  - Hypercalciuria is treated with dietary restriction of calcium intake (plus careful monitoring of bone formation in children). Thiazide diuretic is used where this fails.
- *Hereditary hypercalciuric nephrolithiasis:* Rare disorder associated with proteinuria, nephrocalcinosis, renal stones and frequently renal failure.
- *Familial hypocalciuric hypercalcemia:*
  - An autosomal dominant disorder following a generally benign course, associated with a defective extracellular sensing receptor.
  - Hypocalciuria and hypercalcemia are accompanied by hypermagnesemia with parathyroid hormone levels in normal range.

Aminoacidurias

There are a variety of aminoacidurias, including Hartnup disease, homocystinuria and cystinuria.

- *Hartnup disease:*
  - Rare, autosomal recessive disorder resulting in malabsorption of dietary tryptophan, a pellagra-like syndrome with photosensitive skin lesions, ataxia, and neuropsychiatric disturbances, and aminoaciduria with increased renal clearance of neutral amino acids.
  - Tryptophan malabsorption presents like pellagra, but is less severe.
  - Treatment is with oral nicotinamide.
- *Cystinuria:*
  - Disorder of intestinal absorption and proximal renal tubular reabsorption of the dibasic amino acids, cysteine, ornithine, arginine and lysine.
  - Inheritance is autosomal recessive.
  - Presents with renal calculi causing renal colic, hematuria, urinary obstruction and secondary pyelonephritis, leading to renal failure.
  - Calculi are radiopaque and the cyanide-nitroprusside urine test is positive.
  - Treatment includes a high fluid intake, urinary alkalinization with bicarbonate, D-penicillamine (which reacts with cysteine to form a more soluble compound) and lysine supplementation.

Urinary Tract Infection (UTI)

A UTI is an infection in the urinary tract. Infections are caused by microbes—organisms too small to be seen without a microscope—including fungi, viruses, and bacteria. Bacteria are the most common cause of UTIs. Normally, bacteria that enter the urinary tract are rapidly removed by the body before they cause symptoms. However, sometimes bacteria overcome the body's natural defenses and cause infection. An infection in the urethra is called urethritis. A bladder infection is called cystitis. Bacteria may travel up the ureters to multiply and infect the kidneys. A kidney infection is called pyelonephritis.

The bacterium *Escherichia coli (E. coli)* cause the vast majority of UTIs. Microbes called *Chlamydia* and *Mycoplasma* can infect the urethra and reproductive system but not the bladder.

Test: The person will be asked to give a "clean catch" urine sample by washing the genital area and collecting a "midstream" sample of urine in a sterile container.

Diagnosis is made by the presence of more than 100,000 bacterial colonies/mL of urine.

SELF TEST

1. Name the functions performed by the kidney.
2. List the tests under RFT panel.
3. Define creatinine clearance.
4. Give the formula to calculate creatinine clearance.
5. Give the procedure for performing creatinine clearance.
6. Why is creatinine selected for measuring GFR?
7. State the conditions in which creatinine clearance decreases.
8. State the methods used to determine blood urea concentration.
9. Write the normal values for the following:
   a. Urea
   b. Creatinine
   c. Uric acid.
10. State the causes of decreased urea levels.
11. State the method used for creatinine estimation and write its principle.
12. Write the principle of uric acid estimation by Henry et al method.
13. Which tests are used to measure concentrating and diluting mechanisms of kidney?
14. Write short notes on:
    a. Nephrotic syndrome
    b. Glomerulonephritis.
15. Which tests are used to identify amino acids?
16. Name the test used to detect homocystinuria.
17. Why is the urea clearance test not preferred?
18. Give the normal creatinine clearance value.

MULTIPLE CHOICE QUESTIONS

1. **Nephrotic syndrome is characterized by:**
   a. Massive uricemia
   b. Glycosuria and hyperalbuminemia
   c. Proteinuria and edema
   d. Hypolipidemia and edema
2. **Urea can be determined by:**
   a. DAM method
   b. Zak's method
   c. Jaffe's method
   d. None of the above
3. **All the following are the tests used to detect renal function, *Except:***
   a. Uric acid determination
   b. Urea determination
   c. Creatinine determination
   d. Bilirubin determination
4. **Nitroprusside test detects:**
   a. Alkaptonuria
   b. Homocystinuria
   c. Phenylketonuria
   d. p-OH catabolites
5. **All of the following indicate the Increased total urine amino acids excretion , *Except:***
   a. Alkaptonuria
   b. Phenylketonuria
   c. Cystinosis
   d. Glycosuria
6. **All of the following conditions result in abnormal glomerular filtration rate, *Except:***
   a. Acute tubular necrosis
   b. Dehydration
   c. Glomerulonephritis
   d. Cirrhosis

CASE STUDIES

1. A 45-year-old man was admitted to a hospital following episodes of nausea, vomiting, and abdominal pain. Upon examination, it was discovered that his kidneys were slightly enlarged. Then the physician requested for blood investigation. Following results were obtained from the clinical biochemistry laboratory

Parameter	Result	Reference
Fasting blood sugar	85 mg/dL	(90–110)
Blood urea	80 mg /dL	(8–40)
Creatinine	6.0 mg/dL	(0.8–1.4)
Uric acid	7.0 mg%	(2.5–7.0)
Serum osmolality	380 mOsm/kg	(285–298)
Inorganic phosphorous	5.0 mg/dL	(2.5–4.5)
Potassium	6.0 mEq/L	(3.5–5.0)

   a. What is the most likely diagnosis?
   b. How would you make a definite diagnosis?
   c. Can the diagnosis made using the NPN substance values?

2. A 12-year-female child was brought to the hospital with symptoms of vomiting, anorexia and a sign of swollen face. The pediatrician admitted the child and after physical examination requested for blood and urine tests.
   Results of laboratory test are as follows:

Laboratory test	Result
Total serum protein	5.0 g/dL
Albumin	2.5 g/dL
Globulins	3.0 g/dL
Urine osmolality	1200 mOsm/kg H_2O
Urine albumin	+++

   a. What is the probable diagnosis to be done with the available laboratory results?
   b. How would you make a definite diagnosis?
   c. What is the pathophysiology of this disorder?

3. A 70-year-old woman who lived alone was discovered by her friend in a drowsy, confused state. On admission, she was extremely dirty and her tongue was dry. Immediately she was given fluid with saline through intravenously. After some time, the doctor requested for blood tests which revealed the following results:

Parameter	Result
Sodium	141 mEq/L (normal)
Potassium	5.7 mEq/L (elevated)
Chloride	107 mEq/L (elevated)
Creatinine clearance	80 mL/min (reduced)
Urea	70 mg/dL (elevated)
Creatinine	4.0 mg/dL (elevated)

   a. What is the likely cause of her symptoms?
   b. What is the likely diagnosis?
   c. How would you make a definite diagnosis?

4. A 50-year-old man reported in the adult PCF at government hospital with complaints of abdominal pain, muscle cramps and urinary discomfort. His requested laboratory tests revealed the following results:

Parameter	Result
Urea	100 mg/dL
Creatinine	12 mg/dL
Na^+	170 mEq/L
K^+	6.5 mEq/L
Chloride	120 mEq/L
Phosphorous	6.0 mEq/L
Calcium	5.0 mg/dL
Serum bilirubin	1.0 mg%
Direct bilirubin	0.2 mg%
Indirect bilirubin	0.8 mg%
AST	30 units/L
ALT	25 units/L
Alkaline phosphatase	80 units/L

a. What is your diagnosis and what could be the cause for elevated biochemistry parameters?
b. Why red top tube is preferred for sample collection for electrolyte analysis?
c. List the preanalytical variable that could lead to elevated sodium.
d. Which hormone helps to maintain fluid balance and explain?

5. Steven a 7-year-old boy was brought to a pediatrician by his mother with a history of mousy odor of urine and delay in achieving cognitive functions. On examination, his skin and hair was light in color with hypopigmentation.
   a. What is your diagnosis?
   b. Which enzyme defect causing this disorder?
   c. Which biochemical tests are done to confirm the diagnosis?

18

UNIT

Fluid Balance

LEARNING OBJECTIVES

At the end of this unit, the learner should be able to understand:

- The fluid distribution in ECF and ICF.
- The regulation of fluid balance with two mechanisms.
- The causes and symptoms of hypo- and hypervolemia.

INTRODUCTION

Fluid balance is the concept of human homeostasis that the amount of fluid lost from the body is equal to the amount of fluid taken in. Humans can survive for 4–6 weeks without food, but for only a few days without water. The amount of water varies with the individual, as it depends on the condition of the subject, the amount of physical exercise, and on the environmental temperature and humidity.

- Water constitutes 60% of the total body weight
- The body's water is distributed between two compartments
- That is extracellular fluid and intracellular fluid
- Fluid found within the cells is called intracellular fluid (ICF) and that found outside cells is called extracellular fluid (ECF) **(Fig. 18.1)**
- The ECF is further divided into that which is found as blood plasma within blood vessels, and that which is found in the microscopic spaces between cells called interstitial fluid
- Approximately 2/3rd of body fluid is intracellular and 1/3 is extracellular
- Of the ECF, approximately 80% is interstitial fluid and 20% is blood plasma
- Selectively permeable membranes separate body fluids into distinct compartments.
- Plasma membranes of individual cells separate ICF from ECF and blood vessel walls separate blood plasma from interstitial fluid
- The major components of these fluids include water and solutes
- The solute is mostly comprised of electrolytes—inorganic compounds that dissociate into ions. Electrolytes include cations and anions
- The cations are positively charged atoms Examples are—sodium, potassium, calcium, magnesium
- The anions are negatively charged atoms and examples are chloride, sulfide, phosphate, bicarbonate, and carbonate
- The exchange of interstitial and intracellular fluid is controlled mainly by the presence of the electrolytes sodium, and potassium.

  Potassium is the chief intracellular cation and sodium the chief extracellular cation.

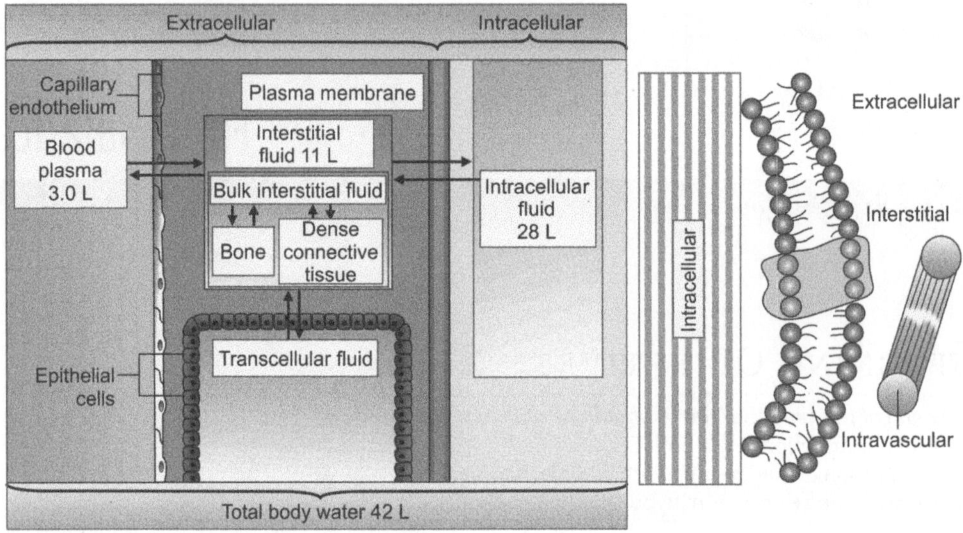

Fig. 18.1: Fluid distribution in different compartments.

Fluid Distribution in Various Compartments (Fig. 18.1)

Fluid distribution	*% of total body weight (70 kg)*	*Volume*
Body water	60%	42 L
1. Intracellular	40%	28 L
2. Extracellular	20%	14 L
• Plasma (blood)	5%	3.0 L
• Interstitial fluid	15%	11 L
– CSF		
– Lymph		
– Synovial fluid		
– Occular fluid		
– Pleural fluid		
– Pericardial fluid		

Fluid Input and Output

Daily intake	*Daily output*
• Liquid intake in the form of water, beverages 1000–1200 mL	• Urine → 1000–1500 mL • Sweat → 400 mL
• Ingested food 700–1000 mL	
• Water produced by metabolism 300 mL	• Respiration → 400 mL • Feces → 200 mL
Total 2000–2500 mL	Total 2000–2500 mL

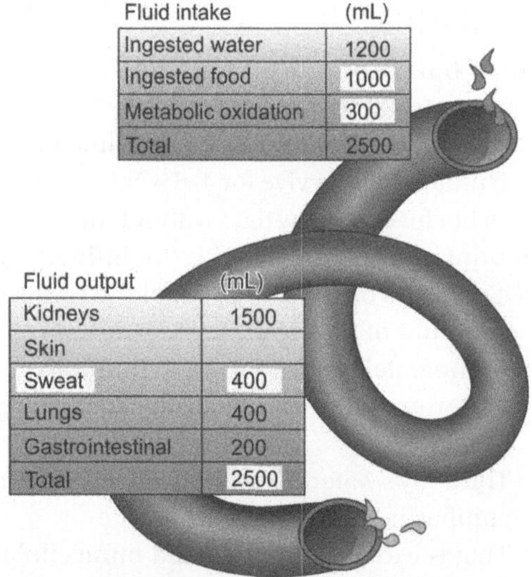

Fluid intake	(mL)
Ingested water	1200
Ingested food	1000
Metabolic oxidation	300
Total	2500

Fluid output	(mL)
Kidneys	1500
Skin	
Sweat	400
Lungs	400
Gastrointestinal	200
Total	2500

Fig. 18.2: Fluid input and output.

The body water is maintained at a constant volume by a regulation between intake and output water as given and shown in **Figure 18.2**.

Regulation of Fluid Balance (Fig. 18.3)

The term fluid balance defines the state where a body's required amount of water is present and proportioned normally among the various compartments.

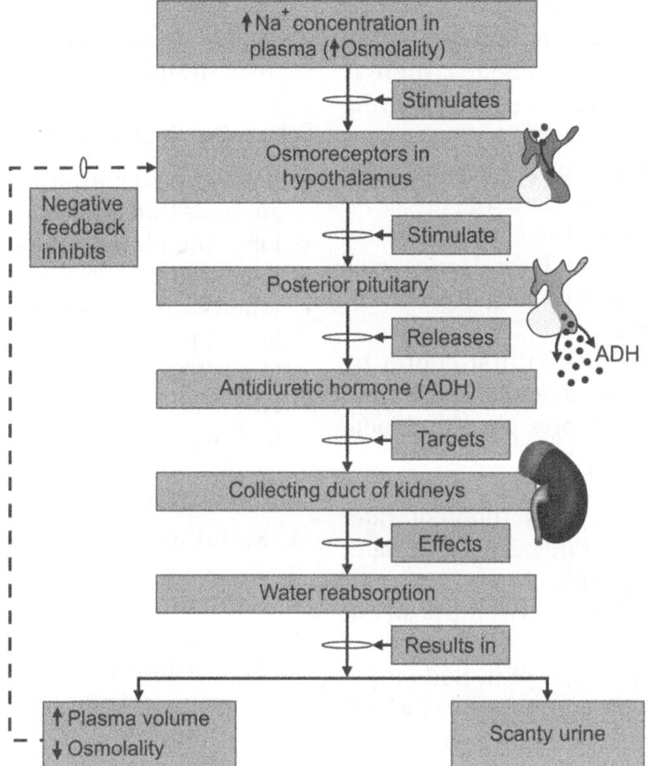

Fig. 18.3: Regulation of fluid balance.

Under normal conditions water loss equals water gain and a body's water volume remains constant.

Water loss takes place through the kidneys, skin, lungs, feces, and menstruation.

Gain water mostly from dietary intake; this is called preformed water.

Metabolic processes, such as cellular respiration and dehydration synthesis reactions generate a small component.

Water is not produced by the body to maintain homeostasis

Metabolic water production is simply a by-product of cellular respiration.

The body regulates water intake via the thirst reflex, which stimulates us to drink. When water loss is greater than water gain the body reaches a state of dehydration, and dehydration stimulates the thirst reflex in three ways:

- Saliva level drops resulting in a dry mucosa in the mouth and pharynx
- Increase in blood osmotic pressure, which stimulates osmoreceptors in the hypothalamus
- There is a drop in blood volume, which leads to the renin/angiotensin II pathway stimulating the thirst center in the hypothalamus.

Mechanism

Thirst Center

- The intake of water is regulated by the thirst center, situated in the brain

- When there is a decrease in the body fluid volume, it leads to increase in the salt concentration; and hence, there is increased osmolality and an increase in the osmotic pressure the ECF
- As a result, the intracellular water comes out and cells become dehydrated
- The dehydration of the cells stimulates the thirst center, which sends messages to tongue and throat causing dryness and drink more water
- Drinking inhibits the thirst center by stretching the stomach and intestines and reducing the osmotic pressure of the blood.

Antidiuretic Hormone (ADH)

The ADH helps in the reabsorption of water from renal tubules and thereby loss of water from the body is regulated.

It is the hormone secreted by the posterior pituitary.

When there is a decrease in body fluid, osmotic pressure of ECF increases which stimulates the cells of the hypothalamus, which in turn stimulates the posterior pituitary to secrete ADH.

The ADH acts on the kidney tubules and increases the reabsorption of water, thus conserving water. When the body fluid content is sufficient, the osmotic pressure of ECF is normal, or low. During this condition, there is no stimulation of the hypothalamic cells or posterior pituitary, so ADH is not secreted. As a result, there is a decrease in the reabsorption of water from the renal tubules and more water is lost in the urine.

Dehydration (Hypovolemia) (Table 18.1)

- Loss of water from the body in excess amounts leads to dehydration
- First, the plasma becomes concentrated followed by the ECF and then the ICF
- When water comes out of the cells, it passes into ECF in exchange of K^+ and Na^+ passes into ICF from ECF
- Loss of more than 20% of body water results in death.

Causes of Dehydration

1. Severe diarrhea and vomiting
2. Excessive heat
3. Difficulty in swallowing and state of unconsciousness
4. Loss of fluid from skin in case of burns
5. Diabetes insipidus (ADH polyurea)
6. Heart stroke
7. Excitement
8. Fever
9. Excessive sweating.

Dehydration induces water to move from the reservoir inside cells into the blood. If dehydration progresses, body tissues begin to dry out and the cells start to shrivel and malfunction. The most susceptible cells to dehydration are the brain cells.

Table 18.1: Observations related to fluid balance.

Observation	*Fluid depletion*	*Fluid overload*
Weight	Loss	Gain
Blood pressure	Lowered smaller pulse pressure	Normal or raised
Respirations	Rapid, shallow	Rapid, moist cough
Pulse	Rapid, weak	Rapid
Urine output	Reduced, concentrated	Increased or decreased if heart is failing
Skin	Dry, less elastic	Edematous
Saliva	Thick, viscous	Copious, frothy
Tongue	Dry, coated	Moist
Thirst	Present	No disturbance
Face	Sunken eyes	Periorbital edema
Temperature	May be raised	No disturbance

Mental confusion, one of the most common signs of severe dehydration, may result and can lead to *coma*. Dehydration can occur when excessive water is lost with such diseases as *diabetes mellitus*, diabetes insipidus, and Addison's disease.

Dehydration is often accompanied by a deficiency of electrolytes, sodium, and potassium in particular. Water does not move as rapidly from the reservoir inside of the cells into the blood when electrolyte concentration is decreased. Blood pressure can decline due to a lower volume of water circulating in the bloodstream. A drop in blood pressure can cause lightheadedness, or a feeling of impending blackout, especially upon standing (orthostatic hypotension). Continued fluid and electrolyte imbalance may further reduce blood pressure, causing *shock* and damage to many internal organs including the brain, kidneys, and *liver*.

Features of Dehydration

1. Dryness of skin, tongue, and throat.
2. Changes in the values of packed cell volume, Hb, plasma protein, plasma electrolytes, urea and decreased blood pressure.

Treatment

- Consuming plenty of plain water or water containing sugar and salt (depends upon the cause of dehydration)
- If the condition is very severe, intravenous infusion of fluids (normal saline) is required.

Water Excess (Hypervolemia) (Table 18.1)

It is a condition in which the body water content is excessive.

Causes

1. Hypersecretion of ADH following the administration of anesthetics.
   This effect occurs for about 12–36 hours after the surgery.
2. Renal failure.
3. SIADH syndrome (inappropriate ADH secretion).
   Here hypersecretion of ADH occurs.

Causes for SIADH: Some malignant conditions, disease of CNS, and side effects of certain drugs.

Overhydration can occur alone or in conjunction with excess blood volume. Distinguishing between the two conditions may be quite complicated. Overhydration induces water accumulation within and around the cells but does not typically show symptoms of fluid accumulation. On the other hand, with excess blood volume, there is an accumulation of sodium and the body cannot transfer water into the reservoir within cells. Conditions, such as heart failure and liver cirrhosis may induce volume overload, whereby fluid accumulates around cells in the abdomen, chest, and lower legs.

Features

1. Mental confusion, incoordination, muscular weakness, nausea
2. Decreased PCV
3. Decreased plasma electrolytes, plasma osmolality, increased urine osmolality and increased blood pressure. When there is increased ADH secretion, more H_2O is absorbed from the renal tubules. As the volume of fluid, increases, the salts get diluted. Hence, the plasma osmolality decreases.

Treatment

1. Withdrawal of fluids
2. Administration of diuretics.

SELF TEST

1. Briefly discuss the regulation of fluid balance in the human body.
2. Give the causes and features of hypovolemia.
3. Write the causes of hypervolemia.

4. How does the thirst mechanism help to gain water?

MULTIPLE CHOICE QUESTIONS

1. The regulation of fluid balance is by:
   a. Antidiuretic hormone
   b. Thyroid hormone
   c. Insulin
   d. Oxytocin

2. All the following are the causes for hypervolemia, *Except:*
   a. Renal failure
   b. SIADH syndrome
   c. Hypersecretion of ADH
   d. Diabetes insipidus

19 UNIT Electrolytes

LEARNING OBJECTIVES

At the end of this unit, the learner should be able to understand:
- The different types of electrolytes with their functions.
- The causes, signs and symptoms of low and high sodium and potassium in the blood.
- The usefulness of determining the serum and urine osmolality.
- The methods for determining the serum electrolytes.

INTRODUCTION

Electrolytes are anions or cations. The major cations are sodium, potassium, calcium, and magnesium (Na^+, K^+, Ca^{2+}, Mg^{2+}). Anions include bicarbonate, phosphates (HCO_3^-, HPO_4^{2}, Cl^-) sulfates, and chloride **(Fig. 19.1)**.

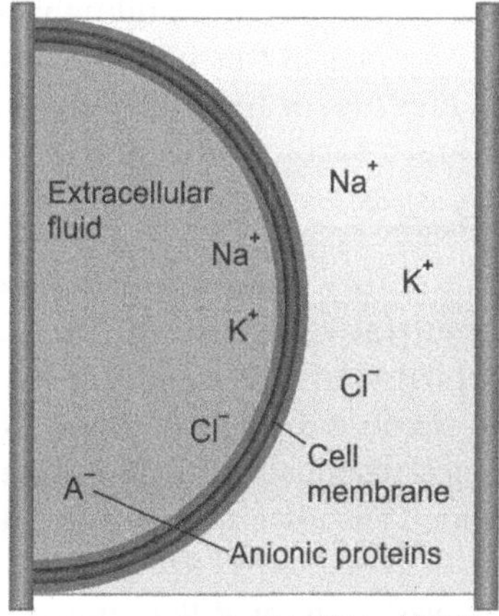

Ion concentration in ICF and ECF

Fig. 19.1: Distribution of electrolytes.

SODIUM (Na^+)

It is the major cation of the extracellular fluid (ECF).

Sources

Salt, pork, sardines, cheese, green olives, corn bread, potato chips, and processed or canned foods.

Average intake from table salt is 5–15 g/day.

Requirement

5 g/day.

Functions

Average serum sodium level is 142 mEq/L (intracellular sodium is 10 mEq/L).

1. Responsible for osmolality of the plasma.
2. Plays a main role in maintaining the normal distribution of water and the osmotic pressure in the ECF compartment.
3. Regulates the electrolyte and pH balance of the extracellular compartment to control the electronic potentials of excitable

tissues such as nerve and muscle, in the active transport of glucose, galactose and amino acids across intestinal mucosa and for Na^+/ K^+-ATPase.

Osmolality

Plasma osmolality/osmolarity measures the body's electrolyte-water balance.

Osmolality and osmolarity are measures that are technically different, but functionally the same for normal use.

Osmolality is a measure of the osmoles (Osm) of solute per kilogram of solvent (osmol/kg or Osm/kg), whereas osmolarity is defined as the number of osmoles of solute per liter (L) of solution (osmol/L or Osm/L)

Osmolality can be measured on an analytical instrument called an *osmometer.*

Clinical Relevance

As cell membranes in general are freely permeable to water, the osmolality of the extracellular fluid (ECF) is approximately equal to that of the intracellular fluid (ICF). Therefore, plasma osmolality is a guide to intracellular osmolality. This is important, as it shows that changes in ECF osmolality have a great effect on ICF osmolality—changes that can cause problems with normal cell functioning and volume. If the ECF was to become too hypotonic, water would readily fill surrounding cells, increasing their volume and potentially lysing them (cytolysis).

Osmolality of blood increases with dehydration and decreases with overhydration. In normal people, increased osmolality in the blood will stimulate secretion of antidiuretic hormone (ADH). This will result in increased water reabsorption, more concentrated urine, and less concentrated blood plasma. A low serum osmolality will suppress the release of ADH, resulting in decreased water reabsorption and more concentrated plasma.

Osmolality of a serum or plasma sample can be measured directly, or it may be calculated if the concentrations of the major solutes are already known. There are many formulae used to calculate the serum osmolality; clinically, the simplest one is:

$$\frac{\text{Serum osmolality}}{\text{(mmol/kg)}} = \frac{2 \times \text{serum (sodium)}}{\text{(mmol/L)}}$$

Clinical Use

Serum osmolality is used in two main circumstances: investigation of hyponatremia and identification of an osmolar gap. Urine osmolality is an important test of renal concentrating ability, for identifying disorders of the ADH mechanism, and identifying causes of hyper- or hyponatremia. Fecal osmolality can be used to assist with diagnosis of the cause of diarrhea.

Serum Osmolality

Serum osmolality is a useful preliminary investigation for identifying the cause of hyponatremia. If a patient with significant hyponatremia (serum sodium <130 mmol/L) has a normal plasma osmolality, the patient may have pseudohyponatremia due to excess lipids or proteins, or the sample may have been collected from a drip arm containing dextrose. If the patient has an increased osmolality it is likely the patient has reactive hyponatremia due to an excess of solute pulling water out of cells. Examples of this include glucose in diabetes mellitus or hyperglycinemia after transurethral resection of the prostate.

Urine Osmolality

Urine osmolality is an important test for the concentrating ability of the kidney. Interpretation of urine osmolality must always be made in the light of the appropriate physiological response to the state of hydration of the patient. The test is useful in the following areas:

- For determining the differential diagnosis of hyper- or hyponatremia.
- For identifying SIADH (urine osmolality >200 mmol/kg, urine sodium >20 mmol/L,

low serum sodium, patient not dehydrated and no renal, adrenal, thyroid, cardiac or liver disease or interfering drugs).

- For differentiating prerenal from renal kidney failure (high urine osmolality is consistent with prerenal impairment, in renal damage the urine osmolality is similar to plasma osmolality).
- For identifying and diagnosing diabetes insipidus.

Atrial Natriuretic Peptide

Atrial natriuretic peptide (ANP) is a potent vasodilator and a protein secreted by cardiac muscle cells. ANP is a circulating hormone regulates atrial blood pressure **(Fig. 19.2)**.

It controls the body water, Na, K, and fat. This hormone is released by muscle cells of upper chamber of heart when BP elevated.

ANP reduces water and sodium and blocks the release of several hormones. ANP produced, pile up, and secreted by myocytes. ANP level usually increase in state of hypertension and excessive of fluids. Human heart secretes ANP and brain natriuretic peptide (BNP). Both BNP and ANP levels increase hypertension, secondary hypertensions, and chronic heart failure during heart pacing, chronic renal failure, an acute myocardial infarction determined. These receptors are having their own functions and purposes. Atrial natriuretic peptide is having four receptors, i.e., renal, vascular, cardiac, and adipose tissues.

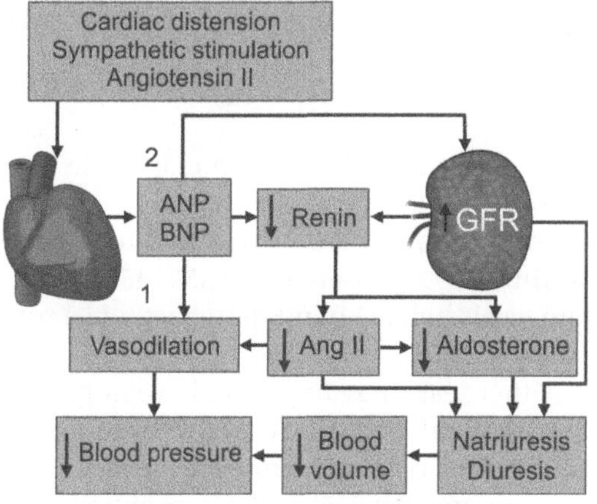

Fig. 19.2: Role of ANP and BNP.

ANP attaches to a specific group of receptors. These receptors are design to cause a reduction in blood volume and reduction in cardiac output and systematic blood pressure. Renal reduces aldosterone secretion by adrenal cortex. Kidneys inhibit rennin secretion. In vascular, it relaxes vascular smooth muscles in arterioles. Adipose tissues increase the release of fatty acids from adipose tissues.

The ANP in combination with the brain natriuretic peptide (BNP) helps in reducing the volume of blood as well as the excessive pressure on the blood which allows keeping everything related to the heart and blood to normal levels. This ensures best control over the blood flow in our body as well as a great control over our entire body and its functions.

Deficiency

- A nutritional deficiency is highly important.
- On a low sodium diet, the kidney decreases the excretion of sodium in urine.
- A low blood sodium triggers the kidney to release angiotensin, which causes the adrenal cortex to secrete aldosterone, the latter induces the renal tubules to reabsorb sodium from the glomerular filtrate.

Hyponatremia

Hyponatremia refers to a lower-than-normal level of sodium in the blood. Sodium is essential for many body functions, including the maintenance of fluid balance, regulation of blood pressure, and normal function of the nervous system. Hyponatremia has sometimes been referred to as "water intoxication", especially when it is due to the consumption of excess water; for example, during strenuous exercise, without adequate replacement of sodium.

Causes: Hyponatremia occurs because of an imbalance of water and sodium. Most frequently it occurs when excessive water dilutes the amount of sodium in the body or when not enough total sodium is present in the body. A common classification of hyponatremia is based on the amount of total body water that is present.

- Decrease in plasma sodium may be due to defect in kidneys or adrenal cortex.
- Sweating, burns, vomiting or diarrhea, which can cause loss of sodium containing fluids.
- In adrenocortical insufficiency (Addison's disease), decrease of serum sodium, and increase in sodium excretion are seen.

Normal Volume (Euvolemic) Hyponatremia

The amount of water in the body is normal, but an antidiuretic hormone is being inappropriately secreted (SIADH = syndrome of inappropriate ADH secretion) from the pituitary gland. This may be seen in patients with pneumonia, small cell lung cancer, bleeding in the brain, or brain tumors.

Excess Volume (Hypervolemic) Hyponatremia

Too much total body water dilutes the amount of sodium contained in the body. This can be seen in heart failure, kidney failure, and liver diseases like cirrhosis. This situation is somewhat misnamed because while there is increased total body water, there may be a relative decrease of fluid within the bloodstream. Because of the underlying disease, fluid leaks into the space between tissues (called the third space) causing swelling of the extremities or ascites, fluid within the abdominal cavity.

Inadequate Volume (Hypovolemic) Hyponatremia

The amount of water in the body is too low as can occur in dehydration. The anti-diuretic hormone is stimulated, causing the kidneys to make very concentrated urine and hold onto water. This may be seen with excessive sweating and exercising in a hot environment. It can also occur in patients with excess fluid loss due to vomiting and diarrhea, pancreatitis, and burns.

Other Specific Situations Hyponatremia Seen

- Hyponatremia may be a side effect of medications, especially diuretics or water pills used to help control blood pressure. This class of drugs can cause excessive loss of sodium in the urine.
- Hormonal diseases such as Addison's disease or adrenal insufficiency and hypothyroidism may be associated with low sodium levels.
- Polydipsia, or excessive water intake, may cause "water intoxication", diluting sodium levels. This is occasionally associated with psychiatric illness.
- In some people who exercise, their concern about the potential for dehydration causes them to drink more water than they lose by perspiration. This may cause significant hyponatremia and has been known to be fatal in marathon participants who drink too much fluid without replacing lost sodium, in excess of what their thirst mechanism dictates.

Symptoms

- Confusion
- Nausea and fatigue
- Seizures
- Some individuals do not show any symptoms.

Diagnosis

The diagnosis of hyponatremia is made by a blood test that measures the concentration of sodium in the bloodstream. The normal sodium level is between 135–145 mEq/L, and levels below 110 mEq/L constitute a true emergency.

Other tests may help decide what type of hyponatremia situation exists. The amount of sodium that is being excreted in the urine may be measured, as well as the concentration of urine.

Hypernatremia

Hypernatremia or hypernatraemia is an electrolyte disturbance with elevated sodium level in the blood.

Hypernatremia is generally not caused by an excess of sodium, but rather by a relative deficit of free water in the body. For this reason, hypernatremia is often synonymous with the less precise term, dehydration.

Water is lost from the body in a variety of ways, including perspiration, imperceptible losses from breathing, and in the feces and urine. If the amount of water ingested consistently falls below the amount of water lost, the serum sodium level will begin to rise, leading to hypernatremia. Rarely, hypernatremia can result from massive salt ingestion.

Even a small rise in the serum sodium concentration above the normal range results in a strong sensation of thirst, an increase in free water intake, and correction of the abnormality. Therefore, hypernatremia most often occurs in people, such as infants, those with impaired mental status, or the elderly, who may have an intact thirst mechanism but are unable to ask for or obtain water.

Causes

Decreased activity of ADH

Hyperactivity of the adrenal cortex (in Cushing's syndrome)

Common causes of hypernatremia include:

- *Hypovolemic:*
  - Inadequate intake of water typically in elderly or otherwise disabled patients who are unable to take in water as their thirst dictates. This is the most common cause of hypernatremia
  - Excessive losses of water from the urinary tract, which may be caused by glycosuria, or other osmotic diuretics
  - Water losses associated with extreme sweating
  - Severe watery diarrhea.
- *Euvolemic:* Excessive excretion of water from the kidneys caused by diabetes insipidus, which involves either inadequate production of the hormone, vasopressin, from the pituitary gland or impaired responsiveness of the kidneys to vasopressin.
- *Hypervolemic:*
  - Intake of a hypertonic fluid (a fluid with a higher concentration of solutes than the remainder of the body). This is relatively uncommon, though it can occur after a vigorous resuscitation where a patient receives a large volume of a concentrated sodium bicarbonate solution. Ingesting seawater also causes hypernatremia because seawater is hypertonic. There are several recorded cases of forced ingestion of concentrated salt solution in exorcism rituals leading to death.
  - Mineralocorticoid excess due to a disease state, such as Conn's syndrome or Cushing's disease.

Signs and Symptoms

- Lethargy
- Restlessness
- Spasticity
- Edema
- Seizures.

Treatment (Fig. 19.3)

The treatment is administration of free water to correct the relative water deficit. Water can be replaced orally or intravenously. Water alone cannot be administered as intravenously rather can be given with addition to dextrose or saline infusion solutions. The body (in particular, the brain) adapts to the higher sodium concentration. Rapid lowering the sodium concentration with free water may cause water to flow into brain cells and causes them to swell. This can lead to cerebral edema, potentially resulting in seizures, permanent brain damage, or death. Therefore, significant hypernatremia should be treated carefully by a physician or

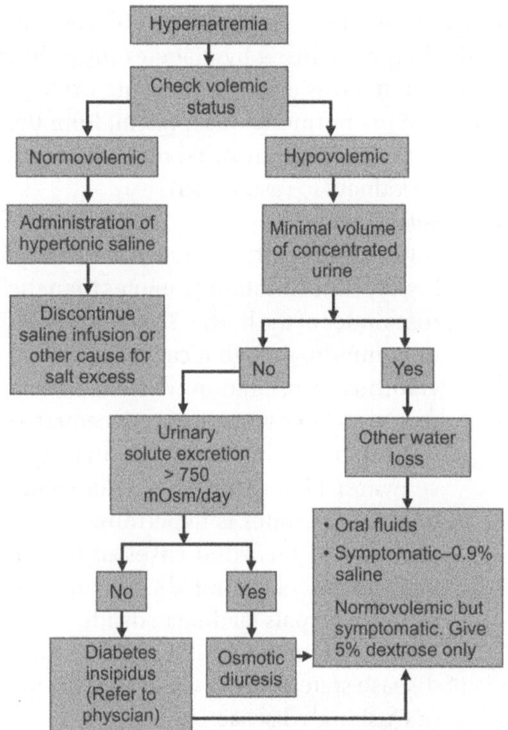

Fig. 19.3: Treatment option for hypernatremia.

other medical professional with experience in treatment of electrolyte imbalances.

Determination of Sodium

Specimen: Serum, heparinized plasma, sweat, urine, feces, or gastrointestinal fluids are used for the assay.

1. Hemolyzed samples are not suitable for electrolyte analysis because RBC releases potassium, which will cause a false increase in the K^+ values. Hemolysis causes a decrease in sodium values also.
2. Urine collection for electrolyte estimation should be made without any preservative.
3. Serum, plasma or urine must be stored at 2–8°C or frozen if the analysis is delayed.

Sodium may be determined by atomic absorption spectrophotometry (AAS), flame emission spectrophotometry (FES), electrochemically with a sodium ion selective electrode (ISE) or spectrophotometrically. FES and ISE assays are currently used because of their accuracy.

Reference intervals serum: 136–145 mEq/L.

POTASSIUM (K^+)

- Potassium (K^+) is the most important cation of intracellular fluid (ICF).
- Average concentration in the intracellular fluid is 150 mEq/L.
- **Extracellular** potassium concentration is normally kept within a tight range of **3.5–5.0 mEq/L.**
- **Extracellular** potassium is important for its controlling influence upon neuromuscular irritability, cardiac muscle (a proper balance between potassium and calcium is essential for the contraction of heart muscle) and the operation of Na^+/K^+-ATPase (Na^+ pump) against the concentration gradient.
- In cells, there is a significant concentration gradient of sodium and potassium across cell membranes.
- The high intracellular potassium is maintained by an energy requiring extrusion of three sodium out of the cell with replacement by two potassium **(Fig. 19.4)**.
- Intracellular potassium is essential for a number of enzyme reactions (such as pyruvate kinase, glycogen synthesis and protein synthesis), for maintaining osmotic and acid-base balance.

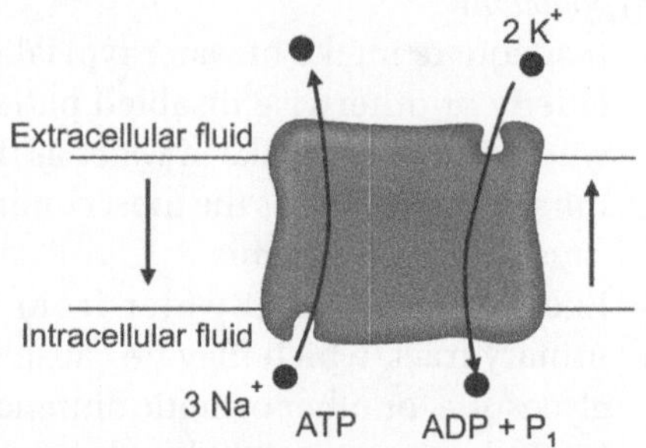

Fig. 19.4: Movement of potassium and sodium across the compartments.

- Nearly all of the total body potassium (98%) is inside cells. If, for example, there is significant tissue damage, the contents of cells, including potassium, leak out into the extracellular compartment, causing potentially dangerous increases in serum potassium.

Sources

Whole and skim milk, bananas, tomatoes, oranges, melons, potatoes, sweet potatoes, prunes, raisins, spinach, turnip greens, collard greens, kale, other green leafy vegetables, most peas and beans, and salt substitutes (potassium chloride).

Functions

1. It is the principal cation of ICF.
2. Potassium is required for the functioning of nerves, skeletal muscle and cardiac muscles. Either decreased potassium or increased potassium levels finally cause cardiac arrest.
3. Potassium is required as a cofactor in several enzymatic reactions in the body.
4. Potassium is involved in acid-base balance.

Hypokalemia

Hypokalemia is a metabolic disorder that occurs when the level of potassium in the blood drops too low.

- It is the condition in which serum potassium is reduced.
- This condition decreases the heartbeat and interferes with vital muscles, such as those involved in respiration.

Possible causes of hypokalemia include:

- Antibiotics (penicillin, nafcillin, carbenicillin, gentamicin, amphotericin B, foscarnet)
- Diarrhea
  - Gastrointestinal loss: A more common cause is excessive loss of potassium, often associated with heavy fluid losses that "flush" potassium out of the body. Typically, this is a consequence of diarrhea, excessive perspiration, or losses associated with surgical procedures. Vomiting can also cause hypokalemia, although not much potassium is lost from the vomitus. Rather, there are heavy urinary losses of K^+ in the setting of post-emetic bicarbonaturia that force urinary potassium excretion. Other GI causes include pancreatic fistulae and the presence of adenoma.
- Diseases that affect the kidneys' ability to retain potassium (Liddle syndrome, Cushing syndrome, hyperaldosteronism, Bartter syndrome, Fanconi syndrome)
- Diuretic medications, which can cause excess urination
- Eating disorders (such as bulimia)
- Magnesium deficiency
  - Magnesium is required for adequate processing of potassium. This may become evident when hypokalemia persists despite potassium supplementation. Other electrolyte abnormalities may also be present
- Sweating
- Vomiting
- Since aldosterone increases the excretion of potassium or administration of cortisone leads to hypokalemia
- Certain diuretics increase the excretion of potassium. It is, therefore, important to supplement enough potassium when these diuretics are used
- Reduced intake of potassium may cause hypokalemia but it is rare. Renal retention of potassium in response to reduced intake ensures that hypokalemia occurs only when intake is severely restricted.

Several factors regulate the distribution of potassium between the intracellular and extracellular space, as follows:

- *Glycoregulatory hormones:* (i) Insulin enhances potassium entry into cells, and (ii) glucagon impairs potassium entry into cells.
- *Adrenergic stimuli:* (i) Beta-adrenergic stimuli enhance potassium entry into cells, and (ii) Alpha-adrenergic stimuli impair potassium entry into cells. Therefore, there is a risk of hypokalemia when insulin given in the treatment of diabetic ketoacidosis.
- *pH:* (i) Alkalosis enhances potassium entry into cells, and (ii) Acidosis impairs potassium entry into cells.
- Alkalosis can cause transient hypokalemia by two mechanisms. First, the alkalosis causes a shift of potassium from the plasma and interstitial fluids into cells; perhaps mediated by stimulation of Na^+-H^+ exchange and a subsequent activation of Na^+/K^+-ATPase activity. Second, an acute rise of plasma HCO_3^- concentration (caused by vomiting, for example) will exceed the capacity of the renal proximal tubule to reabsorb this anion, and potassium will be excreted as an obligate cation partner to the bicarbonate. Metabolic alkalosis is often present in states of volume depletion, so potassium is also lost via aldosterone-mediated mechanisms.

Pseudohypokalemia

Pseudohypokalemia is a decrease in the amount of potassium that occurs due to excessive uptake of potassium by metabolically active cells in a blood sample after it has been drawn. It is a laboratory artifact that may occur when blood samples remain in warm conditions for several hours before processing.

Signs and Symptoms

A small drop in potassium usually does not cause symptoms. However, a big drop in the level can be life threatening.

Symptoms of hypokalemia include:

- Abnormal heart rhythms (dysrhythmias), especially in people with heart disease
- Constipation
- Fatigue
- Muscle damage (rhabdomyolysis)
- Muscle weakness or spasms
- Paralysis (which can include the lungs).

Tests

- Serum potassium determination
- Arterial blood gas
- Basic or comprehensive metabolic panel
- Electrocardiogram (ECG)
- Blood tests to check glucose, magnesium, calcium, sodium, phosphorous, thyroxin, and aldosterone levels.

Treatment

Mild hypokalemia can be treated by taking potassium supplements by mouth. Persons with more severe cases may need to get potassium through a vein (intravenously).

If diuretics used, doctor may try to keeps potassium in the body (such as triamterene, amiloride).

One type of hypokalemia that causes paralysis occurs when there is too much thyroid hormone in the blood (thyrotoxic periodic paralysis). Treatment lowers the thyroid hormone level, and raises the potassium level in the blood.

Hyperkalemia

- Elevated plasma potassium concentration
- It occurs in Addison's disease and in intravenous infusion of potassium at a rate excess of 25 mmol/hr
- Treatment using concentrated potassium solutions.

Causes

- Renal insufficiency (renal failure)
- Medication that interferes with urinary excretion:
  - ACE inhibitors and angiotensin receptor blockers
  - Potassium-sparing diuretics (e.g., amiloride and spironolactone)

- NSAIDs such as ibuprofen, naproxen, or celecoxib
- The calcineurin inhibitor immunosuppressants, cyclosporine and tacrolimus
- The antibiotic trimethoprim
- The antiparasitic drug pentamidine.

- Mineralocorticoid deficiency or resistance, such as:
  - Addison's disease
  - Aldosterone deficiency
  - Some forms of congenital adrenal hyperplasia
  - Type IV renal tubular acidosis (resistance of renal tubules to aldosterone)
- Gordon's syndrome (pseudohypoaldosteronism type II), a rare genetic disorder caused by defective modulators of salt transporters, including the thiazide-sensitive NaCl cotransporter.
- Excessive release from cells
  - Rhabdomyolysis, burns or any cause of rapid tissue necrosis, including tumor lysis syndrome
  - Massive blood transfusion or massive hemolysis
  - Shifts/transport out of cells caused by acidosis, low insulin levels, beta-blocker therapy, digoxin overdose, or the paralyzing agent succinylcholine
- Excessive intake

  Excess intake with salt-substitute, potassium-containing dietary supplements, or potassium chloride (KCl) infusion. Note that for a person with normal kidney function and nothing interfering with normal elimination (see above), hyperkalemia by potassium intake would be seen only with large infusions of KCl or oral doses of several hundred milliequivalents of KCl.

  Pseudohyperkalemia

  Pseudohyperkalemia is a rise in the amount of potassium that occurs due to excessive leakage of potassium from cells, during or after blood is drawn. It is a laboratory artifact rather than a biological abnormality and can be misleading to caregivers. Pseudohyperkalemia is typically caused by hemolysis during venipuncture (by either excessive vacuum of the blood draw or by a collection needle that is of too fine a gauge); excessive tourniquet time or fist clenching during phlebotomy (which presumably leads to efflux of potassium from the muscle cells into the bloodstream); or by a delay in the processing of the blood specimen. It can also occur in specimens from patients with abnormally high numbers of platelets (>500,000/mm^3), leukocytes (>70,000/mm^3), or erythrocytes (hematocrit > 55%)
- Tissue trauma causing the cells to release potassium into the ECF includes burns, traumatic injury and intestinal bleeding.

Signs and Symptoms

- Fatigue
- Weakness
- Tingling
- Numbness
- Paralysis
- Palpitations and difficulty in breathing.

Tests

To gather enough information for diagnosis, the measurement of potassium needs to be repeated, as the elevation can be due to hemolysis in the first sample. The normal serum level of potassium is 3.5–5 mEq/L. Generally, blood tests for renal function and glucose performed. Calculating the transtubular potassium gradient can sometimes help in distinguishing the cause of the hyperkalemia.

In many cases, renal ultrasound will be performed, since hyperkalemia is highly suggestive of renal failure.

Also, electrocardiography (EKG/ECG) may be performed to determine if there is a significant risk of cardiac arrhythmias.

Treatment

Several agents are used to transiently lower K^+ levels. Choice depends on the degree and cause of the hyperkalemia, and other aspects of the patient's condition.

Insulin (e.g., intravenous injection of 10–15 units of regular insulin along with 50 mL of 50% dextrose to prevent hypoglycemia) will lead to a shift of potassium ions into cells, secondary to increased activity of the sodium-potassium ATPase. Its effects last a few hours, so it sometimes needs to be repeated while other measures are taken to suppress potassium levels more permanently.

Severe cases require hemodialysis or hemofiltration, which are the most rapid methods of removing potassium from the body.

Preventing recurrence of hyperkalemia typically involves reduction of dietary potassium, removal of an offending medication, and/or the addition of oral bicarbonate or a diuretic (such as furosemide or hydrochlorothiazide).

Normal range

In serum	3.5–5 mEq/L
In plasma	3.5–4.5 mEq/L

- Serum potassium level above 7 mEq/L and below 2.5 mEq/L is serious, life threatening and requires immediate attention.
  Specimen: Serum, heparinized plasma, sweat, urine, feces, or gastrointestinal fluids are used for the assay.
- Hemolyzed samples are not suitable for electrolyte analysis because of the release of potassium from the RBC, which will cause a false increase in the potassium values.
- Urine collection for electrolyte estimation should be made without any preservative.
- Serum, plasma or urine must be stored at 2–4°C or frozen if the analysis is delayed.

Assay of Potassium

1. Flame emission spectrophotometry (Flame photometry).
2. *Ion selective electrode method (ISE):* Specific electrodes for sodium and potassium are used in this method. The above two methods are more popular and commonly used.
3. Atomic absorption spectrophotometry (AAS).
4. Spectrophotometric methods.

Determination of Sodium and Potassium in Serum using Emission Flame Photometry

Sample: Nonhemolyzed serum.

Principle: Sample is diluted and fed into non-luminous flame in the form of fine spray. Sodium and potassium elements give out characteristic color in the flame. Sodium gives yellow and potassium violet color on ignition in the flame. Yellow or violet flame thus emitted is proportional to the sodium or potassium content. Separate color filters are used for sodium and potassium.

Reagents

1. *Double distilled water:* The method is very sensitive. Water must be free of metal ions. It is recommended to use glass distilled double distilled water.
2. *Stock standard sodium 200 mEq/L:* Keep a little of AR grade sodium chloride at 110°C in an air oven for 2–3 hours. Allow to cool in a desiccator. Weigh 11.69 g of dried sodium chloride and dissolve in water and make up to one liter, mix thoroughly. Store in polythene bottle. Stable at least for 2 weeks.
3. *Stock potassium standard solution 10 mEq/L:* Dry some potassium chloride crystals as given under standard sodium (Reagent 2). Weigh 0.746 g of dried potassium chloride and dissolve in a little water and make up to 1 liter.
   Mix thoroughly. Store in polythene bottle. Keep at least for 2 weeks.
4. *Working standards:* A series of combined sodium-potassium standards are prepared. Mix sodium stock standard and stock potassium standards in the volumes

Table 19.1: Working sodium-potassium standards.

Working stock Na standards	Stock K Sodium solution (mL)	Na content Potassium solution (mL)	K content mEq/L	mEq/L
A	5.5	2.0	1.1	0.02
B	6.0	3.0	1.2	0.03
C	6.5	4.0	1.3	0.04
D	7.0	5.0	1.4	0.05
E	7.5	6.0	1.5	0.06
F	8.0	7.0	1.6	0.07
G	8.5	8.0	1.7	0.08

given in **Table 19.1** and make up to one liter in each instance. Store in separate bottles and label it.

Procedure: Dilute the serum 1 in 100 with double distilled water. That is, dilute 0.2 mL of serum with 19.8 mL of water in a 100 mL conical flask. Mix thoroughly.

Take about 5 mL of working standard A (Na—1.1, K—0.02 mEq/L) in a 10 mL beaker labeled A. Likewise, place 5 mL each of working standard from B, C, D, E, F, and G into 10 mL beaker labeled correspondingly as B, C, D, E, F, and G.

Potassium: Insert the K filter in place in the flame-photometer.

Switch on the galvanometer light. Turn on the knob for the air supply and regulate the air pressure to 12 lb per sq inch. Turn the gas supply on and light the wick and obtain a nonluminous flame. Take about 10 mL distilled water in a small beaker. Dip the end of the tubing connected to the spray intake. Adjust the gas supply in order to obtain a nonluminous flame showing no yellow zone.

Allow a few minutes for the instrument to warm up. Place working standards in the beakers A, B, C, D, E, F, and G in order one after another in a row.

Spray into the flame by dipping the tubing for the spray intake in water.

Operate the zero control to return the galvanometer to zero.

Remove the spray intake tubing from water and dip in high K standard, i.e., beaker G. Adjust the sensitivity knob of the instrument to read 80 on the scale. Check zero with water and the standard again.

The spray potassium standard from B into the flame and note the galvanometer reading. Check with water for zero and the standard again.

Likewise, note galvanometer readings of C, D, E, and F and checking each time with water to zero and the standards.

Spray the diluted serum sample into the flame and note the readings.

Tabulate as follows: Serum diluted 1 in 100.

Beakers	K content mEq/L	Readings
A	0.02	–
B	0.03	–
C	0.04	54
D	0.05	67
E	0.06	–
F	0.07	–
G	0.08	–
Test		62

Calculation It is well understood with an example: Reading of test, say, lies in between the reading of standards, C and D, i.e., the concentration between 0.04 mEq/L and 0.05 mEq/L.

Reading of test = 62
Reading of 0.05 mEq/L standard (C) = 54
Reading of 0.05 mEq/L K standard (D) = 67
Difference in readings of C and D = 67 - 54
= 13 units

Difference in readings of standards C and test
= 62 - 54 = 8

$$\text{Conc. of test} = 0.04 + \frac{8 \times 0.01}{13} = 0.046$$

where 0.01 is the difference in K content between C and D, i.e. (0.05 - 0.04)

Concentration in serum = 0.046 × 100
= 4.60 mEq/L.

where 100 is the dilution factor.

Sodium: Remove K filter and place Na filter into the instrument. Repeat the above procedure with the same series of standard and test solutions. Calculate in the same way as K.

Note: Hemolyzed serum or plasma should not be used as the concentration of potassium is very high inside the cell.

Never refrigerate whole blood prior to separation of plasma.

Determination of Electrolytes using Electrolyte Analyzer

There are different types of electrolyte analyzers are available from different companies to analyze the serum electrolytes.

SELF TEST

1. Name the major extracellular cation and give its function.
2. Give the serum normal values of sodium and potassium.
3. Explain the terms hyponatremia and hypernatremia.
4. Name the major extracellular anion.

MULTIPLE CHOICE QUESTIONS

1. Sodium is an extracellular:
 a. Cation
 b. Anion
 c. Neutral ion
 d. None of the above

2. All the following are the functions of potassium, *Except:*
 a. Functioning of nerves
 b. Acid-base balance
 c. Cofactor for enzymes
 d. Osmotic pressure maintenance

20 UNIT Electrolyte Balance

LEARNING OBJECTIVES

At the end of this unit, the learner should be able to understand:
- The distribution electrolytes and the mechanism to regulate them in the human body.
- The functions and pathological conditions of chloride, calcium, magnesium and phosphorus.

INTRODUCTION

The electrolytes, anions, or cations, which are present either in extracellular fluid or in intracellular fluid, should be maintained in balance otherwise the human body has to face several serious problems.

Distribution of Electrolytes

Solutes	*Plasma (mEq/L)*	
	ECF	*ICF*
Cations		
Na^+	142	10
K^+	5	148
Ca^{++}	5	2
Mg^{++}	3	40
Anions		
Cl^-	103	
HCO_3^-	24	8
HPO_4^{--}	2	136
SO_4^{--}	1	
Protein	15	56
Organic ions	10	

- The sum of *cations* must be equal to the sum of *anions* to maintain electrical neutrality.
- Electrolyte composition of other ECF is similar to that of plasma except that of proteins. Protein concentration is higher in plasma than other extracellular fluid.
- *Sodium* is the major cation of plasma.
- *Chloride* and *bicarbonate* are the major anions of plasma.
- The total electrolyte concentration in ICF is higher than in ECF.
- The major cations in ICF are K^+ and Mg^{++} and these are balanced mainly by the anions PO_4^{--} and proteins.

Sodium Balance

- Kidney is the only organ involved in the excretion of Na^+.
- Kidney helps regulate the body Na^+ content.
- The filtered Na^+ in the glomerular filtrate is reabsorbed in the distal tubule.
- A hormone, namely *aldosterone* secreted by the adrenal cortex is involved in the regulation of sodium reabsorption in the renal tubules.

- Aldosterone increases the reabsorption of Na^+ whenever the plasma Na^+ is low.
- Along with Na^+,Cl^- is also reabsorbed.
- Absorption of Na^+ takes place in exchange for K^+.
- Aldosterone secretion is controlled by the volume of ECF and its Na^+ concentration.

Described in detail below how sodium is balanced in the human body:

- In addition to regulating total volume, the *osmolarity* of bodily fluids is also highly regulated.
- Extreme variation in osmolarity causes cells to shrink or swell, damaging or destroying cellular structure and disrupting normal cellular function.
- Regulation of osmolarity is achieved by balancing the intake and excretion of sodium with that of water.
- Sodium is the major solute in extracellular fluids, so it effectively determines the osmolarity of extracellular fluids.
- An important concept is that regulation of osmolarity must be integrated with regulation of volume, because changes in water volume alone have diluting or concentrating effects on a bodily fluids.
- For example, when a person becomes dehydrated they lose more water than sodium. Then the osmolarity of bodily fluids increases. In this situation the body tries to conserve water but not sodium, thus stemming the rise in osmolarity.
- When a person loses a large amount of blood from trauma or surgery, the losses of sodium and water are proportionate to the composition of bodily fluids. In this situation, the body should conserve both water and sodium.
- As discussed in the previous unit, ADH plays a role in lowering osmolarity by increasing water reabsorption in the kidneys, thus helping to dilute bodily fluids. To prevent osmolarity from decreasing below normal, the kidneys also have a regulated mechanism for reabsorbing sodium in the distal nephron. This mechanism is controlled by *aldosterone,* a steroid hormone produced by the adrenal cortex.
- Aldosterone secretion is controlled in two ways:
  a. When the *osmolarity* increases above normal, aldosterone secretion is inhibited.
     - The lack of aldosterone causes less sodium to be reabsorbed in the distal tubule.
     - ADH secretion will increase to conserve water, thus complementing the effect of low aldosterone levels to decrease the osmolarity of bodily fluids.
     - The net effect on urine excretion is a decrease in the amount of urine excreted, with an increase in the osmolarity of the urine.
  b. The kidneys sense low blood pressure:
     - This triggers a complex response to raise blood pressure and *conserve volume.* Specialized cells in the afferent and efferent arterioles produce *renin,* a peptide hormone that initiates a hormonal cascade that ultimately produces *angiotensin II.*
     - Angiotensin II stimulates the adrenal cortex to produce aldosterone.

Chloride (Cl^-)

- Chloride (Cl^-) is the major extracellular anion.
- Its average serum concentration is 105 mEq/L.

Functions

- It is involved in maintaining osmotic pressure, proper body hydration and electric neutrality.
- Dietary Cl^- is almost completely absorbed by the intestine.

- It is filtered out by the glomerulus and passively reabsorbed in conjunction with Na^+ by the proximal tubules.
- Excess Cl^- is excreted in urine and through sweating.
- Excessive sweating stimulates aldosterone secretion, which acts on the sweat glands to conserve Na^+ and Cl^-.

Hypochloremia

A low serum Cl^- is associated with loss of gastric HCl due to prolonged vomiting, salt-losing renal disease, in metabolic acidosis, etc.

Hyperchloremia

High serum Cl^- is seen in dehydration and decreased renal blood flow.

During the assay of electrolytes high quality of distilled water is recommended for preparation of standards and diluting the samples.

Determination of Chloride

Colorimetric Method

Chloride in the plasma or serum reacts with mercuric thiocyanate to form mercuric chloride and free thiocyanate ions. The thiocyanate ions react with Fe^{3+} ions to form the colored complex with a absorption peak at 480 nm. This method can be done manually or by the autoanalyzer.

1. Mercuric thiocyanate + Chloride → Mercuric chloride + Free thiocyanate $[Fe^2(NO_3)_3]$.
2. Free thiocyanate + Fe^{3+} → Ferric thiocyanate (red colored) → OD at 480 nm

Method of Schales and Schales

Principle

Serum is titrated with mercuric nitrate solution using diphenylcarbazone as indicator, which gives a violet-blue color.

Sample

Serum or plasma.

Reagents

1. *Mercuric nitrate:* Take 20 mL of double distilled water in a beaker. Add 3 mL concentrated nitric acid. Add 3.2 g of mercuric nitrate to the solution in beaker. Dissolve and transfer the solution in the beaker to one liter flask. Make up to 1 liter with water and mix properly.
2. Nitric acid, approximately 1 N: Dilute 6 mL of concentrated HNO_3 to 100 mL with water.
3. Diphenylcarbazone, 0.1%.
   Dissolve 100 mg of diphenylcarbazone in 100 mL of 95% ethyl alcohol. Stored in a brown bottle in refrigerator, keeps indefinitely.
4. Ethyl ether.
5. Standard chloride solution 100 mEq/L.
   Dry some NaCl (AR Grade) crystals at 110°C for 2–3 hours in a hot-air oven. Allow it to cool in a desiccator. Weigh 5.845 g of dry NaCl and dissolve in double distilled water and dilute to one liter.

Procedure

Test: Into a 25 mL conical flask (or test tube) pipette 2 mL water. Add 0.2 mL serum. Add 1 drop of 1 N nitric acid. Add 3 drops of diphenylcarbazone. Add 1 mL of ethyl ether.

Take mercuric nitrate solution in a 2 mL pipette calibrated 0.01 mL, up to '0' mark.

Add mercuric nitrate to the conical flask (or test tube) drop by drop with shaking. A pink color obtained in the beginning disappears. Continue addition till a permanent violet-blue color appears. Note the titer value.

Standard: Pipette 2 mL of water and 0.2 mL of standard into a 25 mL conical flask. Add one drop of 1 N nitric acid. Add 3 drops of diphenylcarbazone. Add 1 mL of ethyl ether. Titrate with mercuric nitrate to get the permanent violet blue color. Note the titer value.

Calculation

$$\text{mEq/L of chloride} = \frac{\text{Titer value of test}}{\text{Titer value of std}} \times 100$$

Note: Use double distilled water. Sodium chloride should be dried before weighing.

Interpretation

The normal level is between 94 and 111 mEq/L. A higher than the normal level may be seen in:
- Dehydration and
- Acute renal failure.

Lower than normal level may be observed in:
- Diarrhea
- Congestive heart failure
- Pyloric obstruction
- Uremia
- Addison's disease
- Pulmonary emphysema
- Diabetic acidosis.

Determination of CSF Chloride by Schales and Schales

Principle

CSF is titrated against mercuric nitrate at the end point of which a permanent pink color is obtained.

Same reagents are used, which are used for serum chloride estimation.

Procedure

Test: Take a test tube and label it Test (T). Pipette 2 mL of water, 0.2 mL of CSF. Add 1 drop of 1 N HNO_3 and 3 drops of diphenylcarbazone. Add 1 mL of ethyl ether, mix. Titrate using mercuric nitrate taken in a 2 mL pipette (calibrated to 0.01 mL) to the appearance of permanent violet color. Note the titration value (mL) of mercuric nitrate.

Standard: Into a tube labeled standard (S), pipette 2 mL water, 0.2 mL standard solution. Add 1 drop 1 N HNO_3 and 3 drops of diphenylcarbazone and mix. Titrate using the same pipette taking mercuric nitrate in it. Note the titration value (mL of mercuric nitrate).

Calculation

$$\text{mEq/L of chloride in CSF} = \frac{\text{Titration of test}}{\text{Titration of std}} \times 100$$

Note: Use double distilled water throughout the work.

Interpretation

- Normal CSF chloride level is between 120 and 130 mEq/L.
- Decrease in CSF chloride found in meningitis.
- In tuberculous meningitis, CSF chloride is lowered.
- It is normal in viral meningitis.

Calcium (Ca^{++})

- Calcium is a mineral
- It is a cation of the ECF
- Calcium is required for the formation of bone and teeth
- Gives hardness and strength to bone and teeth
- Required for blood coagulation process.
- Required for contraction of heart and muscle
- Controls the permeability of cell membranes
- Activates pancreatic lipase in the digestion of fats
- Activates phosphorylase during the break down of glycogen
- Regulates the excitability of nerve fibers
- Releases hormones like insulin from storage granules
- Serves as a second messenger in the action of hormones like adrenaline
- Responses of calcium are mediated by interaction with a receptor protein called calmodulin. This cytosolic protein has calcium-binding sites. Calmodulin-calcium complex activates protein kinases, which in turn activates other enzymes and through these, bring about metabolic effects. In this mechanism, cAMP is also involved
- It is required for the formation of calcium paracaseinate (insoluble curd).

Calcium Content of Body and Blood

Calcium is the major inorganic element comprising nearly 2% of the body weight.

Human body contains 1200 g.

Major amount (99% of this) present in bone and teeth as hydroxyapatite. Remaining 1% is present in blood and soft tissues.

Calcium level of serum in adult is 9–11 mg/100 mL.

Blood calcium present in three different forms:

a. Ionized calcium (Ca^{++}) is the physiologically active form. It constitutes 50% of the total calcium (4.5–5.5 mg%)
b. Protein (albumin) bound form. This is 45% of total level.
c. Calcium complexes with citrate, phosphate and bicarbonate. This fraction is only 5%.

Regulation of Serum Calcium Level

The ionic calcium level is maintained by vitamin D and hormones like parathyroid hormone (PTH) and calcitonin.

Action of Vitamin D

a. Increases the absorption of calcium (and phosphate) from the small intestine.
b. Causes removal of calcium from bone (bone resorption).
   The mechanism by which 1-25-dihydroxy vitamin D_3 increases calcium absorption from intestine is as follows:
   The 1-25-dihydroxy vitamin D_3 enters the intestinal cell and binds to a cytoplasmic receptor. The vitamin D_3 receptor complex then moves to the nucleus where it interacts with DNA. This results in the synthesis of mRNA and this in turn forms a calcium binding protein. The calcium binding protein increases the absorption of calcium from intestine.

Action of PTH on Kidney and Bone (Fig. 20.1)

1. PTH increases the activity of 1 α-hydroxylase in kidney, which increases the synthesis of 1-25-dihydroxy vitamin D_3 and this in turn enhance the absorption of calcium from intestine.
2. It increases the reabsorption of calcium from glomerular filtrate in kidneys.
3. It causes the resorption of calcium from bone.
   These three actions correct the hypocalcemia and bring it to normal level.
4. PTH also causes excretion of phosphate in urine by inhibiting phosphate reabsorption in kidney.

Action of Calcitonin

This is a hormone from C cells of thyroid glands.

Hypercalcemia stimulates its secretion.

Calcitonin inhibits calcium reabsorption from kidneys and resorption from bone. Thus it corrects hypercalcemia.

Normal value ranges from 9 to 10.6 mg per 100 mL serum or 4.5–5.4 mEq/L.

Hypocalcemia

- Hypoparathyroidism
- *Vitamin D deficiency:* Decreased dietary intake, decreased sun exposure, defective vitamin D metabolism, ineffective active vitamin D, intestinal malabsorption
- Magnesium deficiency (hypomagnesemia)
- Eating disorders
- *Chronic renal failure:* The kidney loses its capacity synthesize 1.25 dihydroxycholecalciferol. Increased PTH secretion in response

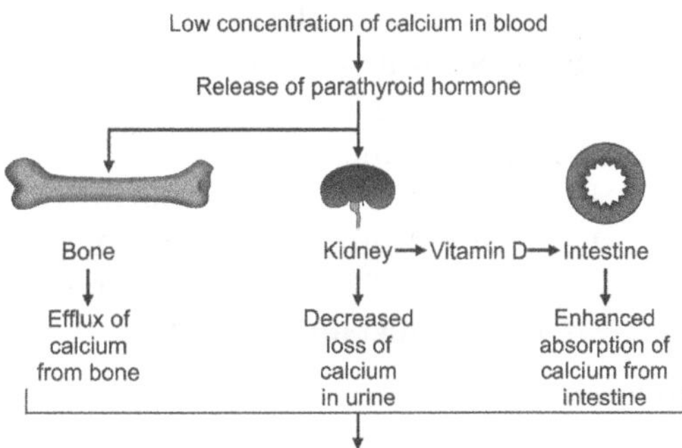

Fig. 20.1: Role of PTH in restoring low plasma calcium to normal.

to hypocalcemia may lead to bone disease if untreated
- *Pseudohypoparathyroidism* is a condition associated primarily with resistance to the parathyroid hormone. Patients have a low serum calcium and high phosphate, but the parathyroid hormone level (PTH) is actually appropriately high (due to the hypocalcemia).

Symptoms

Convulsions, arrhythmias, tetany and numbness/paresthesias in hands, feet, around mouth and lips.
- Petechiae, which appear as on-off spots, then later become confluent, and appear as purpura (larger bruised areas)
- Oral, perioral and acral paresthesias, tingling or 'pins and needles' sensation in and around the mouth and lips, and in the extremities of the hands and feet. This is often the earliest symptom of hypocalcemia
- Carpopedal and generalized tetany are seen
- Latent tetany
  - Trousseau sign of latent tetany (eliciting carpal spasm by inflating the blood pressure cuff and maintaining the cuff pressure above systolic)
  - Chvostek's sign (tapping of the inferior portion of the zygoma will produce facial spasms)
- Tendon reflexes are hyperactive
- Life-threatening complications
  - Laryngospasm
  - Cardiac arrhythmias
- ECG changes include:
  - Intermittent QT prolongation, or intermittent prolongation of the QTc (corrected QT interval) on the EKG (electrocardiogram) is noted.

Treatment

Two ampoules of intravenous calcium gluconate 10% is given slowly in a period of 10 minutes, or if the hypocalcemia is severe, calcium chloride is given instead.

Hypercalcemia

Elevated calcium level in the blood.

Causes

- Primary hyperparathyroidism
  - Solitary parathyroid adenoma
  - Primary parathyroid hyperplasia
  - Parathyroid carcinoma
- Solid tumor with metastasis (e.g., squamous cell carcinoma, which can be PTHrP-mediated)
- Solid tumor with humoral mediation of hypercalcemia (e.g., non-small cell lung cancer or kidney cancer, pheochromocytoma)
- Hematologic malignancy (multiple myeloma, lymphoma, leukemia)
- Hypervitaminosis D (vitamin D intoxication)
- Elevated 1,25$(OH)_2$D (see calcitriol under vitamin D) levels (e.g., sarcoidosis and other granulomatous diseases)
- Idiopathic hypercalcemia of infancy
- Rebound hypercalcemia after rhabdomyolysis
- Renal diseases
- Disorders related to high bone-turnover rates
  - Hyperthyroidism
  - Prolonged immobilization
  - Paget's disease of the bone
  - Multiple myeloma.

Signs and Symptoms

Stones (renal or biliary), bones (bone pain), thrones (sit on throne - polyuria), fatigue, anorexia, and pancreatitis.

Treatment

- Hydration, increasing salt intake, and forced diuresis
- Bisphosphonates are pyrophosphate analogs with high affinity for bone, especially areas of high bone-turnover

Sources

- Milk
- Tofu (with added calcium sulfate)
- Calcium-fortified orange juice
- Soy beverages with added calcium
- Calcium-fortified cereals or breads.

Daily Requirement

Children: 500–800 mg
Adults: 1000–1300 mg

Determination of Serum Calcium by Trinder Method

Principle

Calcium is precipitated with naphthyl hydroxamic acid. The precipitate is dissolved in EDTA and the color is developed with ferric nitrate. The absorbance of color compound is measured in a colorimeter and the calcium level is determined.

Sample

Serum.

Reagents

1. *Calcium reagent:* In a 250 mL beaker add 100 mL water and 5 mL ethanolamine. Add 2 g of tartaric acid and mix. Add 250 mg of naphthyl-hydroxamic acid and dissolve by warming. In a liter flask add 9 g sodium chloride and 500 mL of water. Pour the contents of the beaker into the 1 L flask containing sodium chloride solution. Add water up to 1 L mark. Mix. Filter through Whatman No. 40 filter paper. The reagent is stable for months.
2. *EDTA solution:* Dissolve 2 g of disodium ethylene diamine tetraacetate in 1 L of 0.1 N NaOH.
3. *Color reagent:* Dissolve 60 g of ferric nitrate, in 500 mL of water, add 15 mL of concentrated nitric acid and add water up to 1 liter.
4. Calcium standard, 5 mEq/L.
   Dissolve 125 mg of dry calcium carbonate (dried at 120°C for 30 minutes in a hot-air oven) in 40 mL of 0.1 N hydrochloric acid and dilute to 500 mL with water.

Procedure

Reagents	*B*	*S*	*T*
Serum	–	–	0.2 mL
Standard calcium	–	0.2 mL	–
Calcium reagent	5.0 mL	5.0 mL	5.0 mL
Mix. Stand 30 minutes at room temperature Centrifuge Pour off supernatant			
EDTA solution	1.0 mL	1.0 mL	1.0 mL
Keep in boiling water bath, 10 minutes, Cool			
Color reagent	3.0 mL	3.0 mL	3.0 mL
Read the absorbance at 450 nm or Blue filter			

Calculation

$$\text{Serum calcium in mEq/L} = \frac{\text{OD of T} - \text{OD of B}}{\text{OD of S} - \text{OD of B}} \times 10$$

To convert the result to mg% multiply mEq/L by 2.

Note

The glassware's must be perfectly clean.

O-Cresolphthalein Complexone Method

Principle

Calcium in the serum forms a violet colored complex with O-Cresolphthalein complexone. 8-Hydroxyquinoline included in the reagent prevents interference by magnesium.

Reagents

Reagent A

Transfer 210 g of diethanolamine to about 900 mL of double distilled water into a liter beaker. Dissolve the crystals. Adjust the pH to 11.7 with acetic acid. Transfer to a 1 liter flask and make up to 1 liter with double distilled water. The reagent is stable at least for one month.

Reagent B

Dissolve 64 mg of O-Cresolphthalein complexone, 1.16 g of 8-Hydroxyquinoline and 2.5 mL glacial acetic acid in 250 mL of ethanol. Make up the volume to 1 liter with double distilled water. The reagent is stable for at least one month.

Working Reagent

Mix equal volumes of reagent A and reagent B just before use (calculate the approximate volume of reagent required and prepare the required volume of reagent for the day).

Calcium Standard

10 mg/100 mL or 5 mEq/L. Dissolve 125 mg of dry calcium carbonate in 40 mL of 0.1 N HCl and dilute to 500 mL with water.

Procedure

Pipette 0.2 mL serum and 1.8 mL water to a test tube. Mix. Transfer 0.5 mL from this to a test tube marked test (T). Add 5 mL of working reagent.

To a second test tube add 0.2 mL of calcium standard solution and 1.8 mL of water. Transfer 0.5 mL from this to standard (S). Add 5 mL of working reagent. Mix them.

Label a 3rd test tube as Blank (B) and add 0.5 mL water and 5 mL of working reagent. Mix them.

Read absorbance of B, S and T at 578 nm or using green filter.

Calculation

mg of calcium/100 mL

$$\text{serum} = \frac{\text{OD of T} - \text{OD of B}}{\text{OD of S} - \text{OD of B}} \times 10$$

When mg% is divided by 2, mEq/L is obtained.

Phosphorus

- It is a mineral.
- It is also involved in the release of energy from fat, protein, and carbohydrates during metabolism, and in the formation of genetic material, cell membranes, and many enzymes.
- Helps in the formation of bone and teeth. Inorganic phosphorus is a major constituent of hydroxyapatite in bone, thereby playing an important part in structural support of the body.
- Act as a buffer in blood. Mixture of HPO_4^- and $H_2PO_4^-$ constitutes the phosphate buffer, which plays a role in maintaining the pH of the body fluid.
- Helps in the formation of compounds like nucleic acids, nucleotides like ATP, GTP, ADP, etc. as organic phosphate esters in glycolysis and other metabolic reactions.
- It is also required in energy metabolism, synthesis of phospholipids, cAMP, phosphoproteins, and coenzymes like TPP, etc.
- The phosphorus concentration in serum is inversely proportional to the calcium concentration.
- The normal value for adults is 2.5–4.5 mg% and for children 4–6 mg%.

Hypophosphatemia

Decreased level of phosphorous.

Causes

- Rickets
- Hyperparathyroidism
- Condition associated with decrease in the reabsorption of phosphate from the glomerular filtrate (Fanconi syndrome)
- In the treatment of diabetes, the effect of insulin in causing the shift of glucose into cells also enhances the transport of phosphate into cells, which may result into hypophosphatemia.

Symptoms

Clinical symptoms are muscle pain and weakness with respiratory failure and decreased myocardial output.

Hyperphosphatemia

Increased phosphorus level.

Causes

- Hypoparathyroidism
- Hypervitaminosis D
- Renal failure.

Elevated phosphate may cause a decrease in serum calcium concentration. Therefore, it may lead to tetany and seizures.

Determination of Serum Inorganic Phosphorus by Fiske-Subbarao Method

Specimen

Serum collected from venous blood. Plasma is also suitable.

Principle

Serum proteins are precipitated by trichloroacetic acid. Molybdic acid added to protein-free filtrate converts phosphate to phosphomolybdate. Alpha-naphthol sulfonic acid added reduces phosphomolybdate to a blue colored compound. The intensity of blue color is measured photometrically using red filter or at 660 nm.

Reagents

1. Trichloroacetic acid, 10%. Dissolve 10 g TCA in water and make up to 100 liter.
2. Molybdate reagent: To 200 mL of water add 83 mL sulfuric acid, keeping cold under tap or cold water. Dissolve 25 g of ammonium molybdate in this solution. Dilute to 1 liter with water. Solution is stable.
3. 1,2,4-Amino naphthol sulfonic acid reagent (ANSA).
   Dissolve 0.125 g of 1,2,4-amino naphthol sulfonic acid, 7.28 g of sodium meta bisulfite and 0.25 g of anhydrous sodium sulfite in 50 mL of water. Filter. Store in a brown bottle. There agent is stable for one month kept in refrigerator.
4. Standard phosphorus solution 0.08 mg per mL solution.
   Dissolve 0.351 g of dried potassium dihydrogen phosphate in about 500 mL water in a liter flask. Add 8 mL concentrated HCl and dilute to one liter. Prepare fresh once a month.

Procedure

Reagents	*B*	*S*	*T*
Serum	–	–	1 mL
TCA, 10%	–	–	9 mL
Mix stand for 5 minutes filter			
Water	1 mL	0.5 mL	–
Standard phosphorus solution	–	0.5 mL	–
Filtrate	–	–	5 mL
TCA, 10%	4 mL	4 mL	
Molybdate reagent	1 mL	1 mL	1 mL
ANSA	0.4 mL	0.4 mL	0.4 mL
Mix. stand for 5 minutes			
Water	3.6 mL	3.6 mL	3.6 mL
Read at 660 nm or red filter			

Calculation

$$\text{100 mL serum contains} = \frac{\text{OD of T} - \text{OD of B}}{\text{OD of S} - \text{OD of B}} \times 0.04 \times \frac{100}{1}$$

$$= \frac{T-B}{S-B} \times 4$$

Note

1. The inorganic phosphorus increases when blood is allowed to stand so, determine immediately.
2. Use double distilled water throughout the procedure.
3. The method is employed to determine phosphate in urine, urine is adjusted to pH 5 by adding 1 N HCl. It is diluted to 1 in 10 with water. Proceed same as above. Collect 24-hour sample.

Magnesium (Mg^{++})

- Magnesium is the fourth most abundant cation in the body, with about 50% present in the bones associated with calcium and phosphate.

- Much of the remaining magnesium is intracellular and only a small amount is found in extracellular fluid.
- Magnesium functions as an activator for various physiochemical processes, including phosphorylation, protein synthesis, and DNA metabolism.
- It is also involved in neuromuscular conduction and excitability of skeletal and cardiac muscle.
- Ingested magnesium is absorbed in the intestine and the amount absorbed is inversely related to the total magnesium intake.
- The kidneys effectively control magnesium homeostasis through tubular reabsorption, which conserves magnesium when intake is low and excretes excess when intake is high.

Hypermagnesemia

Causes

- Renal failure
- Acute diabetic acidosis
- Dehydration
- Addison's disease
- Hypermagnesemia has a depressing effect on the central nervous system, causing general anesthesia and respiratory failure. It alters the conduction mechanism of the heart, causing cardiac arrest.

Hypomagnesemia

Causes

- Chronic alcoholism, malabsorption
- Severe diarrhea
- Acute pancreatitis
- Diuretic therapy
- Prolonged parenteral fluid therapy without magnesium supplementation
- Kidney disorders, such as glomerulonephritis
- Tubular reabsorption defects
- Decreased serum magnesium concentrations may result in tetany, convulsions, and cardiac arrhythmias
- Urine magnesium levels are determined in magnesium depletion tests.

Method

Colorimetric method with Chlorophosphonazo III.

SELF TEST

1. Give the normal serum value of chloride.
2. What are the methods available to determine the concentration of sodium and potassium?
3. Name the method used to determine the CSF chloride.
4. State the conditions in which serum calcium increases.
5. Explain the clinical significance of serum inorganic phosphorus estimation.

MULTIPLE CHOICE QUESTIONS

1. The concentration of sodium in the serum is:

a. 130–150 mEq/L
b. 135–140 mEq/L
c. 100–120 mEq/L
d. 150–160 mEq/L

2. The major extracellular anion is:

a. Potassium
b. Chloride
c. Sodium
d. Bicarbonate

3. Reduced calcium levels are seen in all the following conditions, *Except:*
   a. Tetany
   b. Hypoparathyroidism
   c. Acidosis
   d. Childhood rickets

4. Elevated calcium levels are seen in all the following conditions, *Except:*
   a. Primary hyperparathyroidism
   b. Vitamin D over dosage
   c. Bone tumors
   d. Liver disease

5. Elevated phosphorus levels are seen in:
   a. Renal failure
   b. Vitamin D over dosage
   c. Pancreatitis
   d. Liver disease

21 UNIT

Quality Control

LEARNING OBJECTIVES

At the end of this unit, the learner should be able to understand:

- The essentiality of the quality control and quality assurance in the clinical biochemistry laboratory.
- The internal and external quality control program.
- Use of Levey–Jennings chart and westgard rule in the accepting and rejecting the control values.

INTRODUCTION

- The biochemical test results of the laboratory play an important role in the diagnosis and treatment of the disease.
- Any error with the test values may result in wrong diagnosis, unnecessary treatment or prolonged hospitalization.
- The unnecessary hospitalization puts extra-financial burden on the patient.
- Hence, the quality of such tests must be controlled.
- High quality of the biochemical test results can be achieved through adopting standard quality control programs in the laboratory.
- Nowadays, it is necessary to release the tests results after complete review.
- It is necessary for the Clinical Biochemist to check day-to-day error and to take necessary steps to minimize those errors.
- The International Federation of Clinical Chemistry expert panel defines quality control as "the study of errors which are the responsibility of the laboratory and the procedures used to recognize and minimize them".
- All steps should be taken by the laboratory to ensure reliability and the accuracy of laboratory results and reproducibility and compatibility of producers with other laboratories.
- The high quality and accuracy of the tests results are achieved when the following points are taken into consideration:
  - Cleanliness of glassware
  - Daily maintenance of instrument
  - Use of specific and sensitive methods for assays
  - Training of laboratory employees.

International Definitions

Quality Assurance

All those planned and systematic actions necessary to provide adequate confidence that a service will satisfy given requirements for quality.

Trueness

Closeness of the agreement between the average values obtained from a large series of test results and an accepted reference value.

Precision (Fig 21.1)

Closeness of agreement between independent test results obtained under prescribed conditions.

It may or may not be accurate.

Bias

Difference between the expectation of the test results and an accepted reference value.

Accuracy (Fig 21.1)

The measure of the closeness of the estimated value to the true value.

Error

Result of a measurement minus a true value of the measured.

Repeatability Conditions

Conditions where independent test results are obtained with the same method on identical test items in the same laboratory by the same operator using the same equipment within short intervals of time.

Uncertainty of Measurement

Parameter, associated with the result of a measurement that characterizes the dispersion of the values that could reasonably be attributed to the measured.

Quality Control Material

Control material: Material used for the purposes of internal quality control and subjected to the same or part of the same measurement procedure as that used for test materials.

- The pooled and lyophilized normal serum forms the quality control material.

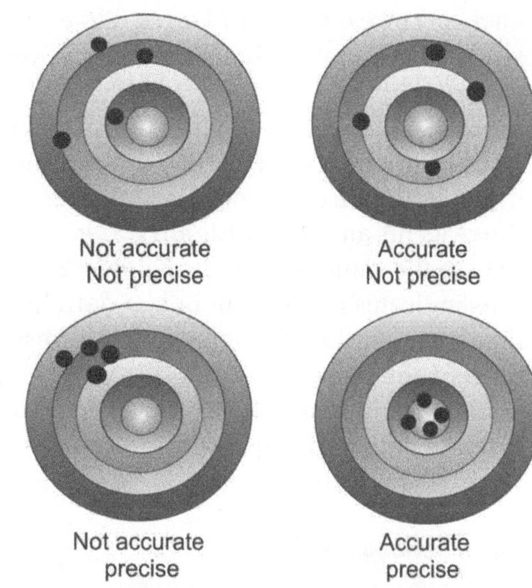

Fig. 21.1: Accuracy and precision.

- These materials can be procured from the suppliers with the analyzed values.
- Quality control materials are mainly available in the powder form.
- Once we dissolve this material to a desired volume it can be distributed into several vials and stored in a refrigerator.
- Each day a vial of low and high quality control material can be used.

Preparation of the Quality Control Material

- The serum samples collected
- Pool the serum samples together (1–2 liters)
- Screen the serum sample for various infective diseases
- Filter the pooled serum through glass wool taken in a funnel and mix thoroughly
- Adjust the pH to 7.5 using concentrated sulfuric acid
- Distribute 10 mL portions of this into several plastic vials and store in the deep freezer and this is stable for three months

- Each day take one vial and bring it to room temperature. Once it liquefies analyze the value
- Enter the value on the quality control chart
- If the value on a specific day falls within ± 2 SD (standard deviation) that indicates all the reagents and standards are good
- In case the value is above or below ± 2 SD. This indicates the reagent or standard has deteriorated. Repeat the assay with fresh reagent and standard
- Sometimes, the control serum itself deteriorates because of improper storage. So, replace with a fresh control.

Standard Deviation (SD)

If a specimen is analyzed several times, the result would be around the mean value. The mean difference of each value from mean is SD.

$$SD = \frac{\varepsilon\,(X - x)^2}{n - 1}$$

X = Individual result
x = Arithmetic mean
n = No. of results
ε = Total of $(X - x)^2$

Coefficient of Variation (CV)

Express dispersion of results
Relates SD to level of measurement

$$CV = \frac{SD \times 100}{Mean}$$

3% - Ideal result
5% - Acceptable
5% - Unacceptable

Is there a need for quality control?

Yes, because each clinical chemist has his or her own goals to achieve something

Goals can be achieved through planned and systematic efforts.

Two primary goals a laboratory must set are:

1. To provide analytical services in useful and convenient manner.
2. To produce consistently precise and accurate data, which are useful in making medical decisions. Quality assurance and quality control are the two tools for achieving goals.

Quality assurance is outlined by 4 points they are plan, practice, procedures, program.

Quality assurance offers three advantages to the laboratory.

1. Conscious among the people about the quality of work.
2. Focuses people's attention on quality goals.
3. Focuses people's attention on analytical goals.

Quality assurance program should have three components to ensure its success.

- Commitment
- Facilities and resources
- Technical competence.

Quality Control

A set of measures useful in detecting errors. Errors can be minimized by exercising control on three factors.

1. *Preanalytical variables*
   - Patient identification and preparation
   - Specimen acquisition and transport
   - Turnaround time
   - Specimen processing
   - Work list preparation and maintenance of work records.
2. *Analytical variables*
   - Selection of appropriate method
   - Standardization and calibration
   - Documentation and verification of procedures
   - Monitoring critical equipment, materials and reports
3. *Control of analytical quality*

   Monitoring quality through the use of control sera, charts and records.

What Quality Goals should We Set for Our Laboratory?

a. To generate consistently reliable, precise and accurate results.
b. To satisfy the medical purposes for which the test designed.
   Common queries a clinician may have in mind while advising tests are:
   - Is a disease present?
   - What is the nature of the disease?
   - Can diagnosis be confirmed?
   - How severe is disease stage reached by the patient?
   - Has a change occurred since last observation?

How Can We Achieve These Goals?

i. Through defining and executing an effective quality assurance program
ii. Designing and implementing effective quality control programs.
   1. Internal QC program
   2. External QC program

Internal QC Program

Set of procedures undertaken by laboratory staff for the continuous monitoring of operation and the results of measurements in order to decide whether results are reliable enough to be released.

Can be designed without much difficulty based upon:

Analysis of Patient Sera

1. Clinical correlation of test with the disease the patient is suspected to be suffered from.
2. *Within-assay variation:* Analyze the same sample twice during an assay and note the results. Ideally, if no random or systemic errors exist, both the results should be identical. A large variation in results indicates the effect of one or more errors.
3. *Correlation with other laboratory results:* The results of a particular test must correlate with the results of other related tests.
   Example: In liver function tests, in a patient whose serum is visibly icteric, and ALT activity is high, total bilirubin concentration must be elevated proportionally. If not, an error is indicated.
4. *Intralaboratory duplicates of days:* Sample can be analyzed in duplicates for two days and the four values studied for reproducibility.
   Variations in the four values indicate one or more random or systemic errors.
5. *Delta checks with previous tests:* The results of a particular test may be compared with the results of previous tests on the patient. If the disease progressing, the values must increase, if the patient is in the recovery phase, the result must show a decrease in the analyte concentration. If not, this indicates errors.
6. *Patient daily and monthly average data:* The law of averages states that the average daily or monthly value for a particular parameter like glucose must lie within a very small range. This can be calculated by the formula:

$$\frac{\text{Sum of concentrations of analyte in all samples}}{\text{No. of samples}}$$

   If the average for a particular day or month varies greatly from the average for other two days or months then it is an indication of an error for that period.
7. Allowable error limit (AEL) for each analyte

$$\%\,\text{AEL} = \frac{0.25 \times \text{Reference range}}{\text{Mean of normal range}} \times 100$$

e.g., Glucose: Normal range = 70–110 mg/dL.

$$\text{Hence, \%AEL} = \frac{\dfrac{0.25 \times 110 - 70}{70 + 110} \times 100}{2}$$

$$\frac{10}{90} \times 100 = 11.11\%$$

If the results fall outside this limit, they must be rejected.

Using Pooled Sera

Samples containing normal and abnormal levels of analytes may be pooled daily until sufficient quantity is collected. Pooled sera are kept in the freezer, filtered, aliquots transferred to small vials, and then frozen.

Use of Commercial Assayed Sera

An assayed control serum may be included in the assay and the result compared with the expected values provided with the control.

External QC Program

Systems of objectively and retrospectively comparing results from different laboratories, by means of surveys organized by an external agency.

Several external quality control programs are available. The participating laboratory is sent vials of controls without reference values. The laboratory may analyze these samples as many times as they wish, and send their best result to these reference laboratories. The reference laboratory then assigns a variance index score (VIS), which is calculated for glucose as shown below:

Reference laboratories' value 120 mg/dL
Participating laboratories' value 95 mg/dL
Difference = 120 - 95 = 25 mg/dL

$$\%\ \text{Variation} = \frac{\text{Difference}}{\text{Ref. mean}} \times 100$$

$$\frac{25}{120} \times 100 = 20.8$$

$$\text{VIS} = \frac{\%\ \text{variation}}{\text{CCV}} \times 100$$

(*CCV = Chosen coefficient of variation)

$$\frac{20.8}{6.8} \times 100 = 30.6 \text{ (less than 50 is good)}$$

Internal QC program is most useful in determining the reproducibility of results (precision). External QC program are useful in determining the closeness of a result to the true value (accuracy).

What are the Types of Quality Control Sera Available?

The three types of QC sera available are listed in the **Table 21.1** along with their characteristics.

While it is entirely up to the laboratory manager to decide upon which type of control material is best suited to his/her own laboratory, a few important characteristics about the control must be considered prior to selection of the control.

Controls should have a matrix similar to the patient's sera. They should be rugged. Controls should be:

- Homogeneous
- Sterile (free from HIV and HbsAg)
- Safe (free from poisons and carcinogens)
- Stable
- Easily available and economic.

How Often Should We Run Controls?

A control or a set of controls (subnormal, normal and abnormal) must be assayed after

Table 21.1: Types of quality control sera and their characteristics.

Criterion	*Frozen*	*Lyophilized*	*Low temperature liquid*
Clarity	Clear	Hazy	Clear
Stability	12 months	12–18 months	12–18 months
Storage	-20°C	2–8°C	-20°C
Cost	Low	High	High

Table 21.2: Criteria to reject and accept result.

Observation	*Decision*	*Action*
1. Both controls are within + 2	SD Approve batch	Release results
2. Both controls are outside +2 SD	Withhold results	1. Inform superior 2. Check calibration error 3. Repeat standards 4. Change control vial 5. Check instrument 6. Repeat tests on controls
3. One control within + 2 SD and one control outside + 2 SD	Withhold results	1. Apply 95% confidence limit rule which states that 1 in 20 results could go wrong 2. Make a decision based on your information

every 20 samples in a continuous run or once in 60 minutes in an interrupted run. Controls should also be used each time the calibrator or one or more reagents are changed. Instances in which the patient's results raise doubts are also ideal times for the use of controls.

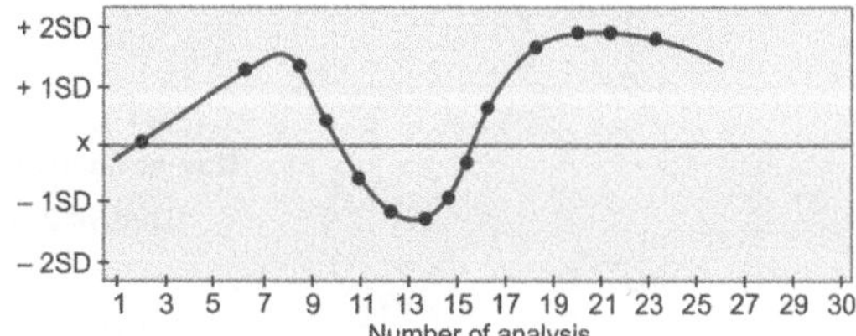

Fig. 21.2: Control chart.

How Do We Reject or Accept Results?

a. *By making a batch analysis decision:* This can be done by analyzing two controls simultaneously and applying the 1:2 SD rule as summarized in **Table 21.2**.
b. Use day control charts on which the reference value is represented by a central line with ± 2 SD and -2 SD lines lying above and below the reference limit. Daily results can be plotted and analyzed periodically to study both accuracy and precision.
c. *Use Levey-Jennings plots:* These charts are useful in long-term monitoring of trends and shifts and thereby the accuracy and precision over extended periods of time.

Control Chart (Levey-Jenning's Chart)

One of the methods of presenting the QC data is plotting Levey-Jenning's charts.

a. Analyze a single batch of control serum for 30 consecutive days.
b. Calculate the mean and SD values.
c. Draw a horizontal line through the mean value.
d. Draw line at 1 SD, 2 SD and 3 SD values above and below the mean line.
e. The value obtained on each day by analysis of control samples is plotted in this chart (separate chart for each parameter).
f. If the analysis is satisfactory, the points will be scattered evenly on either side of the mid line that is within 1 SD limits. The pattern shows that the accuracy is maintained.
g. The values falling within the 2 SD limit are acceptable.
h. Values at 2 SD limit is warning limit, i.e., reanalysis of the control is required.
i. Values at 3 SD limit is action limit.
j. When six consecutive values fall above or below the mean line it shows that the assay is out of control **(Fig. 21.2)**.

WESTGARD RULE (EVALUATING QC RESULTS)

- It detects whether results are "in control" or not.
- It detects the type of laboratory error.
- It is used to diminish the false rejection rate without compromising quality.

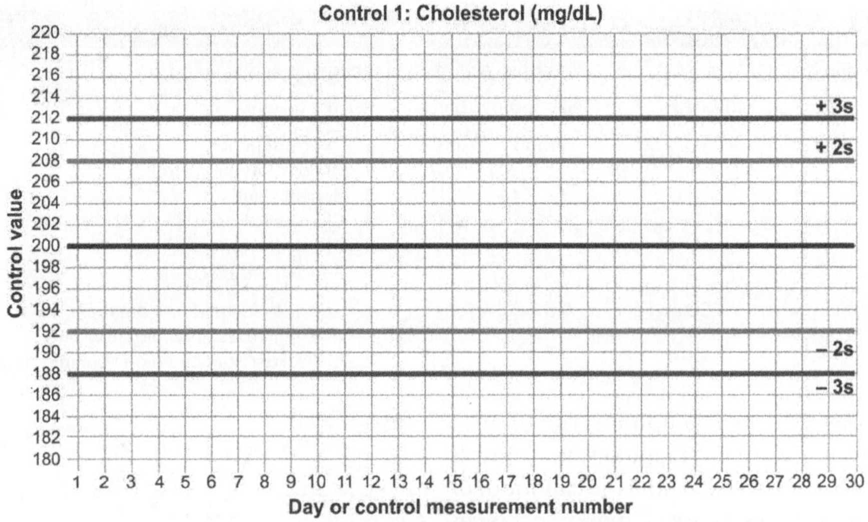

Control 1: Cholesterol (mg/dL)
Control value
220
218
216
214
212
210
208
206
204
202
200
198
196
194
192
190
188
186
184
182
180
+ 3s
+ 2s
– 2s
– 3s
1 2 3 4 5 6 7 8 9 10 11 12 13 14 15 16 17 18 19 20 21 22 23 24 25 26 27 28 29 30
Day or control measurement number

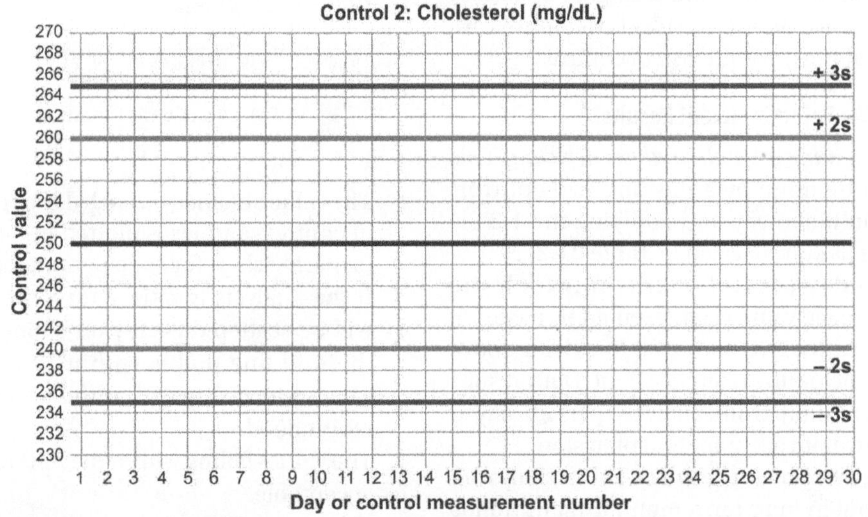

Control 2: Cholesterol (mg/dL)
Control value
270
268
266
264
262
260
258
256
254
252
250
248
246
244
242
240
238
236
234
232
230
+ 3s
+ 2s
– 2s
– 3s
1 2 3 4 5 6 7 8 9 10 11 12 13 14 15 16 17 18 19 20 21 22 23 24 25 26 27 28 29 30
Day or control measurement number

Control data
1 point outside 2 SD
No
In control—report data
Yes
1 point outside 3 SD
No
2 consecutive values outside the same 2 SD
No
Difference between 2 controls within a run exceeds 4 SD
No
4 consecutive control values on one side of the mean and further than 1 SD from the mean
No
10 consecutive values on one side of the mean
No
Yes
Yes
Yes
Yes
Yes
Out of control—reject analytical run

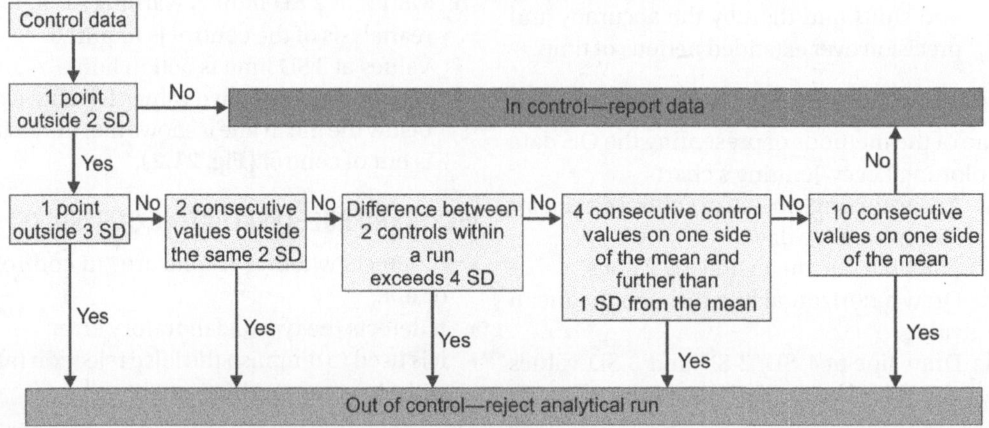

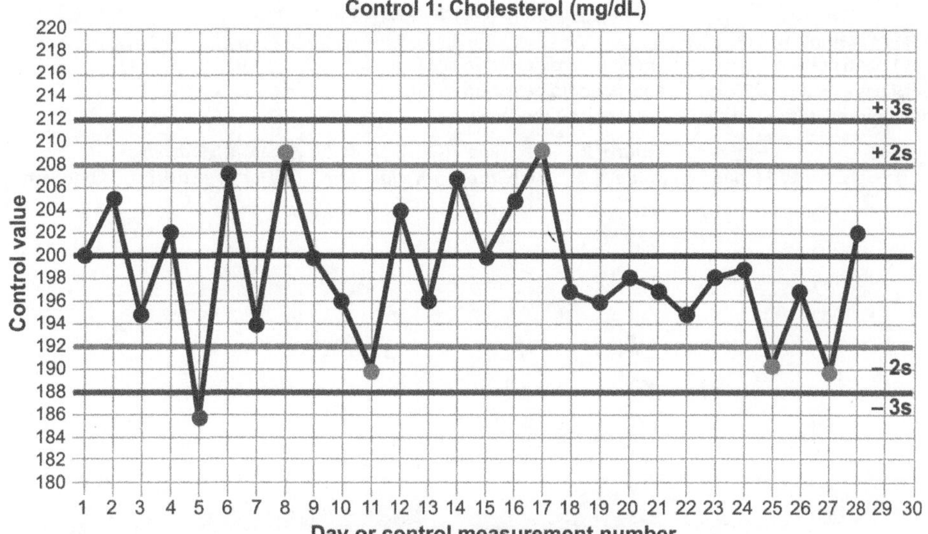
Control 1: Cholesterol (mg/dL)
220
218
216
214
212
210
208
206
204
202
200
198
196
194
192
190
188
186
184
182
180
Control value
+3s
+2s
−2s
−3s
1 2 3 4 5 6 7 8 9 10 11 12 13 14 15 16 17 18 19 20 21 22 23 24 25 26 27 28 29 30
Day or control measurement number

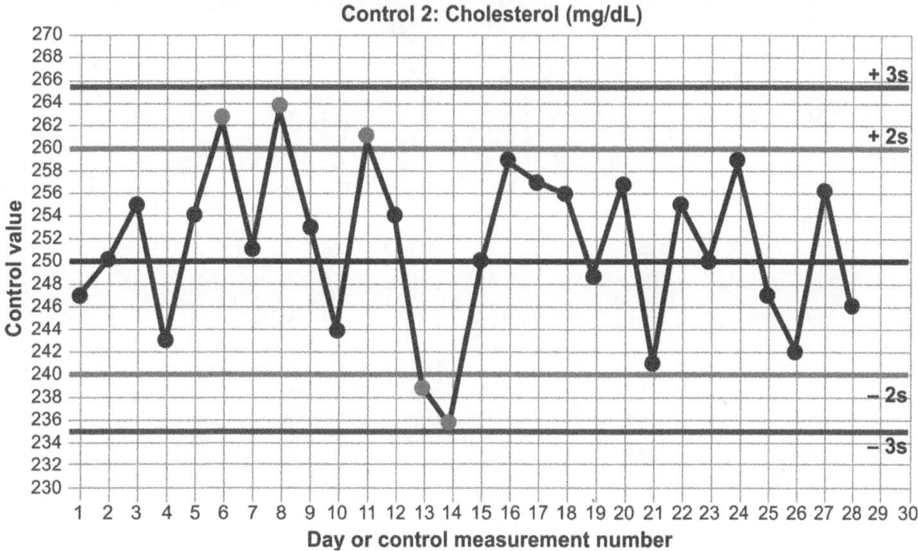
Control 2: Cholesterol (mg/dL)
270
268
266
264
262
260
258
256
254
252
250
248
246
244
242
240
238
236
234
232
230
Control value
+3s
+2s
−2s
−3s
1 2 3 4 5 6 7 8 9 10 11 12 13 14 15 16 17 18 19 20 21 22 23 24 25 26 27 28 29 30
Day or control measurement number

Levey-Jennings QC Exercise Answers:

Cholesterol example where:
Control 1 has a mean of 200 mg/dL and standard deviation of 4.0 mg/dL.
Control 2 has a mean of 250 mg/dL and standard deviation of 5.0 mg/dL.
Prepare appropriate control charts and interpret the results.

Day	***Control 1 value***	***Control 2 value***	***1_{2s} Rule violation***	***1_{3s} Rule violation***	***Accept(A), Warning (W), or Reject(R)?***	***Comments***
1	200	247			A	
2	205	250			A	
3	195	255			A	
4	202	243			A	
5	186	254	-2s	- 3s	R	
6	207	263	+ 2s		W(A)	
7	194	251			A	
8	209	264	+ 2s twice		R	Both exceed + 2s
9	200	253			A	
10	196	244			A	
11	190	261	+ 2s and - 2s		R	Both exceed 2s in opposite directions
12	204	254			A	
13	196	239	- 2s		W(A)	
14	207	236	- 2s		R	2 days in a row exceeding - 2s
15	200	250			A	
16	205	259			A	
17	209	257	+ 2s		W(A)	
18	197	256			A	
19	196	249			A	
20	198	257			A	
21	197	241			A	
22	195	255			A	
23	198	250			A	
24	199	259			A	
25	191	247	- 2s		W(A)	Negative shift
26	197	242			A	
27	190	256	- 2s		W(A)	Follow to see if negative shift continues or worsens
28	202	246			A	

Interpretation of Control Results—With 1_{2s} and 1_{3s} Rules

Use of a 1_{2s} rule as a strict rejection rule would result in rejecting runs on days 5, 6, 8, 11, 13, 14, 17, 25, and 27, for a total of 9 runs, as shown by the check marks in the column for 1_{2s} rule violations.

Use of a 1_{3s} rejection rule would lead to rejection of only one run on day 5, as shown by the single check mark in the column for 1_{3s} rule violations.

It makes a *big* difference what control rule is being applied—9 rejections vs 1 rejection! What if different control rules were used? Given that the 1_{2s} rule is known to cause a high level of false alarms or false rejections, it might be better to interpret the data more carefully, in effect applying additional control rules, such as the 2_{2s} and R_{4s} rules:

- **2_{2s}** indicates a rejection when two consecutive control values exceed the same mean +2s limit or the same mean -2s control limit; this rule is sensitive to shifts in the mean of the distribution, therefore, it is a good indicator of increases in systematic error or changes in the accuracy of the method.
- R_{4s} indicates a rejection when one control measurement in a run exceeds a +2s control limit and another exceeds a -2s control limit. This "range" rule is sensitive to changes in the width of the distribution, therefore, it is a good indicate of increases in random error or changes in the precision of the method.

Use of the 1_{3s} rule together with the 2_{2s} and R_{4s} rules leads to a multi-rule QC procedure in which multiple decision criteria are applied simultaneously. If any single control rule is violated, the run is rejected. Here's how the $1_{3s}/2_{2s}/R_{4s}$ multi-rule procedure would be interpreted for this example set of control results:

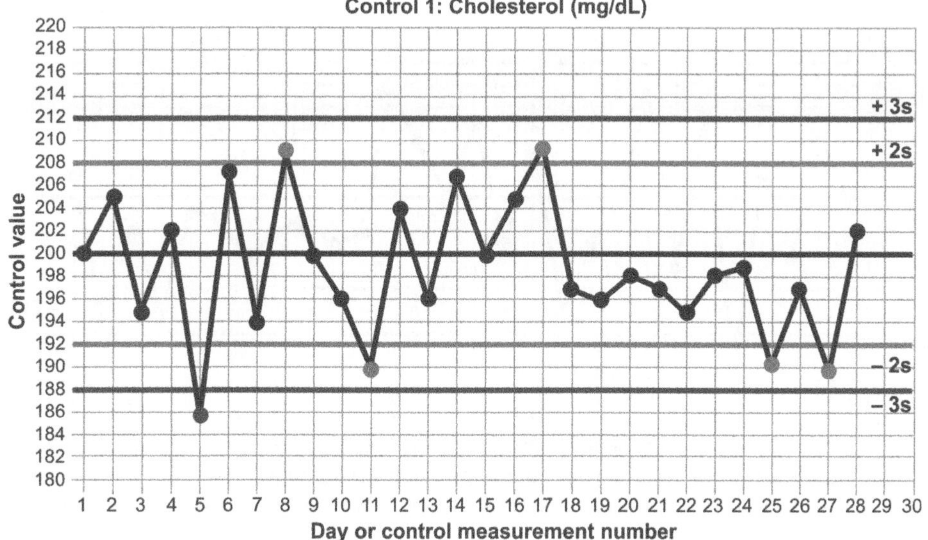

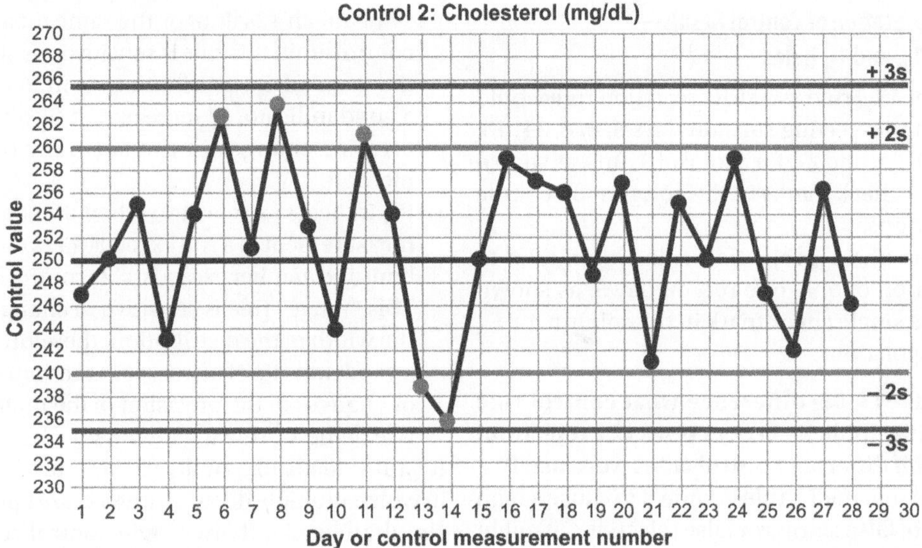

Day 5. The value for Control 1 exceeds a -3s control limit, which is a good indication that there is a problem with the method. Stop, reject the run, trouble-shoot the method, fix the cause of the problem, then restart the method and re-analyze the patient specimens.

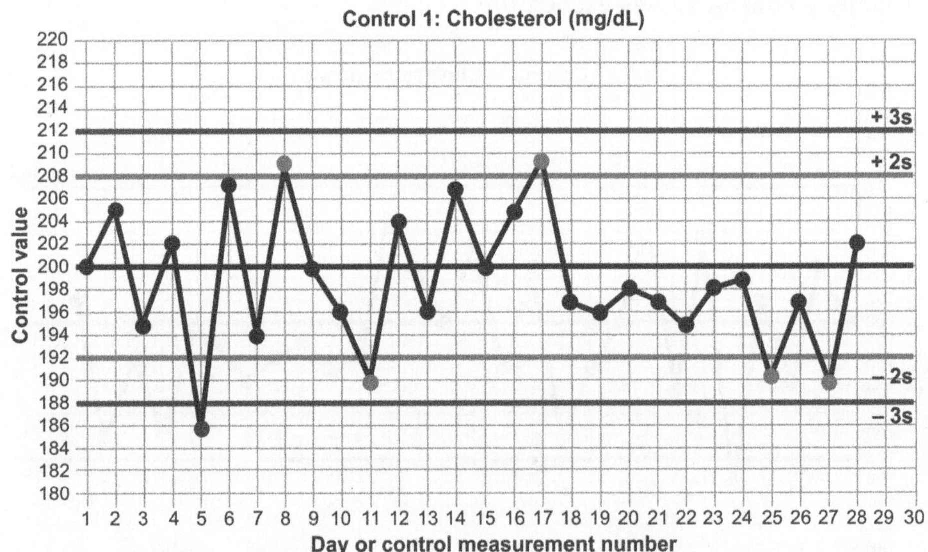

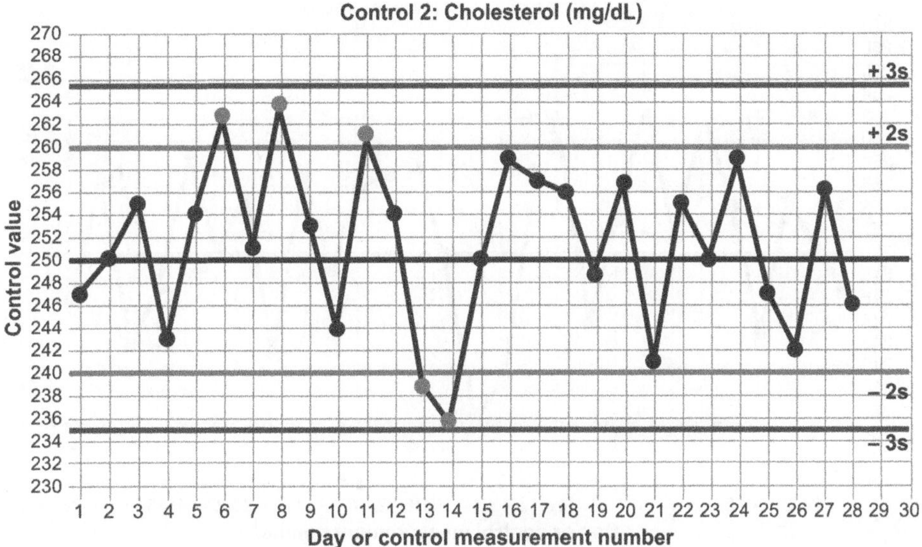

Day 6. The value for Control 2 exceeds a +2s control limit, but doesn't exceed a 3s limit. There might be a problem, but this might also be a false rejection. If a 1_{2s} rule were strictly applied, the run would be rejected. However, because the value for Control 1 is okay, it is likely that this is a false rejection. Accept the run.

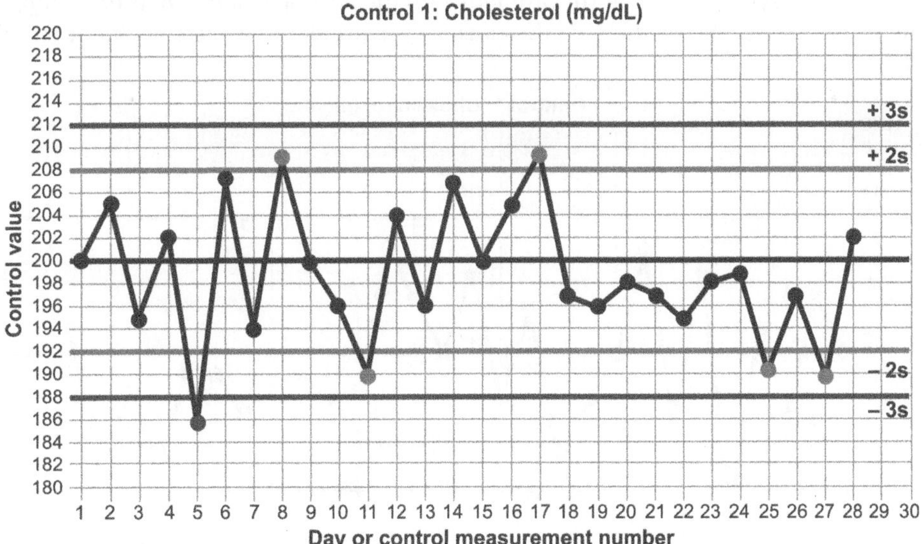

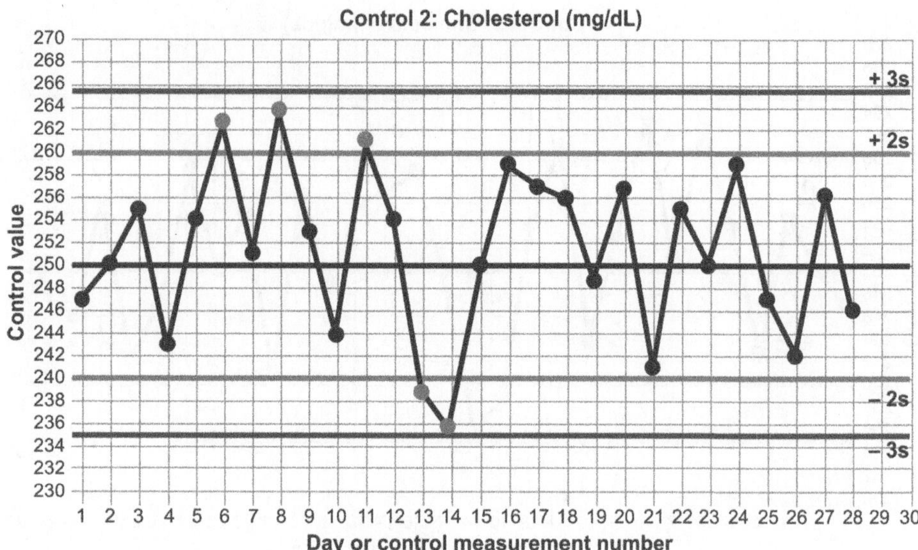

Day 8. Both the values for Control 1 and Control 2 exceed their respective +2s control limits. It is rare to see two values in a row exceed the same +2s limit, therefore this occurrence indicates a problem with the method. Note that this interpretation applies the 2_{2s} control rule, i.e., 2 values in a row exceeding the same control limit. Since both controls are out in the same direction, it is likely there is a systematic error (or problem with the accuracy of the method). Stop, reject the run, trouble-shoot the method, fix the cause of the problem, then restart the method and re-analyze the patient specimens.

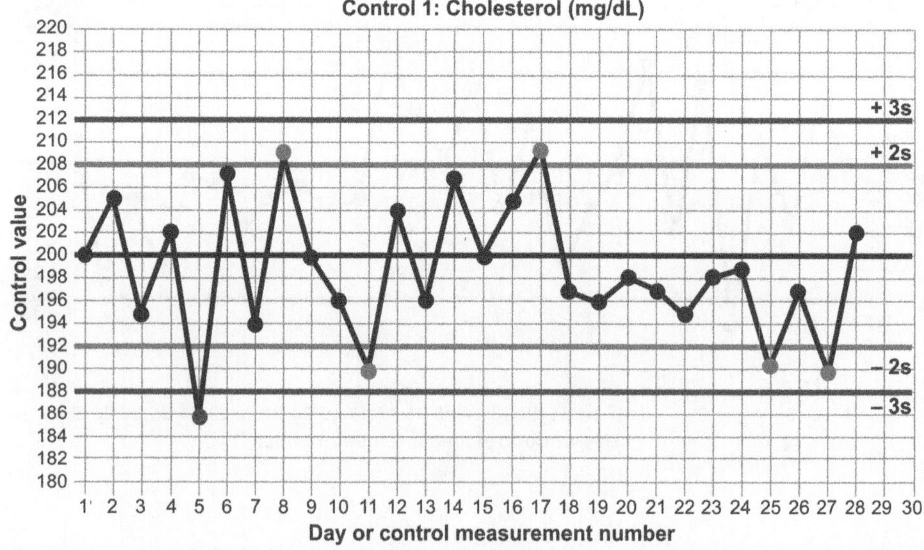

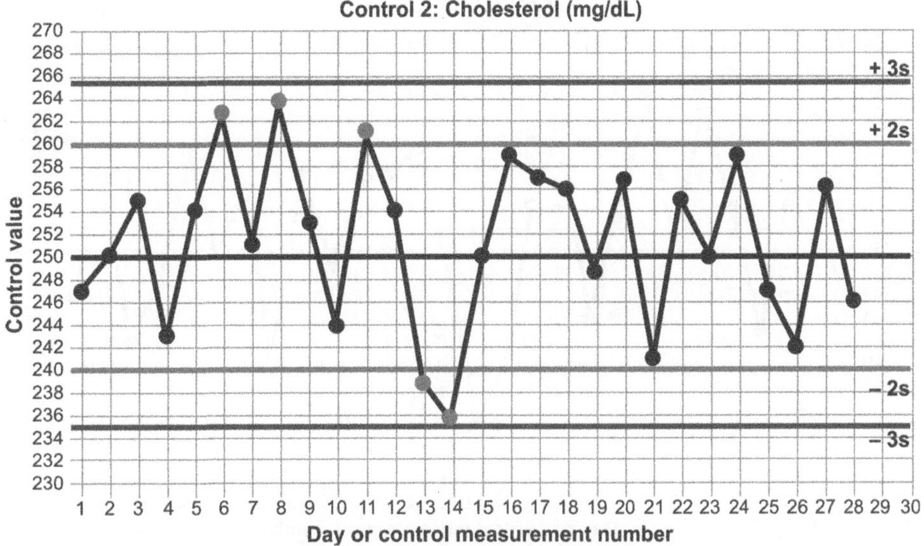

Day 11. Both control values exceed 2s control limits, but one is positive and one is negative. It is a rare occurrence and most likely there is a problem with the method. Since the two controls are out in opposite directions, it is likely that there is a random error (or problem with the precision of the method). Note that this interpretation applies the R_{4s} rule, i.e., the range of the control values exceeds 4s. Stop, reject the run, trouble-shoot the method, fix the cause of the problem, then restart the method and re-analyze the patient specimens.

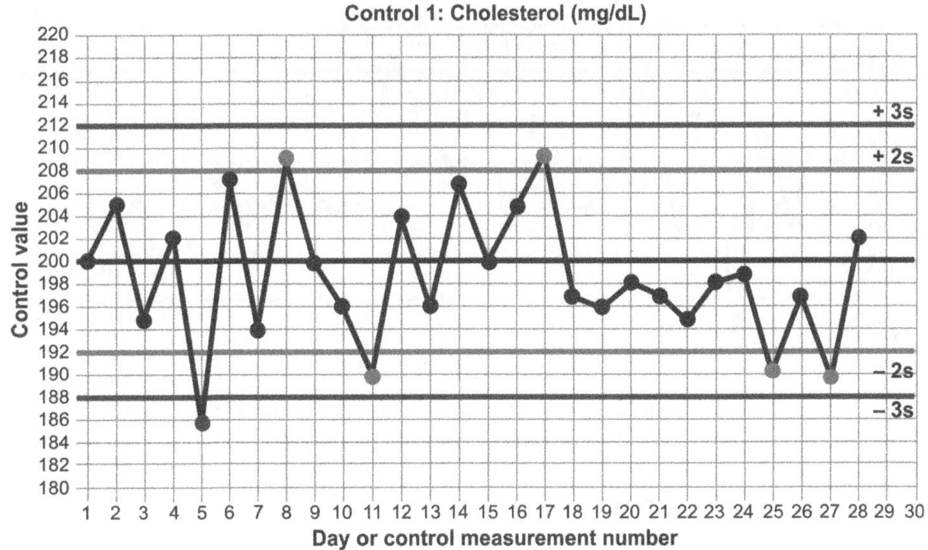

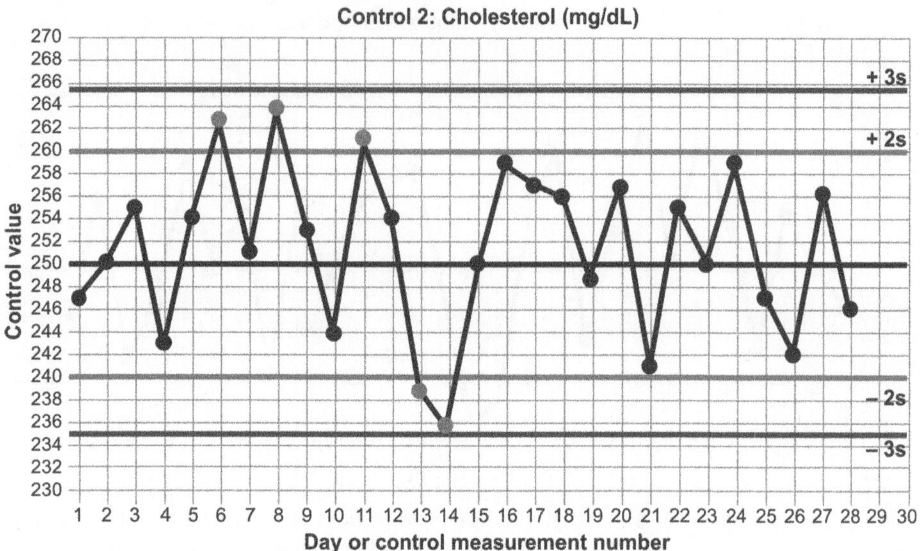

Day 13. The value for Control 2 is outside the low end of the 2s range. There is a warning of a possible problem, but this might also be a false rejection. Accept this run because none of the rejection rules are violated.

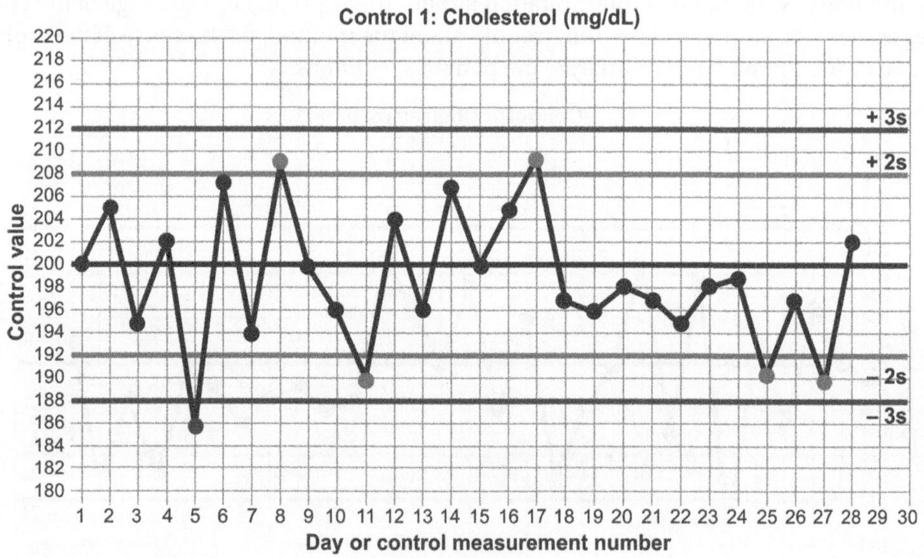

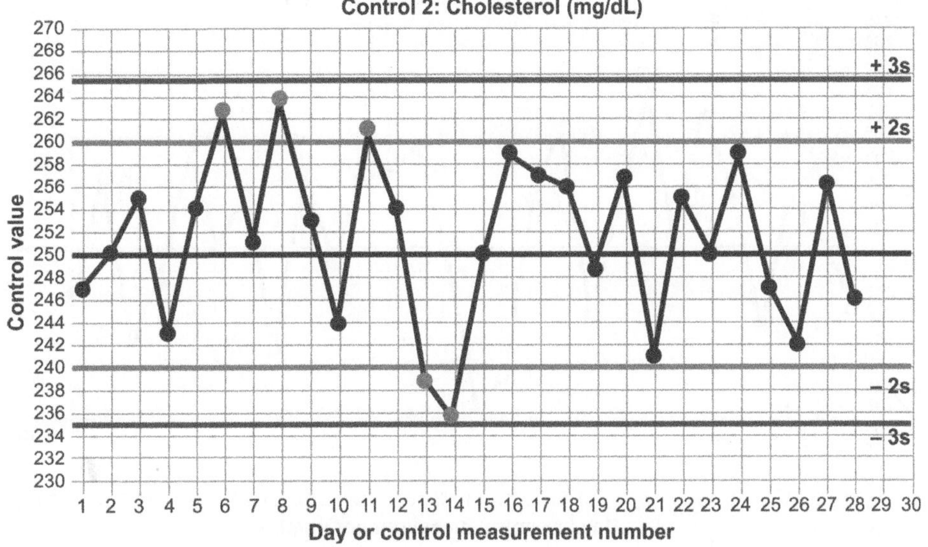

Day 14. The value for Control 2 is again outside the low end of the 2s range. This makes 2 days or 2 runs in a row, which is unusual. Since both values for Control 2 are out in the same direction, it is likely there is a systematic error (or problem with the accuracy of the method). Stop, reject the run, trouble-shoot the method, fix the cause of the problem, then restart the method and re-analyze the patient specimens.

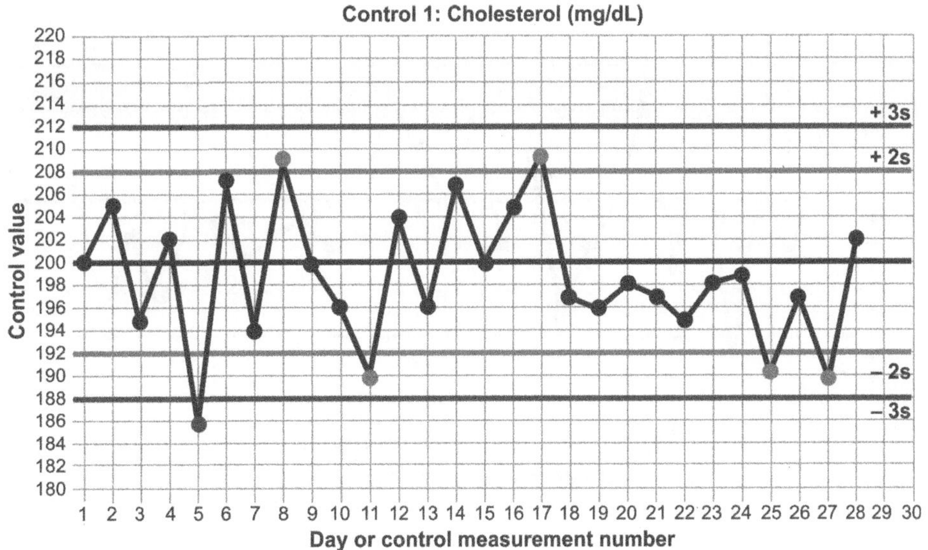

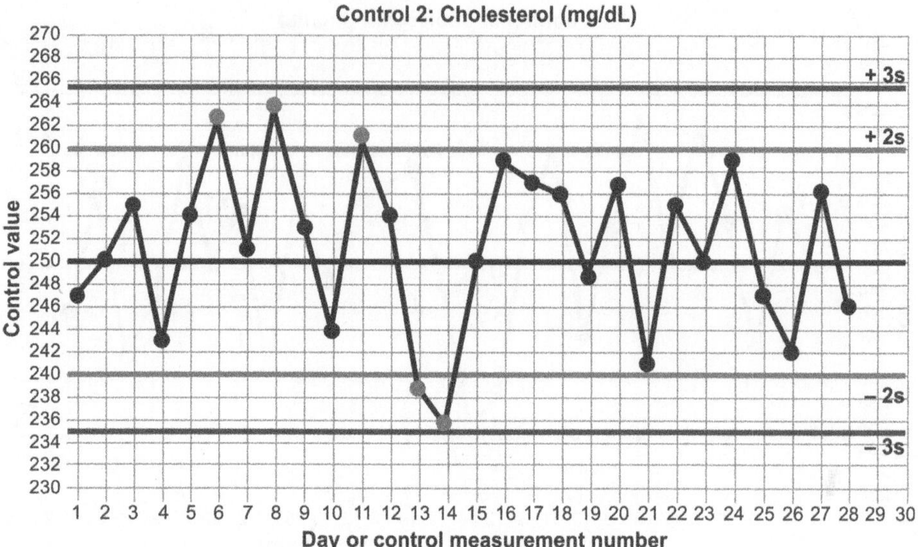

Day 17. Control 1 exceeds the +2s control limit. There might be a problem, but this might also be a false rejection. If a 1_{2s} rule were strictly applied, the run would be rejected. However, because the value for Control 2 is okay, it is likely that this is a false rejection. Accept the run.

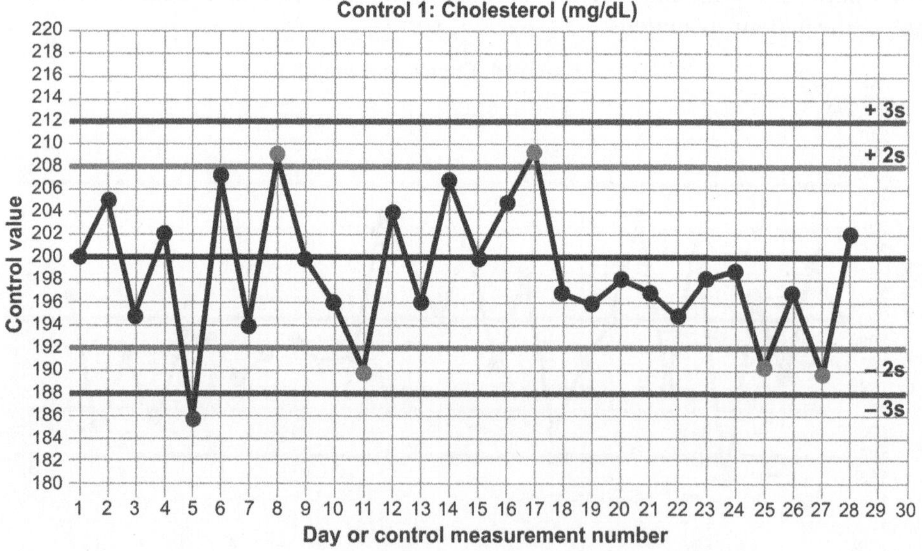

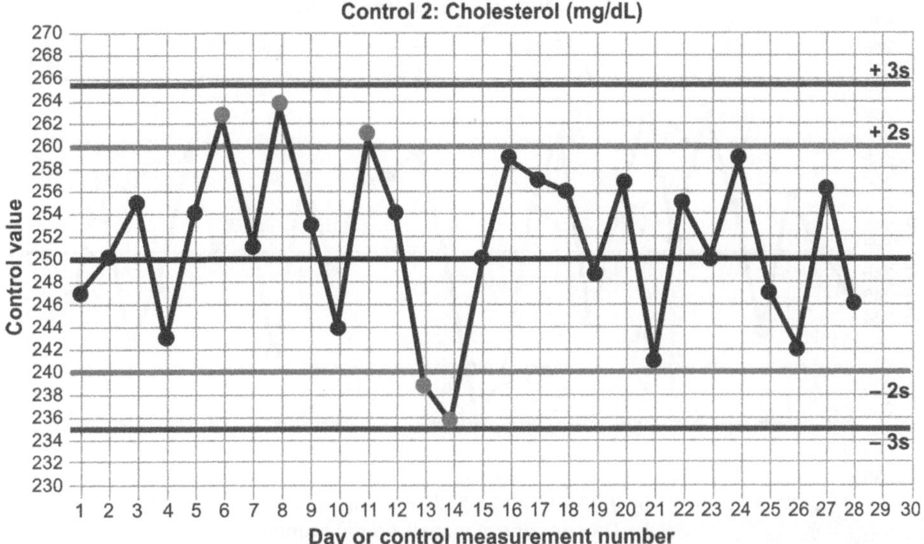

Day 25. Control 1 exceeds the -2s control limit. There might be a problem, but this might also be a false rejection. If a 1_{2s} rule were strictly applied, the run would be rejected. However, because the value for Control 2 is okay, it is likely that this is a false rejection. Accept the run.

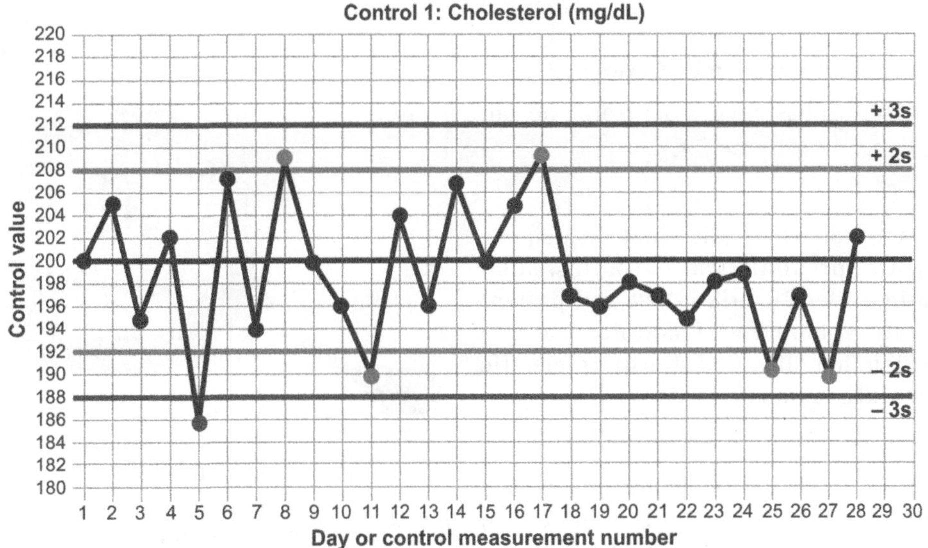

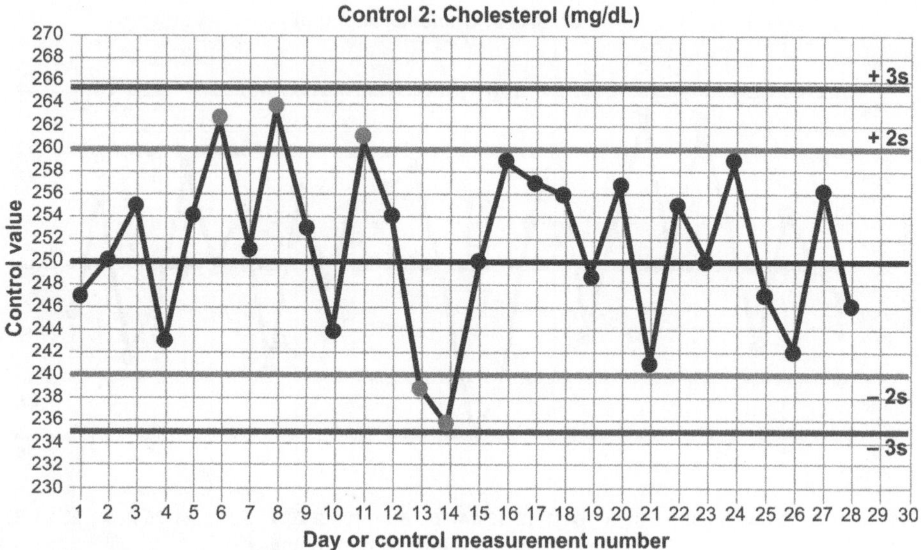

Day 27. Control 1 exceeds the -2s control limit. There might be a problem, but this might also be a false rejection. If a 1_{2s} rule were strictly applied, the run would be rejected. However, because the value for Control 2 is okay, it is likely that this is a false rejection. Accept the run.

What are the Types of Errors We Can Expect?

There are two basic types of errors one can expect.

Random Errors

These are errors, which arise due to inadequate control of preanalytical variables, such as patient identification, test and patient correlation, labeling of samples, sample collection, handling and transport, electric supply and equipment.

Systemic Errors

These are the errors resulting from inadequate control on analytical variables. Systemic errors, most often can be traced to faulty calibration, which includes, use of impure calibration material, erroneous labeling of calibrators, use of wrong unstable or deteriorated calibrators. Unstable reagent blanks and inadequate use of sample blanks are also factors, which contribute to systemic errors **(Fig. 21.3)**.EM

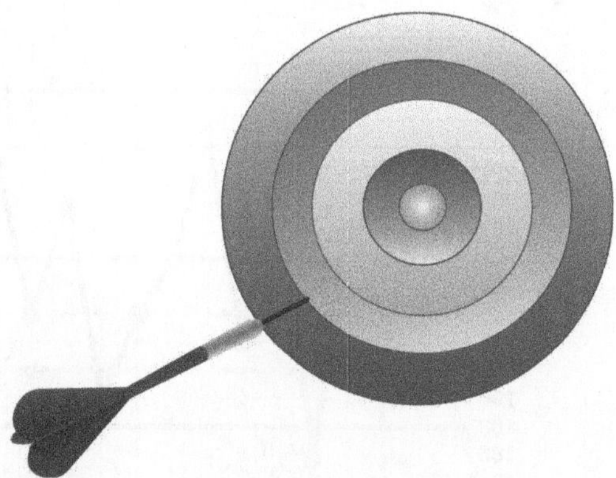

Fig. 21.3: Systemic error.

How Can We Build-up an Effective Troubleshooting System?

Troubleshooting is the ability to detect and identify sources of errors an integral part of quality control. Some of the ways in which an effective troubleshooting system can be developed are by:

1. Identifying and listing possible errors in methods and instruments.
2. Delegating responsibilities to team members in order to improve their skills.
3. Designing preventive programs.
4. Arranging for in-house training
5. Establishing problem-solving teams.

How Do We Select a New Method?

Four important aspects have to be studied carefully before and during selection a new method.

They are:

1. Preliminary facts: Preliminary facts about the product must be studied. These include type of method, manufacturer's claims, cost per test, safety, published references, medical utility of the test and your colleague's opinion.
2. Budget: Important questions relating to budget are: Will it require additional staff, space, time, training or equipment and will the operational costs increase if, we adopt the new method?
3. Performance: The performance of the new method should be analyzed with emphasis on linearity, accuracy, precision, sensitivity and specificity.
4. Dependability: The stability, shelf life, interferences, and analytical recovery and reliability of the method should be studied.

If all four aspects are found satisfactory, you have the green signal to go ahead and adopt the method. It should be noted, however, that few methods will satisfy all the requirements. A laboratory manager, therefore, has to select a method, which best suits his requirements.

SELF TEST

1. Write the procedure for preparation of quality control material in the laboratory.
2. What are external and internal quality control programs?
3. State the preanalytical and analytical variables.
4. What are the types of errors, which may occur in the laboratory?

MULTIPLE CHOICE QUESTIONS

1. **The measure of closeness of the estimated value to the true value is called:**
   a. Precision
   b. Accuracy
   c. Internal quality
   d. External quality
2. **Values at 3 SD limit are:**
   a. Action limit
   b. Warning limit
   c. Assay is satisfactory
   d. None of the above

22

UNIT

Automation in the Clinical Laboratory

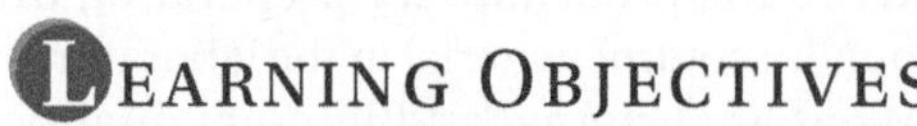

At the end of this unit, the learner should be able to understand:
- The automation and various instruments used in the clinical biochemistry laboratory.
- The right instruments for the laboratory.

INTRODUCTION

- Automation is the mechanization of conventional manual methods.
- Here, analytical instruments perform many tests with less involvement of the analyst.
- With the addition of new tests and as the urgency for reports increases, the workload of the laboratory also increases. When there is a larger workload, manual experiments should be replaced by automated one with the use of autoanalyzers. This will help in dispatching the reports within a shorter time.
- The automation in the laboratory not only improves the standard of the laboratory but also decreases the number of staff members needed.
- Automation of the clinical laboratory helps in performing a larger number of tests with a lower amount of sample.
- Automated methods require less volume reagent when compared to manual procedures.
- Manual procedures are time consuming and make it difficult to handle a large number of samples in a specified time. Therefore, it may be difficult for biochemists to dispatch test results on time.
- All the above advantages of automation and disadvantages of manual procedures made the scientists to introduce automation in 1950s.
- Productivity, quality and safety have subsequently improved dramatically for those laboratories that have properly introduced and managed their automation.
- However, automation increases the demands on the laboratory in many ways.
- Analytical instruments are burdened with an increase in the flow of reagents and specimens to be analyzed.
- Technologists and managers become burdened with managing a high throughput laboratory and processing all the information that results from the automated laboratory.
- Thus, there was a sudden realization that there was a need for information technology to manage the automation process.
- Similarly, the output of analytical data can also cause significant backup in data reduction and interpretation.
- Several manufacturers produce a variety of autoanalyzers.
- The manufacturers provide detailed operational procedures for the instrument they supply.

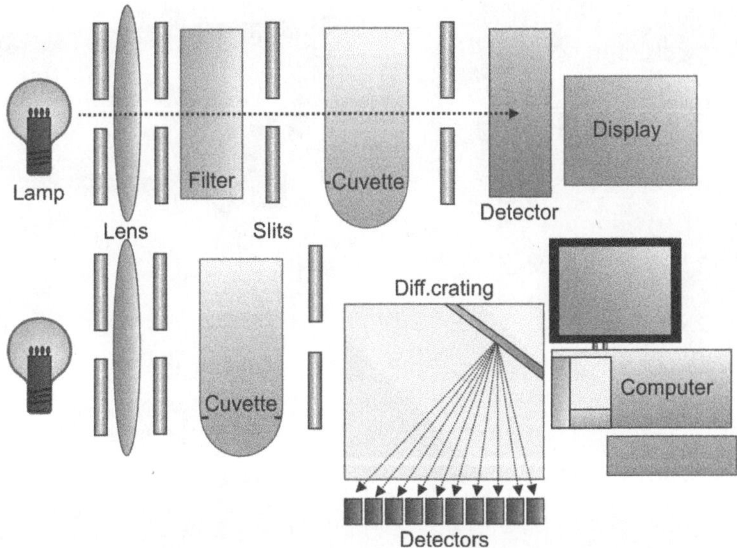

Fig. 22.1: Components of autoanalyzers.

- Automated systems generally incorporate mechanized versions of basic manual laboratory techniques and procedures.
- All autoanalyzers have provisions for reagent placing, feeding the sample or standards of known value, displaying of results and monitor and printing of the values through a recorded printer.
- Basic components of autoanalyzers are shown in **Figure 22.1**.

TYPES OF ANALYZERS (FIG. 22.2)

Semiautoanalyzers

- This type of analyzers were built in such a way that it should read the optical density of the solution contained in the cuvette to produce the concentration of the substance.
- This type of analyzers would be able to read the solution, which has both sample and reagents mixed before.
- Single assay can done at a time using this type of analyzers.
- Setting the unit is automatic with regards to wavelength, time and temperature.
- Suitable for small laboratories, which has sample load of less than 25 per day, e.g., RA 50, ERBA Chem, Transasia, and Stat Fax.

Batch Analyzer

In this type of instrument, the reagent mixture is mixed and fed automatically.

A single reagent can be stored in the machine at a time. So a batch of particular chemistry tests can be performed automatically, e.g., RA 100.

Random Access Autoanalyzers

More than one reagent can be stored in such units.

Samples are kept in the machine and the computer is programed to carry out any number of selected tests on individual samples, e.g., Hitachi 912.

TYPES OF ANALYSIS

It is very difficult to classify automated systems even though the manufacturers focus on the major process in each automated system in order to differentiate one system from the other **(Flowchart 22.1)**.

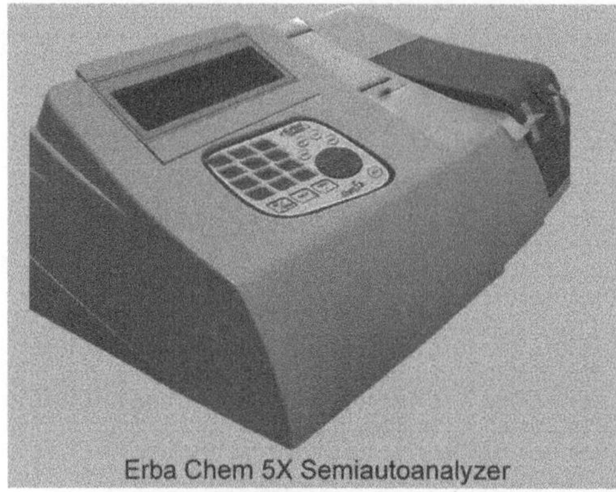
Erba Chem 5X Semiautoanalyzer

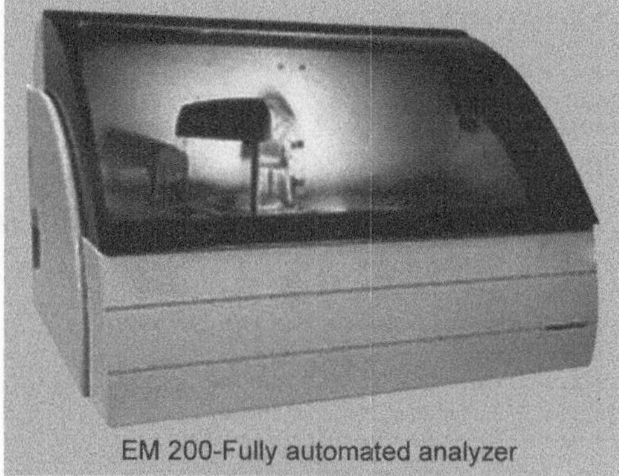
EM 200-Fully automated analyzer

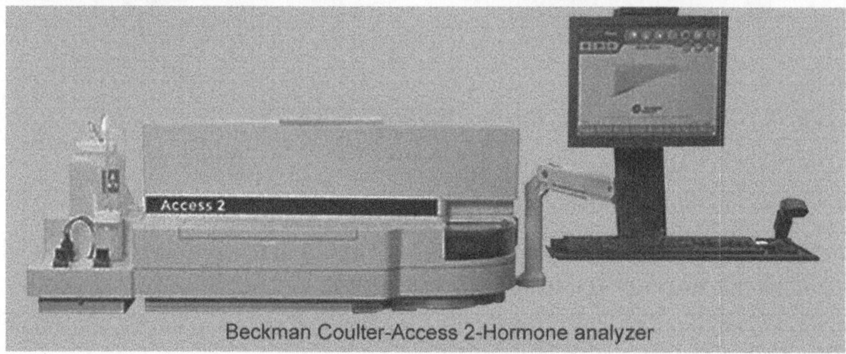

Beckman Coulter-Access 2-Hormone analyzer

Fig. 22.2: Types of autoanalyzer..

It is important to know the meaning of the terms that are commonly used in the autoanalyzers.

Batch Analysis

Many specimens are processed for analysis in the same analytical run.

Sequential Analysis

Each sample in the batch enters the analytical process one after another and the results are printed in the same order as they are fed.

Continuous Flow Analysis

- Each sample in the batch follows one another in a sequence and is subjected to the same analytical reactions as other sample at the same rate.
- In this type of analysis, each sample is separated from the following one with an air bubble.

Discrete Analysis

Each sample has its own separate space. They are separated from one another and are tested in sequence.

Single Channel Analysis

- It is also known as single test analysis.
- Each sample is analyzed by single process.
- So, results of single parameter are produced.

Multiple Channel Analysis

- It is also called multiple test analysis.
- In this type, each sample is subjected to multiple analytical processes and set of test results are obtained.

Flowchart 22.1: Various types of automated equipment.

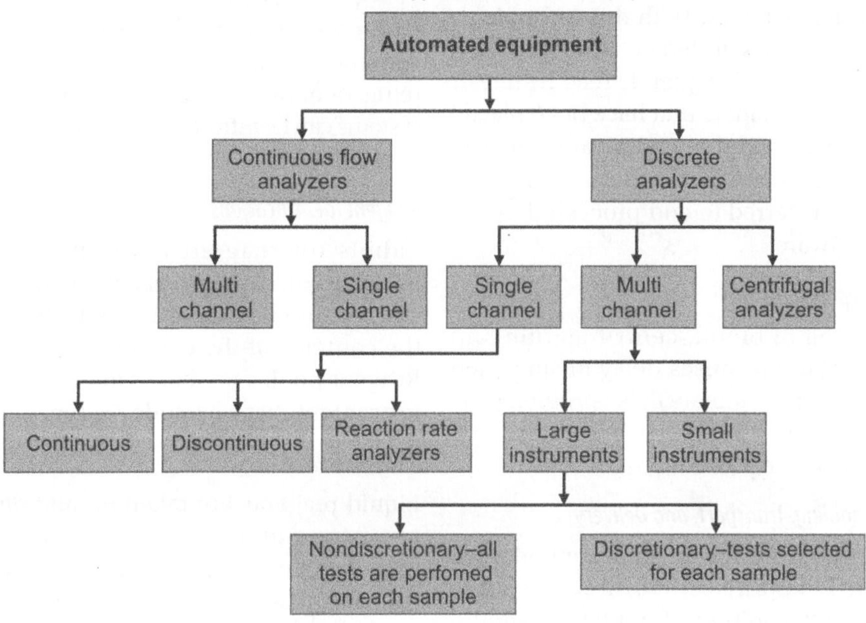

Random Access Analysis

Any sample, by a signal to the processing system, can be analyzed by an available process in or out of sequence with other specimens irrespective of their beginning order.

There are several instruments mainly based on this principle, e.g., Ektachem, COBAS MIRA, immulite Technicon 2000, and Hitachi 912.

Autoanalyzers are divided into floor and bench-top models.

The bench top autoanalyzers use a sequential, batch and discrete type of analysis with samples. The single-channel, continuous-flow batch analyzer provides one result per analyte for each specimen at a rate of 50–60 specimens, e.g., CHEM 1^+.

Steps in the Automated Systems

1. Sample identification
2. Sample preparation
3. Sample handling
4. Sample transport and delivery
5. Sample processing
6. Reagent handling and delivery
7. Chemical reaction
8. Measurement
9. Signal processing and microprocessing.

Sample Identification

A label is affixed to the specimen collection tube when blood is drawn. The specimen on reaching the laboratory is recorded by a computerized procedure. After accessing, specimens undergo the technical handling processes. Those processes, which require physical removal of serum from the original tube, secondary labels bearing the same information as the original label, must be affixed to the secondary tube.

Bar Coding

A major advantage in the automation of specimen identification has been introduction of bar coding technology into several of the analytical systems that are now available to the clinical laboratory. With this technology, a bar coded label is placed onto the specimen container and is subsequently read by one or more bar code readers that have been placed at key positions in the analytical train. The resultant identified and other information are then transferred to and processed by the system software.

Sample Preparation

The clotting of blood, centrifugation and transfer of serum causes delay in specimen preparation. To eliminate these problems the use of whole blood for analysis and automation of specimens can be done.

Sample Handling, Transport, and Delivery

In most cases, the specimen presented to an automated analysis is serum. All cups or tubes containing the solution for analysis should be covered if the assay is delayed. This is to prevent the evaporation of sample. Before the analysis, the sample should be loaded on the loading zone. The loading zone of an analyzer is the area in which specimens are held in the instrument before they are analyzed.

Sample Processing

Automation of the analysis of analytes requires removal of interfering substances or proteins.

Sample Transport and Delivery

The method of sample delivery and transport into the analyzer is the major difference between continuous flow and discrete systems.

In continuous flow, the sample is aspirated to the sample probe into a continuous reagent system, whereas in discrete analyzers, the sample is aspirated into the sample probe and then delivered.

Carry over between the samples can be avoided by setting an adequate flush to—specimen ratio by incorporating wash stations for the sample probe.

Reagent Handling and Storage

Reagents are stored in a plastic or glass containers. They can be stored in laboratory refrigerators if the assay is delayed. Refrigerated systems can be introduced into the instruments as required.

Reagent Identifications

Labels on reagent containers include information, such as reagent identify, volume of the contents or number of tests for which the contents of the containers can be used. Reagent bottles are bar coded, wherever the instruments have barcode readers.

Reagent Delivery

Liquid reagents are taken up and delivered to mixing and then to the reaction chamber by either pumping via tubes or by positive displacement syringe devices.

There are various automated systems available commercially to analyze all blood, CSF and urine parameters. The demand for increased efficiency in healthcare prompted laboratory owners to provide fast service at lower cost. It is necessary for the laboratory directors to plan which type of instruments they should purchase keeping in mind that there should not be any compromise with the accuracy of the test. Systems are selected to fit into a combination of automated, semi-automated, and manual modes of analysis that is suited for any particular laboratory and for the type of work and workload.

Selection of an Autoanalyzer

It is very important to plan the laboratory set up. One who is going to set up a laboratory must survey the surrounding area where planning to open their laboratory. If the area comprises several doctors who are dependent on the laboratory reports for the diagnosis and treatment of patients, it is advisable to discuss with them before starting the laboratory.

It is also advisable to discuss with them for required laboratory tests, which are helpful for them. In this competitive world, one has to improve laboratory standard by concentrating on the cost effectiveness, time consumption and accuracy of the laboratory reports. Before going for an automated laboratory, one has to workout the sample load and types of test one may get. Say, if the sample load is under 20 then it may not be advisable to go for an automated system in the beginning. When sample number exceeds 30 per day, then they can think of installing a semiautomated system in the laboratory. If the sample load crosses more than 100, a fully automated analyzer can be installed. During purchase of any automated instrument one should consider the following factors:

1. The cost of the instrument.
2. Sensitivity, accuracy and reproducibility of the test results.
3. Number of parameters.
4. Time taken for reporting.

SELF TEST

1. Discuss briefly the advantages of automation in the laboratory.
2. What are the different types of analyzers?
3. Name the different steps in the automated systems.

MULTIPLE CHOICE QUESTIONS

1. **The sample analyzed in a process is called:**
   a. Single channel analysis
   b. Double channel analysis
   c. Multiple channel analysis
   d. Discrete analysis
2. **All the following are the steps in automated systems, *except:***
   a. Sample identification
   b. Sample handling
   c. Sample discard
   d. Sample processing

23

UNIT

Special Tests

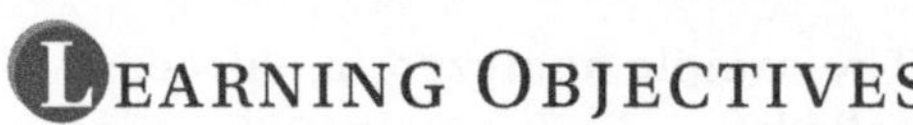

At the end of this unit, the learner should be able to understand:
- The determination and pathophysiology of autoantibodies.
- The inborn errors of metabolism.

INTRODUCTION TO AUTOIMMUNE DISEASE

- The immune system is the body's defense against foreign substances, such as bacteria or viruses, which may be harmful.
- An autoimmune disease is an abnormal condition that occurs when a person's immune system attacks its own tissues as though they were foreign substances.
- Normally, when a foreign substance enters the body, the immune system creates special cells to attack and destroy the foreign substance. These cells include antibodies and white blood cells (lymphocytes).
- In a person with an autoimmune disease, the immune system recognizes some of the person's own tissues as foreign substances. The body makes antibodies and other cells that attack and destroy these tissues. This process often leads to inflammation and eventually, if it continues, scarring and destruction of the organs that are made up of those tissues.
- Autoimmune diseases include lupus, rheumatoid arthritis, scleroderma, and Sjögren's syndrome. Certain types of diabetes and thyroid disease are related to autoimmune reactions. People who have autoimmune diseases are at an increased risk for infections.
- The clinical importance of double stranded deoxyribonucleic acid (dsDNA) antibodies and antinuclear antibodies (ANA) and anticardiolipin antibodies (aCL) estimation in the laboratory.

THE dSDNA ANTIBODIES

Autoimmune diseases occur when damage results from immune reactions against normal body components.

There are two categories of autoimmune diseases:

1. Organ specific: result when immune mediated damage impairs the function of particular target organs (for example, the liver in primary biliary cirrhosis, the thyroid in chronic lymphocytic thyroiditis).
2. Systemic diseases either correlate with, or actually result from immune processes directed against antigens common to all tissues (DNA or snRNP in systemic lupus erythematosus (SLE) and mixed connective tissue disease (MCTD), respectively.

Systemic diseases are characterized by the production of autoantibodies to nuclear antigens (ANA).

Antibodies directed against various components of the cell nucleus are found in serum of many patients suffering from rheumatoid diseases, such as systemic lupus erythematosus, Sjögren's syndrome, progressive systemic sclerosis and polymyositis. Antinuclear antibodies (ANA) comprise antibodies against nucleic acids (ssDNA, dsDNA), nucleoprotein complexes (DNP, RNP), and histones. The presence of dsDNA antibodies is considered to be the most specific marker for the diagnosis of SLE.

Reference Range

- < 50 = Negative
- > 65 = Positive
- 50–65 = Borderline

ANTINUCLEAR ANTIBODIES

The determination of antinuclear antibodies (ANA) is playing a very important role in the diagnosis of rheumatic diseases.

The presence of ANA suggests the possibility of rheumatic autoimmune diseases like:

- Systemic lupus erythematosus
- Polymyositis
- Scleroderma, and
- Mixed connective diseases.

The dsDNA antibodies are considered to be the most specific marker for the diagnosis of SLE. The positive ANA test is considered to be the evidence for systemic rheumatic diseases. Therefore, the ANA test is done to detect:

- Systemic lupus erythematosus
- Scleroderma
- Hashimoto's thyroid disease
- Rheumatoid arthritis
- Sjögren's syndrome.

Reference Value

- < 20 is negative
- > 160 = Positive
- 120–160 = Borderline

Hashimoto's Thyroiditis

- Hashimoto's thyroiditis (chronic autoimmune thyroiditis) is a condition that can cause an underactive thyroid gland (hypothyroidism).
- Hashimoto's thyroiditis develops when the body's immune system makes antibodies that attack and eventually destroy the thyroid gland.
- Hashimoto's thyroiditis is the most common form of autoimmune thyroid disease and occurs most often in women and older adults.
- The disease does not cause any pain and often goes unnoticed for years.
- Hashimoto's thyroiditis is associated with other conditions, including diabetes, Addison's disease, rheumatoid arthritis, pernicious anemia, and premature menopause.
- Symptoms of an underactive thyroid gland include fatigue, thinning hair, dry skin, and brittle nails.

Scleroderma

- Scleroderma is an uncommon disease.
- In this disease, part of the skin, joints, and blood vessels break down and are replaced by fibrous tissue.
- Organ damage may also occur, which can lead to lung, kidney, or heart failure.
- Symptoms of scleroderma include thickening of the skin, joint pain and stiffness and problems in swallowing.

Systemic Lupus Erythematosus (SLE)

- It is a prototypic autoimmune disease characterized by the production of antibodies to components of the cell nucleus in association with a diverse array of clinical manifestations.

- As SLE is a disease of unknown etiology, classification criteria have been devised to diagnose it:
  - Malar rash (rash over the cheeks)
  - Discoid rash (red raised patches)
  - Photosensitivity (reaction to sunlight: development or exacerbation of skin rash)
  - Oral ulcers (ulcers in the nose or mouth, usually painless)
  - Arthritis (nondeforming polyarthritis)
  - Serositis (pleuritis and/or pericarditis)
  - Renal disorder (excessive protein in the urine >0.5 g/day)
  - Neurologic disorder (seizures or psychosis)
  - Hematologic disorder (leukopenia or lymphopenia/hemolytic anemia/thrombocytopenia)
  - Immunologic disorder (anti-DNA/anti-Sm/LE cell/positive antiphospholipid antibody)
  - Antinuclear antibody (positive test for antinuclear antibodies (ANA) in the absence of drugs that can induce it).

Diagnosis

Four of eleven criteria should be fulfilled at the same time or in succession. All organ systems are involved.

Non-erosive and generally nondeforming arthritis and photosensitive rashes occur cumulatively in more than 75% of cases while serositis, central nervous system (CNS) disease, and renal involvement occur in about 50% of cases.

ANTIPHOSPHOLIPID ANTIBODY

- There are several kinds of antiphospholipid antibodies.
- The most widely measured are the lupus anticoagulant and anticardiolipin antibody.
- These antibodies react with phospholipid, a type of fat molecule that is part of the normal cell membrane.
- Lupus anticoagulant and anticardiolipin antibody are closely related, but are not the same antibody.
- Under normal circumstances, antibodies are proteins made by our immune system to fight substances recognized as foreign by our body.
- Examples of foreign substances are bacteria and viruses. Sometimes the body's own cells are recognized as foreign.
- In the antiphospholipid antibody syndrome the body recognizes phospholipids (part of a cell's membrane) as foreign and produces antibodies against them.
- Antibodies to phospholipids (antiphospholipid antibodies) can be found in the blood of some people with lupus, but they are also seen in people without any known illness. Lupus anticoagulant (LAC) and anticardiolipin antibody (ACA) are the two known antiphospholipid antibodies that are associated with recurrent pregnancy miscarriages.

Antiphospholipid Antibody Syndrome

- Positive blood test for either the lupus anticoagulant or the anticardiolipin antibody, on two separate occasions, at least 8 weeks apart.
- In addition to the blood tests, a history of thrombosis (clots within the blood vessels), thrombocytopenia (low platelet count) or recurrent pregnancy loss will be there.
- Among women with recurrent pregnancy losses, antiphospholipid antibodies have been reported to be present in 11–22%.
- Lupus anticoagulant (LAC) high anticardiolipin antibodies (ACA) has been associated with first, second, and third trimester pregnancy losses.
- The association is even higher when the antiphospholipid antibody tests are persistently positive. Although it is unknown exactly how the antiphospholipid antibody syndrome adversely affects pregnancy, one

theory is that it may cause blood clots. These blood clots, which can be microscopic, may occur in the blood vessels of the placenta. The placenta provides nourishment to the baby and any interruption in this process can be harmful to the pregnancy.
- The antiphospholipid syndrome may increase the risk of miscarriage, poor fetal growth, preeclampsia and stillbirth.
- Women who have had a history of recurrent pregnancy losses should be tested for antiphospholipid antibodies in addition to other routine tests.
- A history of unexplained poor fetal growth and or the early onset of severe pre-eclampsia or an unexplained placental abruption are indications for testing
- A history of thrombosis, stroke, heart attack, thrombocytopenia (low platelet count), and presence of other autoimmune disorders, such as lupus, an abnormal VDRL, or PTT blood tests would suggest the need for testing
- The drug of choice for treatment is heparin.

ANTICARDIOLIPIN ANTIBODIES (ACL)

Anticardiolipin antibodies belong to the group of antiphospholipid antibodies (aPLA). The presence was first observed in the sera of syphilis patients. But they have also been described in SLE (systemic lupus erythematosus) patients and in patients with other rheumatic diseases. The antiphospholipid syndrome (APS) or Hughes syndrome is characterized by arterial or venous thrombosis or recurrent miscarriages together with persistently positive tests for aPL. In contrast to secondary antiphospholipid syndrome, which occurs in association with SLE or other rheumatic disorders, there is no evidence for another relevant underlying disease in primary antiphospholipid syndrome.

Anticardiolipin antibodies in infectious diseases and in APS can be distinguished with respect to their dependence on cofactors. In case of patients with infectious diseases, the aCLs recognize the pure phospholipid as antigen, binding of aCL from patients suffering from APS requires beta-2 glycoprotein I as cofactor.

Elevated levels of aCL may be found in patients with cerebrovascular insufficiency or myocardial infarction.

Reference Range

- < 10 = Negative
- > 15 = Positive
- 10–15 = Borderline

Method of estimation: ELISA.

CLINICAL IMPORTANCE OF LACTATE AND PYRUVATE ESTIMATIONS

- Lactate is the end product of carbohydrate metabolism that is produced during anaerobic glycolysis.
- Blood lactate arises from muscle cells and erythrocytes and is metabolized by the liver
- Therefore, the blood lactate levels reflect both production and metabolism.
- The liver can normally remove more lactate than the body can produce; hence, treatment for hypoxia and removal of the initiating condition results in lowering of the blood lactate.
- The measurement of lactate is useful clinically in the diagnosis of angina pectoris or in liver function testing where reduced liver function is suspected.
- Both lactate and pyruvate levels provide an index of severity of circulatory failure.
- The enzymatic method for the estimation is based on the reduction of NAD to NADH by lactate dehydrogenase.
- Severe exercise increases blood lactate levels.
- The common cause for increased blood lactate and pyruvate is anoxia resulting from conditions like shock, pneumonia and congestive heart failure.
- Lactic acidosis may also occur in renal failure and leukemia.

- Diabetic ketoacidosis and thiamine deficiency are associated with increased levels of lactate and pyruvate.
- Lactate levels in CSF are increased in bacterial meningitis, hypocapnia, hydrocephalus, brain abscesses, and cerebral ischemia.

Estimation of Lactate

Principle

$$\text{L-Lactate} + O_2 \xleftrightarrow[\text{Oxidase}]{\text{Lactase}} \text{Pyruvate} + H_2O_2$$

$$H_2O_2 + \text{H donor} + \text{4-aminoantipyrine} \xleftrightarrow{\text{Peroxidase}} \text{Chromogen} + 2H_2O$$

Color intensity is directly proportional to the lactate concentration.

Specimen Required for Estimation

Blood collected in a fluoride-oxalate tube, centrifuged and plasma obtained is used for analysis.

Normal Range

- Venous blood = 5–12 mg/dL (0.5–1.3 mmol/L)
- Arterial blood = 3–7 mg/dL (0.36–0.75 mmol/L)
  mmol/L to mg/dL is obtained by multiplying the value with 9.

Pyruvate Estimation

- Pyruvate is the end product of carbohydrate metabolism.
- It is unstable in blood.

$$\text{Pyruvate} + \text{NADH} + \text{H} \xleftrightarrow{\text{LDH pH 7.5}} \text{Lactate} + \text{NAD}^+$$

At about pH 7.5, the equilibrium constant strongly favors the reaction to the right.

- Venous blood = 0.3–0.9 mg/dL (0.03–0.10 mmol/L)
- Arterial blood = 0.2–0.7 mg/dL (0.02–0.08 mmol/L)
  mmol/L to mg/dL is by multiply by 8.8.

AMMONIA AND ITS CLINICAL IMPORTANCE

Ammonia Estimation

- Ammonia is the end product of amino acid metabolism.
- It is toxic to human body.
- Therefore, it is converted to urea and excreted.
- The individual with urea cycle defects may have elevated blood level of ammonia.
- A newborn with urea cycle defects or organic acidemia may require serial blood ammonia determinations.
- Variety of chemical methods are available for the measurement of ammonia content of plasma.
- The kinetic procedure is based on the reductive amination of α-ketoglutarate using glutamate dehydrogenase and reduced NADH.

$$\alpha\text{-ketoglutarate} + NH_4^+ \text{ NADH} \xleftrightarrow{\text{GLDH}} \text{Glutamate} + \text{NAD}$$

- The enzyme is specific for NH_4^+ and will not react with methylated amines.
- The decrease in absorbance at 340 nm, due to oxidation of NADH, proportional to the concentration of ammonia in the plasma.
- The absorbance is measured by a photometer.
- Hyperammonemia (elevated blood ammonia level) is a feature of disorder of enzymes of the urea cycle and disorders of dibasic branched chain amino acid metabolism.
- Nongenetic causes of hyperammonemia are very rare, but include any cause of severe liver failure due to hepatitis or sepsis of hypoxia.
- Ammonia-free heparin is used as anticoagulant and hemolysis should be avoided.
- Upon drawing, the blood should be placed in an ice bath and plasma should be separated within 30 minutes.

Reference Range

140–490 microgram/L as ammonia nitrogen or 11–35 micromoles/L.

INBORN ERRORS OF METABOLISM (IEM)

- Comprise a large class of genetic diseases involving disorders of metabolism. Majority are due to defects of single genes that code for enzymes that facilitate conversion of various substrates into products.
- Effects are due to toxic accumulations of substrates before the block, intermediates from alternative metabolic pathways, and/or defects in energy production and utilization caused by a deficiency of products beyond the block.
- Most are due to a defect in an enzyme or transport protein, which results in a block in a metabolic pathway.
- Nearly every metabolic disease has several forms that vary in age of onset, clinical severity and, often, mode of inheritance.
- The term inborn error of metabolism was coined by a British physician, Archibald Garrod (1857–1936).
- Inborn errors of metabolism (IEMs) are rare.
- Presentation of the IEM can occur at any time, even in adulthood.
- Diagnosis does not require extensive knowledge of biochemical pathways or individual metabolic diseases.
- An understanding of the broad clinical manifestations of IEMs provides the basis for knowing when to consider diagnosis/testing.

Major Categories of Inherited Metabolic Diseases

Traditionally, the inherited metabolic diseases were categorized as disorders of:

- Carbohydrate metabolism
- Amino acid metabolism
- Organic acid metabolism
- Lysosomal storage diseases.

The following are some of the inborn errors of metabolism:

1. Disorders of carbohydrate metabolism, e.g., glycogen storage disease, carbohydrate intolerance disorder, disorders of gluconeogenesis and glycogenolysis.
2. Disorders of amino acid metabolism, e.g., phenylketonuria, alkaptonuria and maple syrup urine disease, urea cycle defect.
3. Disorders of fatty acid oxidation and mitochondrial metabolism, e.g., medium chain acyl dehydrogenase deficiency.
4. Disorders of porphyrin metabolism, e.g., coproporphyria and acute intermittent porphyria.
5. Disorders of purine or pyrimidine metabolism, e.g., Lesch-Nyhan syndrome.
6. Disorders of steroid metabolism, e.g., congenital adrenal hyperplasia.
7. Disorders of lysosomal storage, e.g., Gauchers' disease.
8. Disorders of mitochondrial function, e.g., Kearns-Sayre syndrome.
9. Disorders of peroxisomal function, e.g., Zellweger syndrome.

Inborn Errors of Amino Acid Metabolism

History

- Developmental delay
- Histories vary by age of presentation and is a function of the age at which various inborn errors of metabolisms manifest clinically
  - Infants and young children (1 month to 5 years) may have a history of recurrent episodes of vomiting, ataxia, seizures, lethargy, coma, and fulminant hepatoencephalopathy.
  - Other findings may include dysmorphic or coarse features, skeletal abnormalities, abnormalities of the hair or skin, poor feeding, failure to thrive, and developmental delay.
  - With routine illnesses, individuals with IEMs may become more severely symptomatic, develop symptoms more

rapidly, or require longer time for recovery than unaffected children.
  - Undiagnosed metabolic disease should be considered in older children (> 5 years), adolescents, or adults with psychiatric abnormalities.
  - Many individuals who actually have an undiagnosed IEM have been diagnosed as having birth injury or atypical forms of psychiatric disorders or medical diseases, such as multiple sclerosis, migraines, or stroke.

Physical examination findings are normal in most patients with IEM.

- Abnormalities may include failure to thrive, dysmorphic features, abnormalities of hair, skin and/or skeleton, abnormal odor, organomegaly, and abnormal muscle tone.
- Clinical symptoms of IEMs tend to be nonspecific and usually relate to major organ dysfunction or failure.
- The same symptoms occur with sepsis, respiratory illness, cardiac disease, GI obstruction, renal disease, and CNS problems.
- Presence of these conditions does not rule out the possibility of an IEM.
- Clinical findings in neonates:
  - Poor feeding
  - Vomiting, diarrhea, and dehydration
  - Temperature instability
  - Tachypnea, apnea
  - Bradycardia, poor perfusion
  - Irritability, involuntary movements or posturing, abnormal tone, seizures, and altered level of consciousness
  - Developmental delay, occasionally with missed milestones
  - Ataxia, hypotonia or hypertonia, and visual and auditory disturbances
  - Symptoms for IEM of substrate and intermediary metabolism develop once there is a significant accumulation of toxic metabolites following the initiation of feeding
  - For IEMs of energy deficiency, symptoms usually develop within 24 hours and often are present at birth.
  - Certain metabolic diseases (including galactosemia during the newborn period), certain organic acidopathies, and congenital adrenal hyperplasia may be associated with an increased risk of sepsis.
  - For neonates with inborn errors of substrate and intermediary metabolism, the physical examination usually is unremarkable.
  - Neonates with inborn errors that result in defects in energy production and utilization often have dysmorphic features, skeletal malformations, cardiopulmonary compromise, organomegaly, and severe generalized hypotonia.
- Clinical findings in older children, adolescents, and adults:
  - Common findings include mild-to-profound mental retardation, autism, learning disorders, behavioral disturbances, hallucinations, delirium, aggressiveness, agitation, anxiety, panic attacks, seizures, dizziness, ataxia, exercise intolerance, muscle weakness, and paraparesis.
  - Some manifestations may be intermittent, precipitated by the stress of illness, or progressive, with worsening over time.
  - While most IEMs diagnosed in this age group are not immediately life threatening, partial ornithine transcarbamylase (OTC) deficiency, a urea cycle defect, can manifest at this time as a life-threatening metabolic catastrophe. This is observed particularly in adolescent females with a history of protein aversion, abdominal pain, and migraine like headaches.

Laboratory Studies

- Laboratory abnormalities can be transient. Therefore, values within the reference range do not rule out an IEM.
- Studies may need to be repeated during other episodes of illness or during provocative testing in a clinical research center.
  - Metabolic acidosis
  - *Hypoglycemia:* Hypoglycemia (plasma glucose <50 mg/dL) is rare in children (0.44% of those tested), even during periods of poor enteral intake. Of the 32 of 40 children with hypoglycemia for whom metabolic workup was performed on initial samples, 28% had a previously undiagnosed fatty acid oxidation defect or endocrine disorder.
  - Hyperammonemia: Early manifestations include anorexia, abdominal pain, headache, irritability, fatigue, latetachypnea, vomiting, lethargy, seizures, coma, and death.
  - Major exceptions include congenital adrenal hyperplasia (hyponatremia and hyperkalemia in a child with apparent sepsis), nonketotic hyperglycinemia (lethargy, coma, seizures, hypotonia, spasticity, hiccups, apnea), and pyridoxine deficiency (encephalopathy, intractable seizures).
- Initial laboratory evaluation
  - Complete blood count (CBC) to screen for neutropenia, anemia, and thrombocytopenia.
  - Serum electrolytes, bicarbonate, and blood gases to detect electrolyte imbalances and evaluate anion gap (usually elevated) and acid/base status.
  - Blood urea nitrogen and creatinine to evaluate renal function.
  - Bilirubin, transaminases, prothrombin time, and partial thrombin time to evaluate hepatic function.
  - *Ammonia:* Obtain if altered level of consciousness, persistent or recurrent vomiting, primary metabolic acidosis with increased anion gap, or primary respiratory alkalosis in the absence of toxic ingestion. Preferably, use an arterial sample, as skeletal muscle releases ammonia. If venous sample is obtained, the sample must be free flowing (no tourniquet). Ice the sample immediately, and assay promptly. Normal values are less than 100 μg/dL in the neonate and less than 80 μg/dL in those older than 1 month.
  - *Metabolic screening:* Where one or more specific enzymes needed in body metabolism are absent or abnormal. The result is an increased blood level of one or more of the amino acids, sugars or lipid fractions. These and their metabolites are then excreted in the urine. Qualitative screening tests are done on the urine to detect excess excretion of these substances.

Reference Values

pH	=	5–9
Protein	=	Negative
Glucose	=	Negative
Ketones	=	Negative
Bilirubin	=	Negative
Blood	=	Negative
Urobilinogen	=	Negative
Mucopolysaccharides	=	Negative
Nitroprusside test (Cysteine and homocysteine)	=	Negative
Dinitrophenylhydrazine (alpha-keto acids)	=	Negative
Ferric chloride (Phenyl pyruvic acid which indirectly detects phenylalanine)	=	Negative
Nitrosonaphthol (P-OH catabolites like tyrosine)	=	Negative
Silver nitrate test (Homogentisic acid)	=	Negative
Reducing sugars	=	Negative

For details of the test, refer Unit 17.

- Blood glucose and urine pH, ketones, and reducing substances.
  - False-positive results for reducing substances are caused by penicillin and glucuronides.
  - Neonates—inappropriate ketones (i.e., ketonuria).
  - Child—Ketonuria with normal glucose or low/absent ketones with hypoglycemia.
- Obtain lactate dehydrogenase, aldolase, creatinine kinase, and urine myoglobin levels in patients with evidence of neuromyopathy.

Other Tests

- Enzyme assay or DNA analysis in leukocytes, erythrocytes, skin fibroblasts, liver, or other tissues.
- Histologic evaluation of affected tissues, such as skin, liver, brain, heart, kidney, and skeletal muscle.
- Secondary studies
  - If initial test results are abnormal, consider consultation with an IEM specialist to determine, which tests are appropriate, how specimens are to be collected and stored, and where they should be sent.
  - Plasma or serum lactate, pyruvate, albumin, triglycerides, uric acid, amino acids, organic acids, quantitative carnitine, and qualitative carnitine [1–2 cc in ethylenediaminetetraacetic acid (EDTA) or heparin tube, on ice.
  - Urine amino acids, organic acids, orotic acid, and/or acylglycine (10–20 cc, freeze immediately).
  - Cerebrospinal fluid (CSF) lactate, pyruvate, and/or glycine collected at the same time as plasma (1–2 cc).
- If a child has died, attempting to diagnose a metabolic disease is still important because of the possibility that presently asymptomatic siblings are affected or that future children will be affected.
  - Plasma, serum, urine, and possibly CSF, skin, and selected organ specimens should be collected and frozen.
  - A metabolic specialist may be helpful in directing the evaluation of patients with suspected metabolic disease.

D-dimer

- Thrombin converts D-dimer to soluble fibrin by cleaving the fibrinopeptides A and B.
- The fibrin monomers polymerize spontaneously.
- Active factor XIII links two D-domains and generates a solid fibrin clot.
- A new plasmin-resistant antigenic determinant ("D-dimer") is produced. Fragments containing D-dimer are accordingly formed during the degradation of a fibrin clot by plasmin.
- A large proportion of the fibrin degradation products consists of high molecular weight X-oligomers.
- Only in vitro or during lysis therapy does complete degradation to D-dimer molecules take place.
- D-dimer is a blood test performed in the medical laboratory to diagnose thrombosis.
- D-dimer may be ordered when a patient has symptoms of DVT, such as leg pain, tenderness, swelling, discoloration, edema; or symptoms of PE, such as labored breathing, coughing, and lung-related chest pain.
- When a patient has symptoms of disseminated intravascular coagulation (DIC) such as nausea, vomiting, severe muscle and abdominal pain, seizures and oliguria, a D-dimer test may be ordered, along with a PT, aPTT, fibrinogen, FDP, and platelet count to help diagnose the condition.
- D-dimer may also be ordered at intervals when a patient is undergoing treatment for DIC to help monitor its progress.

- In patients suspected of disseminated intravascular coagulation, D-dimers may aid in the diagnosis.

Principles of D-dimer Testing

- Fibrin degradation products (FDPs) are formed whenever fibrin is broken down by enzymes (e.g., plasmin). Determining FDPs is not considered useful, as this does not indicate whether the fibrin is part of a blood clot (or being generated as part of inflammation).
- D-dimers are unique in that they are the breakdown products of a fibrin mesh that has been stabilized by factor XIII.
- This factor crosslinks the E-element to *two* D-elements. This is the final step in the generation of a thrombus.
- Plasmin is a natural fibrinolytic enzyme that organizes clots and breaks down the fibrin mesh.
- However, it cannot break down the bonds between one E and two D units.
- The protein fragment thus left over is a D-dimer **(Fig. 23.1)**.

Reference Range

Most sampling kits have 0–300 ng/mL as normal range.

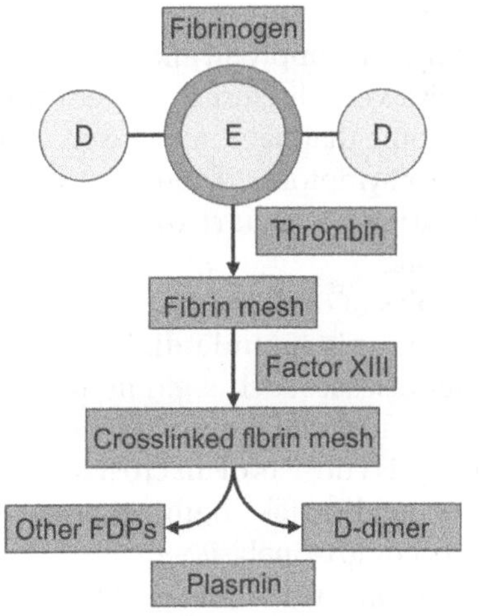

Fig. 23.1: D-dimer testing.

Values exceeding 250, 300 or 500 ng/mL (different for various kits) are considered positive.

Lower Limb Deep Venous Thrombosis/ Pulmonary Embolism

When D-dimer values below the cutoff are obtained, deep venous thrombosis (DVT) of the lower limb and pulmonary embolism can be excluded with the respective test-specific sensitivity.

Complications in Pregnancy

Determination of the fibrin degradation products as part of "gestosis screening" permits the detection of severe pregnancy complications.

Supplementary Tumor Diagnosis

For solid malignant tumors, a positive correlation between fibrin degradation products and the degree of tumor progression has been found in some studies.

D-dimer values are distinctly higher with metastasizing tumors and indicate a poor prognosis for the course of the disease.

Types of Assays

- ELISA
- Latex turbidimetric assay (automated immunoassay, e.g., Roche Tina-quant)
- Enhanced microlatex
- Latex-enhanced photometric
- False-positive readings can be due to various causes: liver disease, high rheumatoid factor, inflammation, malignancy, trauma, pregnancy, recent surgery as well as advanced age
- False-negative readings can occur either if the sample is taken too early after thrombus formation or if testing is delayed for several days. Additionally, the presence of anticoagulation can render the test negative because it prevents thrombus extension.

Kidney Stone

- A kidney stone is a hard mineral and crystalline material formed within the kidney or urinary tract.
- Kidney stones are a common cause of blood in the urine and pain in the abdomen, flank, or groin. Kidney stones are sometimes called renal calculi.
- The condition of having kidney stones is termed nephrolithiasis or urolithiasis.
- Kidney stones form when there is a decrease in urine volume or an excess of stone-forming substances in the urine.
- The most common type of kidney stone contains calcium in combination with either oxalate or phosphate.
- Other chemical compounds that can form stones in the urinary tract include uric acid and the amino acid cystine.
- Dehydration through reduced fluid intake or strenuous exercise without adequate fluid replacement increases the risk of kidney stones.
- Obstruction to the flow of urine can also lead to stone formation.
- Kidney stones associated with infection in the urinary tract are known as infection stones.
- A number of different conditions can lead to kidney stones:
  - *Gout* results in an increased amount of uric acid in the urine and can lead to the formation of uric acid stones.
  - *Hypercalciuria* (high calcium in the urine), another inherited condition, causes stones in more than half of cases. In this condition, too much calcium is absorbed from food and excreted into the urine, where it may form calcium phosphate or calcium oxalate stones.
  - *Other conditions* associated with an increased risk of kidney stones include hyperparathyroidism, kidney diseases such as renal tubular acidosis, and some inherited metabolic conditions including cystinuria and hyperoxaluria.
  - *People with inflammatory bowel disease* or who have had an intestinal bypass or ostomy surgery are also more likely to develop kidney stones.
- It is better to send the kidney stone to biochemistry laboratory to know the constituent of the stone.
- The report may help the surgeon to advise the patient for future care.

Symptoms of Kidney Stone

- Sudden onset of excruciating cramping pain in their low back and/or side, groin, or abdomen. Changes in body position do not relieve this pain.
- It may be so severe that it is often accompanied by nausea and vomiting.
- Kidney stones also characteristically cause blood in the urine.
- If infection is present in the urinary tract along with the stones, there may be fever and chills.
- Nowadays, the laboratories use urine analysis as a screening test to detect the crystals, microorganisms, blood, ketone bodies, pH, glucose and protein.

Urinanalysis

- Urinalysis is simply an analysis of the urine.
- Urinalysis can disclose evidence of diseases, even some that have not caused significant signs or symptoms. Therefore, a urinalysis is commonly a part of routine health screening.
- Examples of diseases that can be detected by urinalysis include diabetes mellitus, kidney diseases such as glomerulonephritis, and chronic infections of the urinary tract.
- Urinalysis consists of macroscopic urinalysis, urine dipstick chemical analysis, and microscopic urinalysis.
- Macroscopic urinalysis is the direct visual observation of the urine, noting its quantity, color, clarity or cloudiness, etc.

- This microchemistry system permits qualitative (yes/no) and semiquantitative analysis within a minute by simple observation. The color change occurring on each segment of a dipstick is read by being compared to a color chart.
- Dipsticks can, for example, be used to determine the urine's pH (acidity), specific gravity (density), protein content, glucose, ketones, nitrite content.
- Dipsticks, whether they be paper or plastic, have many advantages. They are simple, fast, convenient, easy to use, and they are the most cost-effective way to screen urine.
- However, what can be learned from a dipstick is limited by the design of the dipstick.
- Examination is then performed through the microscope at high power to further identify any cells, bacteria and clumps of cells or debris called casts.

GASTRIC FUNCTION TESTS

The healthy functioning of our digestive system is very important for the body. Our stomach is a reservoir of ingested food, and it is through digestion that food breaks down and becomes a source of nourishment. One of the tests which are done to get evaluate how well the digestive system is functioning is the gastric function test. The test is done to assess the acid secretory potential of the stomach by evaluating gastric juices the body produces. The tests help to diagnose chronic problems such as diarrhea, constipation, bloating, and other gastrointestinal disorders. Gastric juice is a variable mixture of water, hydrochloric acid, electrolytes, and mucus.

Gastric juice is a clear, pale yellow, odorless fluid with a strong acidic pH (around 1) and a specific gravity of approximately 1.007.

Composition of Gastric Juice

- Pepsinogen secreted by chief cells
- Hydrochloric acid secreted by parietal cells
- Rennin
- Haemopoietic factor
- Mucus secreted by mucous cells
- Organic acids
- Water 98–99%

Functions of Gastric Juice

- Water liquefies the food swallowed
- HCl
- Acidifies the food and stop the action of salivary amylase
- Kills ingested microbes
- Provides the acidic environment required for action of salivary amylase
- Digestive enzymes (Rennin, Pepsin and lipase) act on food
- Intrinsic factor helps in absorption of Vitamin B12

Important Gastric Function Tests

- Examination of resting contents in resting juice (gastric residuum)
- Fractional gastric analysis using a test 'meal'
- Examination of the contents after stimulation:
  - Alcohol stimulation
  - Caffeine stimulation
  - Histamine stimulation
  - Augmented histamine test
  - Insulin stimulation
  - Pentagastrin test
- Tubeless gastric analysis

Gastric secretion may be caused by:

- Factor such as sight, taste or smell
- Hormone (gastrin)
- Insulin stimulating the vagus
- Histamine a powerful stimulant
- Alcohol (in moderate concentration)

Gastric Juice Analysis

Fractional Test Meal

Collection of stomach contents with Ryle's tube. Ryle's tube is a long thin rubber tube 4 mm in diameter. It has a lead piece at the tip of the tube and perforations at a short distance away from the tip. The tube is passed into the stomach, and gastric juice is collected periodically. After the samples are thus collected, they are examined for free and total acidity.

Pentagastrin Stimulation Test

Pentagastrin is an artificial peptide that can stimulate gastric secretion. Here, the contents of the stomach are aspirated with the Ryle's tube, collected at 15-minute intervals, and further analyzed for the next hour.

Augment Histamine Test Meal

One of the most powerful stimulants for gastric secretion, this is also aspirated at 15-minute intervals and collected for a detailed analysis. Through the test samples, the levels of acid content are measured.

Insulin Test Meal

It is mainly done to assess the results of vagotomy. Vagotomy is the process of cutting a branch of the vagus nerve to reduce stomach acid secretion. This test involves delivering electrical impulses to the vagus nerve in the brain. This is also known as Hollander's test and in this test, insulin is intravenously administered to the patient.

Tubeless Gastric Analysis

The test is helpful to ascertain the levels of gastric acidity without the use of complicated or cumbersome chemical procedures and intubation. This gastric acidity analysis is helpful to diagnose problems such as duodenal ulcers, achlorhydria, and pernicious anemia.

Preparation for the Test

There is no special preparation for the test besides fasting. The patient will have to fast for 12 hours overnight through the next morning till the test is completed. In most of the above types of testing, the patient is asked to swallow the bulbous end of the Ryle tube into the throat. When the first mark is at the level of the incisor teeth, the tip is at the esophagus. When the second mark is at the level of the incisor teeth, the tip has reached the stomach's pyloric region. When the third mark is at the level of the incisor teeth, the tip is at the duodenum.

Gastric Juice Analysis—Qualitative

- *Physical examination:*
  - Volume: 30–60 mL
  - Appearance: Clear and watery liquid
  - Color: Pale yellow (normal), brownish red (presence of excess blood), yellow (presence of fresh bile), greenish (presence of old bile), red (presence of small amount of blood)
  - Odor: Odorless (normal) typical odour in case of presence of pathological constituents.
- *Chemical examination:*
  - Test for chloride
  - Gunzberg's test for HCl
  - Ufflemann's test for presence of lactic acid
  - Iodine test for starch
  - Benzidine test for blood
  - Test for pepsin.

Preparation of the Patient

- The patient will take light evening meal and fast for 12 hours overnight and also on the next morning till the test is completed.
- Introduction of the tube.
- On the next morning, the patient is asked to swallow the bulbous end of the Ryle tube into the throat and the process of swallowing will be continued till the third marking reaches the teeth.

Aspiration of Gastric Juice

- The fasting contents will be completely withdrawn by means of syringe, measured and kept for analysis. This is total resting juice.

- The patient is now administered 50–80 cc liquid meal (7% alcohol) into the stomach with the help of a syringe.
- 10–15 mL of gastric juice is aspirated at every 15 minutes up to 2:30 hours (10 samples).

Analysis of Gastric Juice

Each aspirated fasting sample along with 10 samples after the test meal are tested separately.

Physical Examination

Amount: Resting juice 15–50 mL. Increase resting juice indicates pyloric stenosis, peptic ulcer or gastric malignancy.

Examination of Resting Contents

Volume

In most normal cases after a night's fast only 20 to 50 mL of resting contents is obtained. Volume greater than 100 to 120 mL is considered abnormal.

An increase in volume of resting contents may be due to:

- Hypersecretion of gastric juice
- Retention of gastric contents due to delayed emptying of the stomach
- Due to regurgitation of the duodenal contents.

Consistency

The normal resting gastric juice is fluid in consistency and does not contain food residues. It may contain small amounts of mucus. Food residues are present in carcinoma of the stomach.

Colour

In more than 50 per cent of normal individuals, the gastric residuum is clear or colourless, or it may be slightly yellow or greenish due to regurgitation of bile from duodenum.

A bright red or dark red or brown color in the residuum is due to presence of blood-fresh/or altered blood.

Bile

Bile may be found occasionally but is not usually of any particular significance. A small amount may be regurgitated from the duodenum as stated, as a result of nausea which some people may experience in swallowing the tube. Increase quantities of bile is abnormal which may result from intestinal obstruction or ileal stasis.

Blood

Normally blood should not be present. amount of fresh bright blood may be traumatic. Mucus: A small Normally mucus is present in only small amounts. Increased mucus is found in gastritis and in gastric carcinoma. Presence of mucus is inversely proportional to the amount of HCl present.

Gastric Juice Analysis: Quantitative

Determination of Free and Total Acidity

- Free acidity- Acidity due to HCl acid
- Combined acidity- acidity due to organic acids like lactic acid, citric acid, butyric acid, other fatty acids
- Total acidity = Free acidity + Combined acidity

Reagents

- (0.01 N) NaOH soln.
- Topfer reagent (0.1% methyl orange in Abs. alcohol)
- Phenolphthalein soln.

Determination

- Determination of acidity by titration and plotting graph:
- Method: 1ml of filtered gastric fluid is treated with 2drops of Topfer s reagent and titrated with 0.01 N NaOH solution.

- The end point is indicated by the disappearance of all traces of red colour and appearance of yellow, orange colour or canary yellow. Note the burette reading.

Interpretation

- In normal condition
  - The total acidity varies from 50–70
  - Free acidity: 35–55
  - Combined acidity: 10–15

Hyperchlorhydria

- High total acidity: - 100–110
- High free acidity: - 60–100
- But combined acidity: - 10–15
- Resting juice: Increase

Caused by - Chronic duodenal ulcer - Chronic appendicitis - Chronic colitis - Chronic amoebic dysentery.

Hypochlorhydria

- Decrease of free acidity.
- Caused by: Chronic gastritis and chronic gastric ulcer.

Achlorhydria

- This term is used when there is no secretion of free acidity (HCl). But pepsin may still be present.
  Caused by: Gastric carcinoma, with pyloric obstruction (stenosis) and pernicious anemia.
- Under microscope malignant cells, RBC, acid fast bacilli and other can be identified.

CLINICAL SIGNIFICANCE

Zollinger–Ellison Syndrome

The defect in this condition is carcinoma of the gastrin-producing cells. Excess gastrin causes a persistent stimulation of the parietal cells, resulting in marked increase in the acid output even in the unstimulated state. Consequently, the ratio of the basal acid output and the maximum acid output rises up to 0.6% (Normal: BAO, 0–17 mmol/h; MAO, 4.7–58.4 mmol/h). In pernicious anemia, the basic pathology is gastric mucosal atrophy with lack of intrinsic factor and in great majority of cases "true" achlorhydria. Some occasional young persons with pernicious anemia have been found to have acid secretion. Following gastrectomy entails removal of a portion of the acid-secreting stomach wall. It is performed for treating acid hypersecretion.

SELF TEST

1. Discuss the clinical importance of ANA and dsDNA determination.
2. What is D-dimer and when it is ordered?
3. State the clinical significance of D-dimer determination.
4. What are inborn errors of metabolism? Explain with examples.
5. What is lactate? Briefly explain its clinical importance.
6. State the conditions in which ammonia estimation is necessary.

MULTIPLE CHOICE QUESTIONS

1. All the following may lead to formation of a kidney stone, *except:*

a. Gout
b. Hypercalciuria
c. Bowel disease
d. Thyroid abnormality

2. Which of the following tests detects the presence of alkaptonuria?

a. Phenyl hydrazine test
b. Ferric chloride test
c. Hay's test
d. Nitrosonaphthol test

3. **All the following statements are correct regarding autoimmune disease, *except:***
   a. The immune system is the body's defense against foreign substances, such as bacteria or viruses, which may be harmful
   b. An autoimmune disease is an abnormal condition that occurs when a person's immune system attacks its own tissues as though they were foreign substances
   c. Normally, when a foreign substance enters the body, the immune system creates special cells to attack and destroy the foreign substance
   d. The immune system does not have any relation with autoantibodies

24

UNIT

Organization and Management of Diagnostic Laboratory

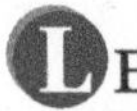

LEARNING OBJECTIVES

At the end of this unit, the learner should be able to understand:
- Management of the diagnostic laboratory.
- The safety procedures to be implemented in the diagnostic laboratory.

INTRODUCTION

Laboratory medicine is the base of the modern-day healthcare system. The advance in technology, better understanding of the various disease processes, advancement of medical research and the growing demand for reliable test results has greatly revolutionized the area of laboratory medicine.

Most of the present-day laboratories are now equipped with, to a varying degree, sophisticated automated instruments, with test results, which are accurate and reproducible. There is more emphasis on the quality control programs.

Today, in larger hospitals, major sections of the laboratory are specialized to the extent that they engage specialized staff and perform all the tests relating to their disciplines within sections. In smaller hospitals, the staff may be required to work in more than one section. It is usual for these smaller hospitals to establish and staff some sections and send the specimens to the other larger institutions.

Presently, there is no prevailing legislation to check the laboratories, which do not satisfy the minimum standards and hence do not provide quality results, which is a cause for great concern. The ministry has established an accreditation board to fix some rules and regulations for the small laboratories, which do not even have the recommended instruments and qualified persons.

In this changed scenario, organization and management of laboratory services is not only a complicated and complex process but also a great challenge.

Objectives

After studying this unit, one should know the following to organize and manage their laboratories:

1. Facilities and general laboratory design.
2. Designing and requirements of the various sections in the laboratory.
3. Laboratory operational flow.
4. Work force/staffing.
5. Equipment, instruments and reagents used.
6. Laboratory safety.
7. Quality control, quality assurance, and accreditation.
8. Reporting laboratory results and record keeping.
9. Financial considerations in laboratory planning.
10. Medicolegal concerns.

Purposes of the Laboratory Medicine

The laboratory results assist the clinicians in:

a. Diagnosing the disease.
b. Providing guidelines in patient management.
c. Establishing prognosis.
d. Monitoring follow-up therapy.

MAIN OBJECTIVES OF LABORATORY ORGANIZATION AND MANAGEMENT

The prime objective should be to ensure accuracy and precision of the laboratory results through quality assurance and to provide accurate results for good patient care.

There are several tools required for achieving this objective:

1. Good planning and designing of the laboratory.
2. Implementing appropriate quality assurance programs.
3. Maximum utilization of the equipment.
4. Utilization of high quality reagents.
5. Training qualified staff.
6. Employing sound management practices.
7. Providing a safe and healthy environment.

It is important to adhere to the basic laboratory principles through proper collection, handling and processing of the patients specimens.

FACILITIES AND DESIGN

Good planning and design to meet the current and foreseeable needs pertaining to personnel, equipment, space and tasks to be performed is very important for establishing a cost effective and successful laboratory service.

The steps in the design process are as follows:

Preparation

Assess the needs of the laboratory staff requirement; technology (current and future) committee may be formed involving laboratory staff, an architect, medical staff, and an interior designer.

Functions

- Define the activities that are to be performed
- Consider the flow of the people and material
- **Storage:** Reagents, stationary and equipment spare
- Utilities
- Specific needs of each individual section in the laboratory.

Schematic Design

- Structural design
- Architectural design
- System options like plumbing, electricity, heating, ventilation and air conditioning
- Cost estimation.

Design Development

Interior designing—color, texture, finish, and furnishings.

Construction

Bidding and negotiations, legal documentation, actual construction, completion and occupancy.

Considerations in Laboratory Design

- *Location of the laboratory:* In a hospital, the laboratory should ideally be located close to the emergency department, outpatient department, intensive care units and operating rooms. The laboratory should be very near to the doctor as well as the city.
- *Space requirement:* The laboratory should be spacious to comfortably house the equipment and laboratory personnel. There should be no hindrance for the movement of the personnel **(Flowchart 24.1)**.
- Adequate lighting, good ventilation, temperature control (equipment should be kept in AC rooms to increase their life), electrical power (including emergency

Flowchart 24.1: Laboratory design.

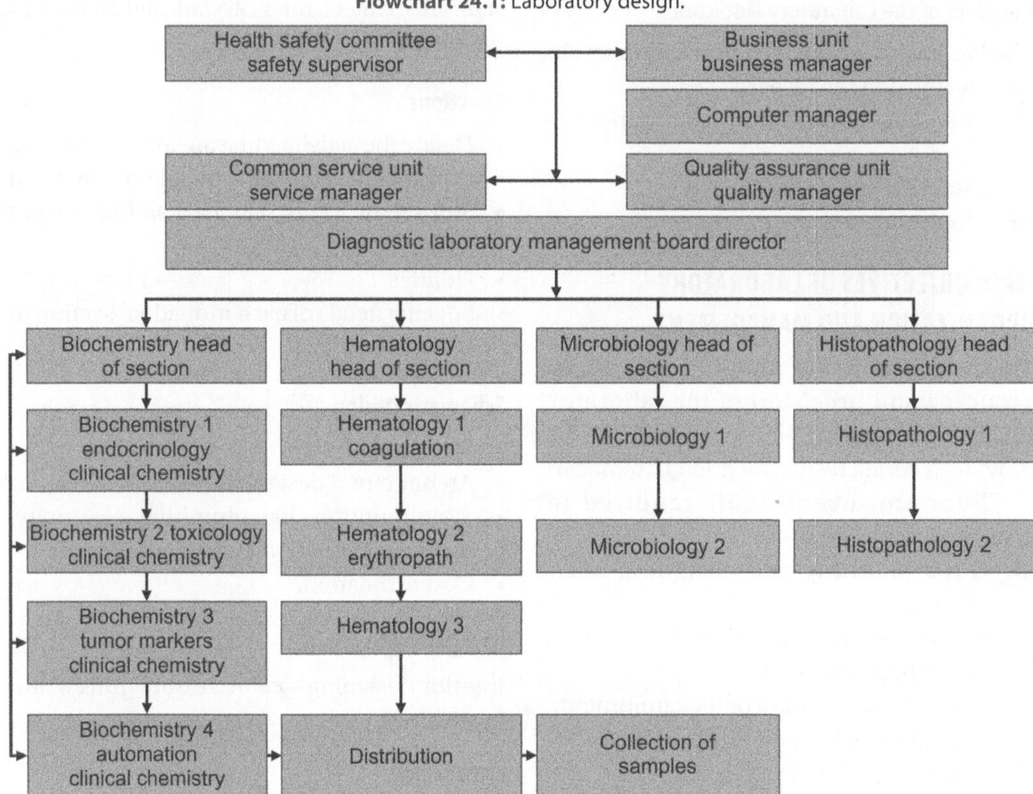

power/generators), continuous water supply and good sanitation should be provided to the laboratory.

- Noise control in the open laboratories is achieved by installing a drop ceiling. This in addition can be used for installation of utilities like power cables and computer cables, which adds flexibility to the design.
- Fume hoods and biological safety cabinets are required and should be located away from high traffic areas and doorways.
- It is advisable to have movable partitions instead of permanent brick walls between various sections of the laboratory, as it adds to the flexibility for any future expansions or alterations.
- The workbenches, used for tasks performed while sitting should be 2.5 ft in height and those to be used for tasks, which are performed while standing should be 3 ft high. The width of these workbenches should be at least 2'6". Wood surface with acid proofing, smooth cement surface or cement surface with ceramic tiles are the recommended work surfaces.
- Base cabinets (under the laboratory counters/work benches are preferred over the suspended cabinets, as they provide 30% extra storage space.
- Installation of a fire extinguisher is mandatory. It should be located at an easily reachable position and maintained in good working condition.
- Emergency exit, which opens to the corridor, should be provided.
- Separate rest rooms should be provided for the laboratory staff.

- Choose the furniture; modular furniture (detachable, movable, and foldable), though expensive but allows more flexibility.

LABORATORY MANAGEMENT

It is not expected that the candidate for the laboratory will have had the opportunity to become fully conversant with all details of laboratory management. The clinical biochemist should, however, have a reasonable knowledge of the important aspects of the following:

- Organization of a clinical biochemistry laboratory, including routine and emergency services, screening and profiling, staff training, performance management, and work assignment
- Laboratory safety including chemical, radiation, physical and biological hazards
- Reagents and apparatus, their selection, sources of supply, and techniques for assessing the quality of equipment and reagents
- Budget preparation and monitoring
- Presentation of results of biochemical analysis, reports of results.

The head of the laboratory should be convergent with many of the accreditation standards and governmental regulations. One should not just take up the job of managing a clinical laboratory attracted by the monetary benefits but also one should realize its vast responsibility as those laboratory reports have a direct impact on the healthcare of patients.

Clinical laboratory management requires expertise in medical, scientific and technical areas. The person should have resources in the form of personnel, equipment, supplies; facilities and skills in organization, management and communication.

A clinical laboratory should stand on firm goals and objectives. In order to achieve these objectives, the clinical laboratory should have adequate facilities, equipment, supplies and personnel.

The objective of a clinical laboratory to assist the medical professionals with reliable reports of tests is a vital component of excellent healthcare delivery system. Such being the case every effort is made at maintenance and improvement of quality of work through the following:

- Quality control implementation, monitoring, performance evaluation
- Quality management systems
- International standardized organization (ISO) guide 25, ISO 9002 systems
- Efficiency of laboratory testing strategies
- Diagnostic sensitivity, specificity and efficiency of tests
- Evidence-based medicine.

Functions and Tasks, Responsibilities and Competencies

Clinical chemistry departments have:

- Business/financial unit
- Common service and maintenance unit.
- Health and safety unit
- Quality committee.

These provide supporting services for the clinical chemistry department. Each of these units and committees has a manager or supervisor.

Management Board

The management board of the clinical chemistry department is composed as follows:

- Laboratory manager
- Heads of sections
- Quality manager
- Business manager
- Common service manager.

Head of Sections

In departments with more than one consultant pathologist or scientist, the headship is held on a rotating basis.

The managers are responsible directly to the director.

Laboratory Specialists

The professional staffs are specialized in the following areas: (laboratory specialists):

Biochemistry
- Endocrinology
- Toxicology
- Tumor markers
- General biochemistry

The staff have a defined individual responsibility for consultation, choice of methodology and assay quality. These responsibilities are included in the specific job description.

Business Manager

The business manager is full time responsible for the laboratory's business and computing systems.

The computer manager reports to the business manager.

Common Service Manager

The common service manager is full time responsible for the reception, secretarial and clerical services, blood collection, transport, maintenance, and purchasing.

Quality Officer

The quality officer is employed half-time on quality assurance and half-time as the safety officer.

As quality officer, he/she maintain the quality system and manual, and reporting directly to the head of the department.

He or she is responsible for ensuring that the requirements of the National Accreditation System Standards are met on a day-to-day basis and for management of the health, safety and environmental management systems, in consultation with the health and safety manuals.

Security/Safety Officer

The quality officer is also the health, safety and environmental management officer. The safety officer attends the management board as required.

Sections within the Clinical Biochemistry Laboratory

The following are the various sections within the clinical biochemistry section:

Reception

The reception is meant to receive the test request forms and handle the incoming specimens. There should be a pass through opening to receive the specimens.

Once a sample is received it should be labeled properly with an appropriate ID. Then the requested tests are entered into computer. Then it is transferred to the centrifugation area.

Centrifugation and Separation of Samples for Various Tests

After centrifuging, the sample serum or plasma removed and sent for the investigation to the appropriate section.

Autoanalyzer Section

Nowadays, most of the laboratories have analyzers for routine biochemistry investigation purposes. These may vary from semi to fully automated analyzers. Modern analyzers are structured to perform glucose tests, including profiles like lipid, cardiac, renal, thyroid, and pancreatic. It is advisable to have sophisticated instruments for the purpose of hormone analysis. Along with fluoropolarization, and radioimmunoassay, chemiluminescence assay, ELISA are one of the modern methods used to estimate hormones, including autoimmune antibodies. To handle these instruments, staff should be trained in such a way that if minor error occurs, one should be able to correct the problem without much difficulty. The recent automation advances in biochemical parameter testing allow laboratories to increase efficiency of sample handling. Many of today's analyzers are available with a sample handling system that allows laboratory personnel to place the bar-coded samples on a device that continually feeds samples to the analytical portion of the instrument. This improvement in sample handling frees up technologists to perform tests in other areas.

A number of companies manufacture these analyzers, such as Stat Fax, Erbachem, Photometer 5010, and Stat 21 (Semiautomated analyzers), Hitachi 911 and 912, RA 2000 (Fully automated analyzers). The choice depends upon the workload and affordability. They are available on rental basis also from these companies.

Endocrinology

As explained above, it is advisable to have special areas and special instruments for the purpose of hormone analysis. Because nowadays, it is one of the parameters required for the clinicians to diagnose and treat the patient correctly. For example, endocrine hormones are the fluctuating hormones in the body in some of the serious problems. So, clinicians need the patient's particular hormone value for further treatment. Enough space should be allotted to host the instrument as well as to accommodate the staff to work freely without any hindrance.

Toxicology

The separate section of toxicology assay of drugs like phenobarbital, phenytoin, digoxin and so on.

Tumor Markers

Tumor marker estimation values help clinicians diagnose the disease of particular organ, treatment, and prognosis. The recent automation advances in tumor marker testing allow laboratories to increase efficiency of sample handling. Many of today's analyzers are available with a sample handling system that allows laboratory personnel to place the bar-coded samples on a device that continually feeds samples to the analytical portion of the instrument. This improvement in sample handling frees up technologists to perform tests in other areas.

A number of companies manufacture these tumor marker analyzers, such as Axsym and Elecsys. The choice depends upon the workload and affordability.

Electrophoresis Section

Hemoglobin, serum protein, and lipoprotein electrophoresis are the advanced tests, which provide the information to the clinicians about the clinical status of the patient regarding hemoglobin, protein as well as hyperlipoproteinemias. Here, most of the work is manually performed. Some of the laboratories can quantitate with the help of a scanner. It is advisable to have separate air-conditioned room to keep the electrophoresis apparatus in a good working condition. Along with this deputation of a trained staff for this section is necessary.

Laboratory Operational Flow

The functional plan of a clinical laboratory is based on the flow of the specimens, people and the materials. This is an important step in designing the laboratory.

Flow of Specimens

This includes the specimen collection, organization, and distribution, testing and reporting.

- *Specimen collection, organization, and distribution:* The specimens are brought in by the phlebotomist, collected by the laboratory staff from outpatients, mailed in, or brought in by the messenger is received at the central receiving station. The clerk stationed there identifies the specimen by appropriate ID number and organizes the specimens, which are later dispatched to the various sections of the laboratory for testing **(Flowchart 24.2)**.

Flowchart 24.2: Specimen management.

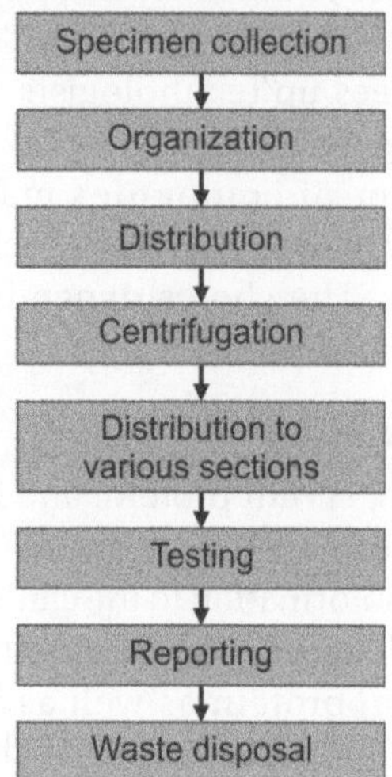

- *Testing and reporting of results:* The choice of the equipment and methodology determines the rate at which the testing can be done. The test results are documented.
- *Waste disposal*
  - The specimens not saved after the testing are to be properly disposed.
    Blood, urine and stool samples should be decontaminated before disposal.
  - Radioactive waste samples should be stored in shielded containers and disposed in accordance with the rules of the nuclear regulatory commission.
  - Contaminated samples, which pose danger to the staff and general public, should be decontaminated in a sterilizer, located in the laboratory or in the central decontamination facility.
  - A soiled collection room should be provided at the periphery of the laboratory, having access to the corridor. Here the liquid waste is flushed and the solid waste is accumulated for disposal. This room should not accumulate more than a day's waste.

General equipment, instruments and reagents used.

Equipment and Instruments

Equipment selection is a key area where difficulties are often encountered. As a general rule, the equipment should be durable.

a. Chemical balances should be checked for accuracy and sensitivity periodically. This is done with a sophisticated balance with high sensitivity, if available, or by comparing with a set of standard weights.
b. pH meters should be checked monthly for correct performance. This is done with standard buffers prepared fresh. The electrode is washed with an organic solvent like alcohol occasionally.
c. Colorimeters and spectrophotometers are checked periodically for correct performance at different wavelengths using different solutions of known OD. The phototube is replaced when decreases, shows sensitivity by low OD- for the known standard solutions.
d. Water baths and oven temperatures should be checked often.
e. Distilled water should be checked for ions like chloride, sulfate, phosphate, calcium, etc.
f. Voltage fluctuations in the mains are better overcome with the use of stabilizers.
g. Perfect cleanliness and discipline should be maintained in the laboratory.

Basic instrument and equipment requirements should be made available. So far as possible, some of the vital instruments should be in duplicates.

One should decide what supplies one needs, and in what quantities. Much time can be wasted unless a systematic procurement system is developed. For this, the addresses of various manufacturers must be procured.

Equipment, chemicals and other supply-markets are so competitive that only through product investigations can the best product be selected within the available funds. This is best done in consultation with several other clinical laboratories.

Maintenance is very important for successful operation of the equipment and so it is essential to either have a maintenance contract with the vendor or to have local trained maintenance staff who are familiar with the equipment and can attend to the repairs in case of emergencies.

The instruments should be calibrated and standardized before being used.

All the staff should be aware of proper handling of the equipment.

All the instruments should be properly maintained, regularly cleaned and monitored.

The various centrifuges in use should be regularly checked for the rotor speed and time and if corrective measures are required, calibration should be done immediately.

The glassware should be thoroughly cleaned to avoid any hemolysis or faulty results.

Validation results of all the instruments should be maintained.

Reagents

Reagents should be purchased from good companies, which really provide the quality of kits or reagents to meet the accuracy. The analar or guaranteed grade chemicals are good enough for the manual assays to carry in the laboratory.

Every personnel in a laboratory should be thoroughly familiar with storage specifications irrespective of chemicals reagents or instruments.

A constant check is maintained on expiration dates. Chemicals and reagents after the expiration dates should be disposed of without delay to prevent impending hazards.

Storage specifications mentioned for the chemicals by the manufacturer and the expiration of dates are strictly followed.

Note: All the reagents and supplies used in the laboratory should be stored at proper temperature in a safe and hygienic place and in accordance with the instructions provided by the manufacturer.

Washing Room

1. Autoclave with temperature and pressure indicator, hot air oven
2. Distillation plant
3. Ultrasonic cleaner
4. Detergent and other agents for cleaning laboratory glasswares.

Office

- Telephones and telex
- Filing cabinets
- Computer with printer (typewriter)
- Stationary items.

Accessories

Gauze, solution jars, waste disposal containers, soaps, detergents, paper napkins, towels, incinerator, first aid kits and stand by generator.

Workforce/Staffing

The following staff positions are required:

1. Medical officer—A medical officer with a recognized degree with having suitable experience.
2. Laboratory technicians—Possessing recognized diploma or degree in medical laboratory technology.
3. Scientific assistant.
4. Laboratory assistants.
5. Laboratory attender.
6. Secretary/clerk-cum-typist.

Personnel

a. Qualified persons should be recruited.
b. A good rapport should maintain between the person incharge and the working staff.
c. Basic needs and comforts should be provided.
d. The staffs are given the job description.
e. Duty allotment schedule among the staffs should be carefully prepared.
f. Opportunities should be provided for betterment of skills and position.

The candidate should attend the following activities as an adjunct to higher own studies and practical experience:

a. Regular seminars on clinical biochemistry run by the association.
b. Appropriate lectures, seminars, discussions or case presentations held in hospitals or other institutions.
c. Use of the Internet.
d. Use of Medline and other searches.

The professional duties of the specialists in clinical chemistry differ from country to country. One of the main goals is to promote a high scientific and professional standard in the field of clinical chemistry and laboratory medicine. This can be stimulated by the knowledge of the local conditions in each country and by striving towards a strong and harmonized position in all the countries.

Reporting Laboratory Test Results and Record Keeping

a. Standardization in the reporting of the laboratory test contributes to the efficiency of laboratory services and is of a great value when the patients are referred from one place to the other.
   Request forms should provide provision for entering all the relevant patient information and the other laboratory-printed stationary should be prepared and issued by a central stationary office.
   The top portion of the test request form must prominently give the name, address, age, sex, and name of the referring doctor, hospital number, laboratory reference number and the date. The title of the report should be mentioned, e.g., hematology, biochemistry, or microbiology.
   Then the investigations requested for should be stated. Below this the patient's value followed by the normal reference value are to be stated.
   The report form or the copy of the report taken should provide space for the signature of the biochemist.
b. *Record:* A record of all the test results performed each day should be entered in the report form as well as in the computer and the data should be retained at least for 6 months. The clinicians if they have networking facility on his computer can access the test report, which is entered onto the computer in the laboratory.

Standard Operating Procedures Equipment and Instruments (SOPs)

Operating manuals for equipment should be readily available and staff handling such equipment must be able to check the critical operating characteristics and should do so at intervals appropriate to the equipment and its workload.

1. Name of the instrument
2. Purpose
3. Principle—A brief description of the principle is sufficient
4. Specimen type
5. Operating procedure—A stepwise detailed procedure is required
6. Any special precautions to be observed should be clearly indicated
7. Special safety considerations
8. Procedure for preventive maintenance
9. Job assignments and personnel for maintenance
10. Surveillance of maintenance procedures
11. Service requirements
12. Service intervals and remainder system
13. Authorized personnel for operation and maintenance
14. The SOP for operating procedure should be retained in a master file with a copy at the site of the instrument
15. The SOP should be authorized by a technical staff member and the head of the unit along with the signatures and date. Any amendments should be carried out only by the above personnel, again with signature and date.

Standard Operating Procedures

The preparation of test procedures comes under the broad heading of standard operating procedures (SOPs). SOP is a clear, concise and comprehensive written instruction of a method or procedure, which has been agreed upon and authorized as the operating policy of the department.

In general, SOPs, which mainly contain detailed descriptions of each analytical method, are essential for maintaining the same analytical quality over a long period. The procedures are a prerequisite to correct transfer of methods from one laboratory to another. The contents of SOP are as follows:

- Introduction
- Principle of method
- Specimen types, collection and storage
- Reagents, standards and control—preparation and storage
- Equipment, glassware and other accessories
- Detailed procedure
- Calculations, calibration curve
- Analytical reliabilities (QC and statistical assessment)
- Hazardous reagents
- Reference range and clinical interpretation
- Limitations of method (e.g., interfering substances and troubleshooting)
- References, and
- Signature of authorization.

Quality Control, Quality Assurance, and Accreditation

Each laboratory should establish and maintain a quality control and quality assurance program that is 'adequate and appropriate' for validity and reliability of the procedures performed in the laboratory. Some of the steps to be taken are:

- All the calibrations must be performed at the manufacturers' recommendations and must be documented.
- When a problem surfaces, it should be investigated, corrected and steps should be taken to prevent its recurrence. If the problems are recurrent, the methodology or the instrument should be considered for replacement.
- Controls are used to document the reproducibility and must be performed according to the manufacturers' recommendations. At least two levels a normal and abnormal should be performed in each run. Repetitive testing and use of statistical methods determine target values for the controls.
- A minimum of 20 replicate tests is needed to establish statistical limits.
- If the control results detect drift or error, remedial action must be performed and documented.
- The patient's test results obtained in unacceptable run should be evaluated to see if the patient's test results have been adversely affected, and corrected results must be issued promptly if such are identified.
- QC results should be analyzed by a computer such that each result is compared with the expected and the previous result. Prompt action must be taken if deviation or trends appear.
- Record of the QC activities should be retained for a period of 2 years. For details, refer, Unit 21.

Quality Assurance

Quality assurance is necessary for moderate and high complexity laboratories to access various facts of their technical and non-technical performance. This involves setting a quality target, measuring if the target has been reached, and instituting corrective action if it has not. Potential areas of quality assurance monitoring include assessment of specimen quality, identification and handling, timeliness and accuracy of the reporting system, as well as timeliness of the personnel evaluation. For details, refer to Unit 21.

Accreditation

Accreditation is the assessment of the laboratory by national or international body (like ISO) for the competence. The laboratory will be evaluated for sufficient space, personnel training, continuing medical education of the staff; appropriate methodologies followed in the laboratory, records, preventive maintenance and QC programs. Once the laboratory fulfills the criteria, the certificate of accreditation will be awarded to the laboratory.

Laboratory Safety

Handling of potentially infectious samples (HIV and hepatitis), handling of noxious chemicals and isotopes, mechanical and electrical safety, fire free cautions, dealing with an accident.

The following precautions are to be given all the laboratory personnel to avoid the accidents:

1. The bottles containing chemicals and reagents should be clearly labeled and the hazard noted.
2. Always carry large bottles by holding with both the hands.
3. Keep bottles in use on shelves lower than eye level.
4. Take great care while opening the bottles or pouring from the bottles containing corrosive chemicals like nitric, sulfuric and hydrochloric acids, sodium, and potassium hydroxide.
5. Always add contents slowly to water, preferably while cooling and stirring.
6. Never keep acids and alkalis in bottles with ground glass stoppers as they may be stuck.
7. Whenever possible use small measuring cylinders for measuring acids and alkalies. If more accurate measurement is required use a pipette plugged with non-absorbent cotton wool or with a rubber tube attached.
8. Toxic chemicals include cyanide and barbiturates. Keep these locked in a cupboard. Mouth pipetting for these should be totally forbidden.
9. Organic solvents may have toxic properties. Thus, benzene is toxic to bone marrow. Carbon tetrachloride and other halogenated hydrocarbons are toxic to the liver.
10. So, keep exposure to the minimum. Carry out procedures including distillation in a fume-hood.
11. Many chemicals have the potential to cause cancer and the most commonly carcinogenic chemicals used are aromatic amines such as benzidine and ortho-toluidine. Precautions include keeping them in well-closed bottles labeled 'Carcinogenic' and avoiding any contact with skin. When handling carcinogens, rubber or plastic gloves should be used, which must be washed well afterwards under cold running water.
12. Picric acid, when dry explodes on percussion. It should not be stored underground glass stopper. It should be stored underwater, in a container closed by a rubber stopper.
13. Always keep ether in brown bottles.

Fire

1. Flammable gases like hydrogen, propane and acetylene, stored in cylinders, constitute fire hazards. Keep cylinders, not in use, in a storeroom, which is outside the laboratory.
2. Smoking should be prohibited in the laboratory.
3. All connections to flammable gases to instruments, such as the flame photometer must be leak proof.
4. Never store flammable solvents in a refrigerator or deep freeze in which the thermostat is inside the compartment.

Infection

The hospital is always filled with sick people, some of whom have contagious diseases. Sometimes, laboratory may receive high-risk samples. The infection hazards are viral hepatitis and acquired immunodeficiency syndrome (AIDS).

Infectious hepatitis can be contracted by entrance of the virus through breaks in the skin or through the entrance of contaminated material into the gastrointestinal tract. The precautions to handle these samples are same. The following precautions should be taken to reduce the chances of infection of any type:

1. Mouth pipetting should be avoided.
2. When processing all blood sera, serum should not be poured from one tube to another because a drop of the serum may roll down the outside of the tube and contaminate all who handle it. So always use pasteur pipettes should be used for transferring the serum.
3. No raw blood material should be poured down the sink. It should be autoclaved before washing.
4. Frequent handwashing with an antiseptic soap after handling blood specimens is a good habit to cultivate.

The AIDS virus can spread through the use of syringes, needles and instruments, which have been in contact with the blood of a person who is carrying the AIDS virus. So, sterilize the needles and equipment. The virus is very fragile and dies at 60°C. Sterilization can be done either by boiling the equipment for 20 minutes or by steam or pressure-cooking, autoclaving or by soaking for 20 minutes.

For details of precautions to be taken about corrosive chemicals, toxic fumes, broken glassware burns caused by heat and carcinogens, refer, Unit 1.

Legal and Ethical Regulations

Laws, guidelines and recommendations on work in clinical laboratories: In particular, accident prevention and hygiene regulations, handling of isotopes, calibration, quality control, education regulations, labor laws and occupational diseases should be followed according to the laws and guideline.

Important Ten Laboratory Safety Rules

- **Follow the instructions:** Whether it's listening to your instructor or lab supervisor or following a procedure in a book, it's critical to listen, pay attention, and be familiar with all the steps, from start to finish, *before* you begin. If you are unclear about any point or have questions, get them answered before starting, even if it's a question about a step later on in the protocol. Know how to use all of the lab equipment before you begin.
- **Keep snacks out of the lab:** Food and drinks should *never* be consumed in a lab. There is a chance that they could become contaminated by the chemicals used in the lab. There is also a chance that the food and drinks could spill and contaminate an experiment. If you need to eat or drink, make sure you do it before you enter a lab or wait until you leave.
- **Don't sniff the chemicals:** Not only should you not bring in food or drinks, but you shouldn't taste or smell chemicals or biological cultures already in the lab. Tasting or smelling some chemicals can be dangerous or even deadly. The best way to know what's in a container is to label it, so get in the habit of making a label for glassware before adding the chemical.
- **Dispose of waste properly:** Much of the waste created in a lab needs to be disposed of in something other than just the regular waste bin. You also need to avoid dumping most chemicals down a drain since it could be bad for the plumbing system and potentially the environment. Make sure you know how to dispose of everything you plan on using in the lab before you start your next experiment.

- **Identify safety equipment:** If something goes wrong while you're in the lab, you need to know where the safety equipment is located so that you can start using it right away. From the location of the fire extinguisher to the location of the eye wash, you should make sure the safety equipment is present and point out where it is before you begin an experiment.
- **Think safety first:** If a chemical were to spill in the lab, what would you do? Or if you were injured while doing an experiment, what would be your next move? It's impossible to eliminate all accidents from a lab, but you can take the right steps to prepare yourself for one. It could prevent a small problem from turning into a larger one.
- **Dress for the lab:** From the moment you walk into a lab, you need to be dressed properly from head to toe. This means wearing long pants, a lab coat, safety goggles, covered shoes, and any other protective gear required by the lab. You should also put your hair up if you have long hair and wear gloves and hearing protection if the experiment you are conducting calls for them.
- **Don't play the mad scientist:** Another important safety rule is to act responsibly in the lab. Don't play Mad Scientist, randomly mixing chemicals to see what happens. The result could be an explosion, fire, or release of toxic gases. Similarly, the laboratory is not the place for horseplay.
- **Leave experiments at the lab:** It's important, for your safety and the safety of others, to leave your experiment in the lab. Don't take it home with you. You could have a spill or lose a specimen or have an accident. This is how science fiction films start. In real life, you can hurt someone, cause a fire, or lose your job.
- **Don't experiment on yourself:** The plot of many science fiction films starts with a scientist conducting an experiment on him or herself. However, you would not gain superpowers or discover the secret to eternal youth. More than likely, whatever you accomplish will be at great personal risk **(Fig. 24.1)**.

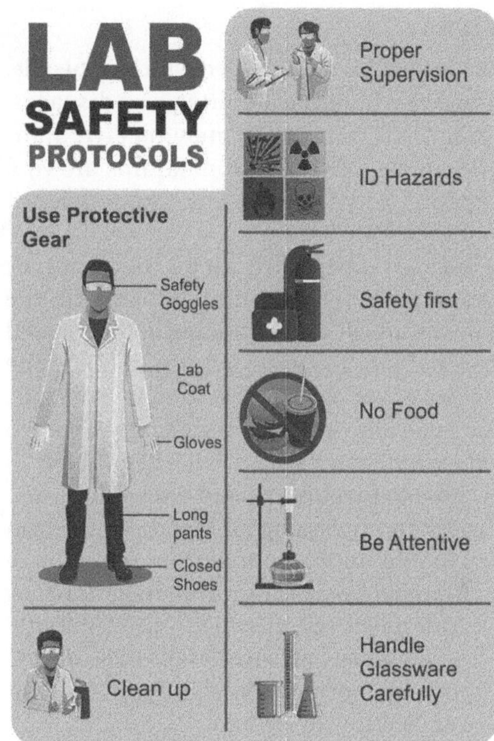

Fig. 24.1: Lab safety protocols.

POINT-OF-CARE TESTING (POCT)

Author Christopher Price says, POCT is "the provision of a test when the result will be used to make a decision and to take appropriate action, which will lead to an improved health outcome." The key objective of POCT is to produce a result more quickly, so the utility of POCT is in the immediacy of response.

The POCT is defined as medical testing at or near the site of patient care. The driving notion behind POCT is to bring the test conveniently and immediately to the patient. This increases the likelihood that the patient, physician, and care team will receive the results quicker, which allows immediate clinical management decisions to be made. The POCT includes blood glucose testing, blood gas and electrolytes analysis, rapid coagulation testing (PT/INR), rapid cardiac markers diagnostics, drugs of abuse screening, urine strips testing, pregnancy testing, fecal occult blood analysis, food pathogens screening, hemoglobin diagnostics, infectious disease testing and cholesterol screening.

- POCT includes a range of testing of various analytes.
- Capable of delivering results in a timely manner for clinical decisions to take quickly and better clinical outcome.
- The use of diagnostic laboratory procedures has central role in the practice of medicine and it is possible that >60% of diagnosis depend upon laboratory tests.
- POCT covers a broad range of laboratory testing.

Definition

The POCT is a laboratory test performed in the clinical setting by a member of the healthcare team or by nonlaboratory healthcare professionals.

It varies by test and equipment. This comprises:

Noninstrumental systems: Disposable systems or devices that vary from reagent test strips for a single analyte to sophisticated multi-analyte reagent strip incorporating procedural controls.

Small analyzers: Usually hand- or palm-held devices, such as blood glucose meters, (although they vary in size) **(Fig. 24.2)**.

Desktop analyzers: These are larger and include systems designed for use in clinics/ small laboratories **(Fig. 24.3)**.

i-STAT blood gas analyzer

- POCT may be undertaken by diagnostic laboratory personnel and by non-laboratory trained healthcare professionals for personal or commercial purposes. The user may be the person who is responsible for the patient care or otherwise acting on the caregiver's behalf.
- Users of POCT should receive a formal training in the operation of devices to ensure quality results, and have understanding of the results obtained appropriate to their medical use.

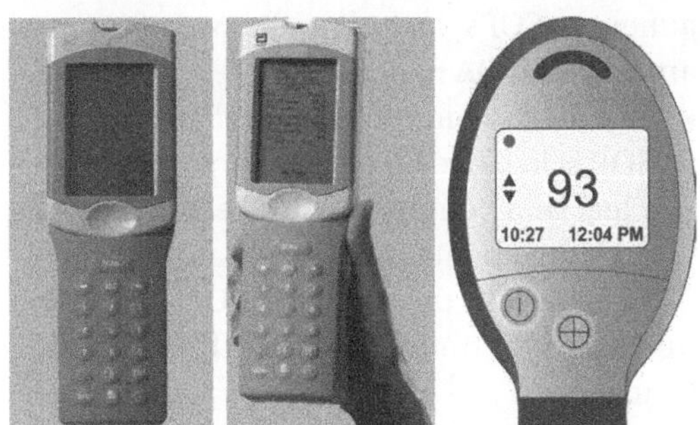

Fig. 24.2: Small analyzers: blood glucose meter.

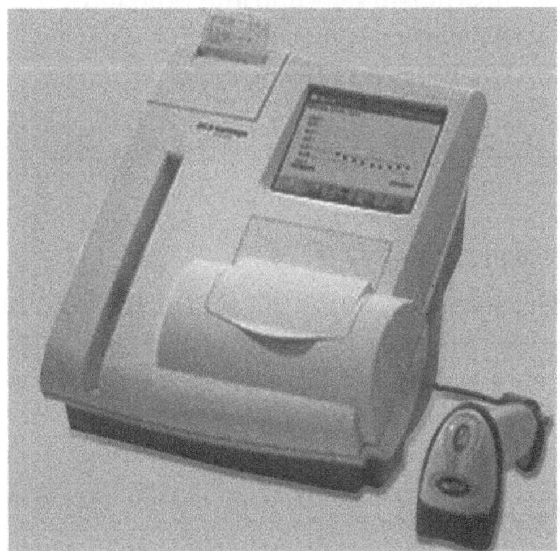

Fig. 24.3: Desktop analyzer.

All users of POCT devices must be trained in the function and use of the devices as described in the SOPs, and no user should be allowed to perform test that will alter clinical management. They must be registered and sign that they recognize the legal responsibilities of the tests that they undertake. They must adhere to SOPs, including the use of internal and external QA material.

- The POCT committee should ensure that a SOP is in place for each device.
- Clear and comprehensive record-keeping and documentation is mandatory.

To maintain the effective POCT program one should concentrate on the following factors:

1. Administration
2. Communication
3. Education and training
4. Instrument selection and validation
5. Policies and procedures
6. Quality management
7. Connectivity and IT
8. Regulations associated with the practice of POCT.

Administration

The administration of a POCT program involves not only the technical oversight of the performance of POCT devices or kits but also the working relationships between the area performing POCT and the laboratory.

Communication

Effective communication skills result in specific benefit that allow the POCT to:

- Reduce conflict of stress
- Increase accuracy of POCT
- Get result without demanding
- Develop people who want to help
- Encourage more understanding
- Stimulate open and frank discussion.

Education and Training

Educational process contributes to all other results and outcomes associated with the POC program.

Instrument Selection and Validation

Instrumentation for POCT must be simple to use, capable of producing results consistent with clinical requirements, and safe in storage, use and disposal.

During instrument selection, the factors to concentrate are:

- Who is requesting the implementation of a new POCT?
- Where will this test be used and by whom?
- Why is it necessary to have this test at the POC?
- How it cost to implement and maintain?
- What is the current throughput of this test?

Validation is the other important aspect, which requires the evaluations of accuracy, precision, reportable range of test results for the test system and verification of the manufacturer's reference intervals as they relate to the local patient population. Validation studies should be reviewed and approved by the laboratory or medical director responsible for the testing.

Policies and Procedures

Well-written policies and procedures should be available at the POCT.

Connectivity and IT

Each type of POCT device may be directly interface with a host LIS/HIS, but due to high interface, may POCT programs are looking to utilize connectivity platforms that can connect to multiple POCT from different manufacturers through a single interface connection to the LIS/HIS.

Quality Management

Quality management can be done through training and competency in:

Preanalytical: Patient identification, preparation, labeling and specimen collection.

Analytical: Timely testing, instrumentation and methodology, quality control (liquid QCs, QC frequency: at least daily, new shipment of reagent, every analyzer prior to use, if patient result do not correlate with the clinical condition), calibration and maintenance.

Postanalytical: Reporting results, accreditation (important quality indicator) and proficiency testing is required by regulatory and accrediting agencies.

SELF TEST

1. What are the main objectives of laboratory organization and management?
2. What considerations one should take during laboratory design?
3. Draw the general schematic diagram of laboratory design.
4. List the four specialized areas of the biochemistry.
5. Write a note on various sections of a clinical biochemistry laboratory.
6. Draw a flowchart to show the operational flow.
7. Explain the importance of quality control and quality assurance in the laboratory.
8. What are the precautions to be taken to avoid the accidents in the laboratory?
9. What precautions do you take during handling of corrosive chemicals?

MULTIPLE CHOICE QUESTIONS

1. **All the following are purposes of laboratory medicine, *except:***
   a. Diagnosis of the disease
   b. Guidelines to patient management
   c. Prognosis
   d. None of the above
2. **All the following are considered during laboratory design, *except:***
   a. Adequate lighting
   b. Good ventilation
   c. Location of the laboratory
   d. Dark fully closed room
3. **One of the following is not necessary for schematic design of the laboratory:**
   a. Structural design
   b. Laboratory manager area
   c. System options like plumbing, electricity, heating, ventilation and air conditioning
   d. Cost estimation

25 UNIT

Case Studies and Laboratory Values

LEARNING OBJECTIVES

At the end of this unit, the learner should be able to understand:
- About the different cases and answering those with proper diagnosis.
- The normal values of different blood and urine parameters.

Case 1. *Oral glucose tolerance test was performed with a 48-year-old person and the results are given below. What is your interpretation?*

Time	Blood glucose (mg%)	Urine sugar
0 (Fasting sample)	60	Blue
0.5	90	Blue
1.0	130	Blue
1.5	90	Blue
2.0	60	Blue

Case 2. *Following are the values of oral glucose tolerance test performed on an individual. Indicate the probable diagnosis.*

Time (Hours)	Blood glucose (mg%)	Urine sugar
0 (Fasting)	60	Blue
0.5	110	Blue
1.0	150	Blue
1.5	120	Blue
2.0	110	Blue

Case 3. *The oral glucose test tolerance of a pregnant woman showed the following values. What is your interpretation?*

Time (Hours)	Blood glucose (mg%)	Urine sugar
0 (Fasting)	120	Blue
0.5	190	Green
1.0	230	Yellow
1.5	210	Yellow
2.0	180	Green

Case 4. *The following are the biochemical results of a 45-year-old person visited nephrology clinic. What is your probable diagnosis?*

Blood fasting glucose	180 mg%
Urine sugar	Positive
Serum creatinine	3.0 mg%
Blood urea	80 mg %

Case 5. *Depending on the following laboratory findings of gastric juice analysis, give your interpretation.*

Free acidity	10 mEq/L
Total acidity	50 mEq/L
Benzidine test	Positive
Lactic acid test	Positive

Case 6. *A 40-year-old person voluntarily came to the laboratory and was requested the laboratory technician to do his LFT. Give your*

probable diagnosis depending on the following laboratory findings.

Serum bilirubin	1.0 mg%
Direct bilirubin	0.2 mg%
Indirect bilirubin	0.8 mg%
AST	18 units/L
ALT	10 units/L
Alkaline phosphatase	25 KA units
Urine bile pigments	Negative
Urine bile salts	Negative
Urobilinogen	Trace
Feces	Normal color

Case 7. *The sample received from a nephrology ward showed the following biochemical findings, what is your interpretation?*

Blood urea	30 mg%
Serum creatinine	2.0 mg%
Serum cholesterol	560 mg%
Total serum protein	4.0 mg%
Albumin	1.0 g%
Globulin	3.0 g%
Urinary protein	10 g/L

Case 8. *A 50-year-old person was brought to the hospital with a complaint of swelling in the face and abdominal pain. Depending on the following biochemical findings, give your probable diagnosis.*

Blood urea	120 mg%
Serum creatinine	6.0 mg%
Serum uric acid	9.0 mg%
Serum inorganic phosphorous	6.0 mg%

Case 9. *A 30-year-old patient was brought to a hospital with a complaint of weakness, swelling in the face and abdominal pain. His blood and urine sample was sent to the laboratory. The following are the laboratory findings. What is your probable diagnosis?*

Blood urea	90 mg%
Serum creatinine	4.2 mg%
Serum cholesterol	560 mg%
Total plasma protein	4.0 mg%
Albumin	1.2 g%
Globulin	3.0 g%
Urinary protein	6 g/L

Case 10. *A 36-year-old man consulted the physician seeking a treatment for his illness. The physician after through checkup ordered a LET. Give your probable diagnosis depending on the following laboratory findings.*

Serum bilirubin	4.0 mg%
Direct bilirubin	2.2 mg%
Indirect bilirubin	1.8 mg/L%
AST	78 units
ALT	99 units
Alkaline phosphatase	25 KA units
GGT	105 units

Case 11. *The patient visited doctor with a complaint of yellowish skin and sclera of the eye. The doctor suggested him to have blood and urine test in the biochemistry laboratory. The following are the biochemical findings. What is your probable diagnosis?*

Serum bilirubin	12 mg%
Direct bilirubin	0.4 mg%
Indirect bilirubin	11.6 mg%
AST	18 units
ALT	9 units
Alkaline phosphatase	7 KA units
Urine bile pigments	Negative
Urine bile salts	Negative
Urobilinogen	+++
Feces- stercobilinogen	+++

Case 12. *The following are the biochemical findings of a patient. What is your interpretation?*

Serum bilirubin	12 mg%
Direct bilirubin	7.0 mg%
Indirect bilirubin	5.0 mg%
AST	280 units/L
ALT	300 units/L
Alkaline phosphatase	25 KA units
Urine bile pigments	++
Bile salts	+
Urobilinogen	+

Case 13. *The following are the biochemical findings of a 20-year-old boy admitted to the hospital. What is your interpretation?*

Serum bilirubin	12 mg%
Direct bilirubin	11.6 mg%

Indirect bilirubin	0.4 mg%
AST	60 units/L
ALT	70 units/L
Alkaline phosphatase	30KA units
Urine bile pigments	++
Urine bile salts	++
Urobilinogen	Negative
Feces- stercobilinogen	Negative

Case 14. *The patient's blood after acid-base analysis showed the following results. With the following results, name the acid-base status of the person.*

Blood pH	7.4
pCO_2	40 mm Hg
Plasma HCO_3^-	27 mEq/L
H_2CO_3	1.35 mEq/L

Case 15. *Name the acid-base status of the patient with the following data.*

Blood pH	7.1
pCO_2	40 mm Hg
Plasma HCO_3^-	17 mEq/L
H_2CO_3	1.30 mEq/L

Case 16. *From the following data, name the acid-base status of the patient.*

Blood pH	7.55
pCO_2	40 mm Hg
Plasma HCO_3^-	37 mEq/L
H_2CO_3	1.32 mEq/L

Case 17. *Name the acid-base status of a patient with the following data*

Blood pH	7.1
pCO_2	70 mm Hg
Plasma HCO_3^-	27 mEq/L
H_2CO_3	2.6 mEq/L

Case 18. *From the following data obtained after the blood gas analysis of the patient sample, name the acid-base status of the patient.*

Blood pH	7.55
pCO_2	20 mm Hg
Plasma HCO_3^-	27 mEq/L
H_2CO_3	0.7 mEq/L

Case 19. *A child was brought to a doctor with a complaint of poor growth and milestones of the child were delayed. On examination, the child was found to have cataract in the eye and hepatomegaly (enlargement of liver) urine examination showed reduction with Benedict's reagent but not with glucose oxidase method. What is the probable diagnosis and give reasons?*

Case 20. *A child was brought to the hospital with a complaint of swelling in the abdomen and history of reeling sensation. On examination, liver was found to be enlarged. The biochemistry results showed the increased serum uric acid and free fatty acid and associated with hypoglycemia. There was no increase in blood glucose even after intravenous administration of glucagon. What is your probable diagnosis?*

Case 21. *Following are the laboratory findings of a person aged 50. What is your interpretation?*

FBS:	200 mg%
Glycated hemoglobin	14% glycosylated Hb
Benedicts test with urine	Yellow

Case 22. *Following are the laboratory findings of a patient admitted in the nephrology ward. What is your probable diagnosis?*

Blood urea	150 mg%
Serum creatinine	7.0 mg%
Serum calcium	5.0 mg%
Serum inorganic phosphorus	6.0 mg%
Serum sodium	120 mEq/L
Albumin	2.0 g%

Case 23. *The sugar factory workers went on hunger strike. One of the employees was brought to the hospital in an unconscious state. Immediately his blood was sent to the laboratory. From the following laboratory findings what is your probable diagnosis?*

Blood sugar	40 mg%
Blood pH	7.20
Serum bicarbonate	14 mEq/L
Rothera's test with urine for ketone bodies	Positive

Case 24. *The patient was brought to the hospital in the coma condition. Following are the laboratory findings of the patient. What is your probable interpretation?*

Blood sugar	280 mg%
Benedicts test with urine	Red
Blood pH	7.20
Serum bicarbonate	14 mEq/L
Rothera's test with urine for ketone bodies	Positive

Case 25. *A fair chubby boy was brought to hospital with a complaint of mental retardation. The following are laboratory findings of the boy. What is your probable diagnosis?*

Serum phenylalanine Very high Dinitrophenylhydrazine test with urine for phenylacetate, phenyllactate and phenylpyruvate Positive

Case 26. *A mother sought medical help for her child with a complaint that the diapers used for the child stained black. Blackening of urine was observed on exposure. The doctor immediately asked the child's mother to give the urine and blood samples for the laboratory test. Following are the laboratory findings. What is your diagnosis?*

Benedicts test with urine	Positive
Glucose oxidase test	Negative
Ferric chloride test	Positive

Case 27. *The following are the biochemical findings of a 8-year old child. What is your probable diagnosis?*

Blood urea	16 mg%
Serum creatinine	1.4 mg%
Serum calcium	7.5 mg%
Serum inorganic phosphorus	1.8 mg%
Serum alkaline phosphatase	670 U/L

Case 28. *A 40-year-old patient was brought to the hospital with a complaint of chest pain radiating to left arm. Following are the laboratory findings. What is your probable diagnosis?*

AST	80 U/L
CK	830 U/L
CKMB	900 U/L
LDH	800 U/L
LD1	700 U/L

Case 29. *The following are the biochemical findings of a patient. What is your probable diagnosis?*

Urinary creatine	Very high
Serum creatine kinase	Elevated

Case 30. *The patient was brought to the hospital with a complaint of acute abdominal pain. His serum amylase, lipase and urinary amylase were increased. What is your probable diagnosis?*

Case 31. *The CSF analysis of a person showed the following laboratory findings. What is your opinion?*

Color	Clear, colorless
Cells	2 × 106 cells/L
Protein	30 mg%
Sugar	60 mg%

Case 32. *A child was admitted with a high fever and rigidity of neck. On examination of CSF, showed the following results. Give your opinion.*

Color	Turbid
Cells	800 × 106 cells/L
Protein	30 mg%
Sugar	25 mg%

Case 33. *A 40-year-old woman visits the doctor with a complaint of sleepiness, constipation and sensitivity to cold. The doctor noticed a slow heart rate and advised her to have a blood test. Following are the biochemical findings. What is your probable interpretation?*

TSH	10 mIU/L
T_3	0.2 ng/mL
T_4	2.0 µg/mL

Case 34. *A 40-year-old woman visits the doctor with a complaint of sleeplessness, weight loss, weakness and excessive sweating. The doctor noticed a rapid heart rate and nervousness and advised her to have a blood test. Following are*

the biochemical findings. What is your probable interpretation?

TSH	0.1 mIU/L
T_3	7.0 ng/mL
T_4	20 μg/mL

Case 35. *A 50-year-old woman was admitted to the hospital due to increased heart rate, severe weakness, weight loss and exophthalmos (abnormal protrusion of the eye). She was extremely irritable, could not tolerate heat and was short of breath. Physical examination revealed bilateral eyelid lag. The plasma levels of T_3 and T_4 showed high value. What is your probable diagnosis?*

Case 36. *A 30-year-old man was brought to the hospital with multiple symptoms of hypoglycemia, sensitivity to insulin, severe weakness, intolerance to stress and weight loss. The serum and urinary cortisol was also found to be very low. What is your diagnosis?*

Case 37. *A 30-year-old man was brought to the hospital with the symptoms of hyperglycemia, muscle wasting, peculiar redistribution fat, obesity and typical buffalo hump. The serum and urinary cortisol was also found to be very high. What is your diagnosis?*

Case 38. *A 50-year-old chronic smoker visits the cardiologist with a complaint of indigestion after a meal. He was admitted and ECG was done and it showed an abnormal pattern. The laboratory findings are as shown below. What is your probable interpretation?*

ALT	25 U/L
AST	70 U/L
LDH	600 U/L
LD1	400 U/L

Case 39. *A 25-year-old man was admitted to the hospital with the symptoms of headache, pain in the flanks, anorexia (loss of appetite). He passed red colored urine and had edema around his eyes. Results of laboratory test are as follows:*

What is your probable diagnosis?

Laboratory test	Result
Blood pressure	60/110 mm Hg
Serum electrolytes	
• Sodium	160 mmol/L
• Potassium	5.5 mmol/L
• Calcium	7.0 mg/dL
Phosphate	5.6 mg/dL
Total protein	7.0 g/dL
Albumin	4.5 g/dL
Globulins	2.5 g/dL
BUN	45 mg/dL
Creatinine	3.0 mg/dL
Hb	9 g/dL
Urine specific gravity	1.010
Creatinine clearance	50 mL/min

Clinically, this is characterized by a generalized edema, mild hypertension with headache, pain in the flanks and oliguria. Edema, noticeable around eyes is because of diminished glomerular filtration. Tubular function is abnormal, resulting in retention of water and electrolytes.

Case 40. *A 30-year-old man was admitted to the hospital. His blood sample was sent to the laboratory. Following are the laboratory findings. What is your probable diagnosis?*

Total serum protein	10 g%
Albumin	3.5 g%
Globulin	6.5 g%
Electrophoresis showed	"M" band
Bence-Jones protein in urine	Positive

Case 41. *A 40-year-old man was admitted to the hospital with a complaint of abdominal pain. His blood investigation showed following results. What is your interpretation?*

Total serum protein	6.5 g%
Albumin	2.5 g%
Globulin	4.0 g%
ALT	60 units/L
Serum electrophoresis	β-γ bridge

Answers

1. It is a normal response.
2. Mild diabetes mellitus.
3. Diabetes mellitus.
4. Diabetic nephropathy.
5. Gastric carcinoma.
6. Normal liver function.
7. Nephrotic syndrome.
8. Chronic renal failure.
9. Nephrotic syndrome leading to renal failure.
10. Liver cirrhosis.
11. Hemolytic jaundice.
12. Hepatic jaundice.
13. Obstructive jaundice.
14. Normal acid-base status.
15. Metabolic acidosis.
16. Metabolic alkalosis.
17. Respiratory acidosis.
18. Respiratory alkalosis.
19. Galactosemia.
    Reason: The galactose converted to galactose-1-phosphate that is then converted to uridine diphosphate glucose with the help of an enzyme galactose-1-phosphate uridyltransferase. Because of the deficiency of this galactose accumulates; galactose, which is reduced to galactitol, may accumulate and leads to cataract.
20. Von Geirke's disease.
21. Uncontrolled diabetes.
22. Chronic renal failure.
23. Starvation leading to ketoacidosis.
24. Diabetic ketoacidosis.
25. Phenylketonuria.
26. Alkaptonuria.
    The homogentisate oxidase deficiency leads the accumulation of the metabolite homogentisic acid (reducing substance).
27. Rickets.
28. Myocardial infarction.
29. Muscular disease.
30. Acute pancreatitis.
31. Normal CSF analysis.
32. Meningitis.
33. Primary hypothyroidism.
34. Hyperthyroidism.
35. Hyperthyroidism (Grave's disease)
36. Addison's disease.
37. Cushing's syndrome.
38. An episode of ischemia.
    Ischemia is the situation, in which an organ has an inadequate blood supply to maintain its essential function. Patients with an inadequate blood supply to heart often complain of a constricting central chest pressure or pain (angina), which comes on with exertion and is relieved by rest.
39. Glomerulonephritis.
40. Multiple myeloma.
41. Liver cirrhosis.

LABORATORY VALUES

Blood

Tests	*Normal values*	*To diagnose*
Fasting glucose	60–110 mg/dL	Diabetes
Postprandial glucose	90–140 mg/dL	Diabetes
Random glucose	90–150 mg/dL	Diabetes
Urea (UN)	8–40 mg/dL	Prerenal and renal disorder
BUN	7–25 mg/dL	Prerenal and renal disorder
Creatinine	0.6–1.4 mg/dL	Renal disease and muscle degeneration
Sodium	130–143 mEq/L	Renal and cardiac disorder
Potassium	3.5–5.0 mEq/L	Renal and cardiac disorder
Chloride	93–110 mEq/L	Renal disorder
Total CO_2	22–26 mEq/L	Renal and acid base disorder
Anion gap	10–20	Acid-base disorder
Osmolality	270–285 mOsm/kg	Renal disorder
Uric acid	3–7 mg/dL	Renal disorder and Gout
Calcium	8.5–10.6 mg/dL 4.5–5.4 mEq/dL	Renal and bone disorder
Phosphate	2.5–4.5 mg/dL	Renal disorder
Cholesterol	170–220 mg/dL	Atherosclerosis, diabetes, and hypothyroidism
Triglycerides	40–160 mg/dL	Atherosclerosis, hypothyroidism, liver disease, pancreatitis, myocardial infarction, metabolic disorders
HDL-cholesterol	45–70 mg/dL	High value indicates healthy metabolic system. Low in liver disease
LDL- cholesterol	60–140 mg/dL	Atherosclerosis
Total bilirubin	0.2–1.2 mg/dL	Jaundice and liver disease
Direct bilirubin	0–0.2 mg/dL	Jaundice and liver disease
Total protein	6.0–8.0 g/dL	Liver disease, malabsorption lupus, chronic infections, alcoholism, leukemia

Contd...

Albumin	3.5–5.0 g/dL	Liver disorder, shock, multiple myeloma
Globulin	1.8–3.4 g/dL	Liver disease and chronic infections, multiple myeloma, rheumatoid arthritis
A/G ratio	0.8–2.0	Liver disease and chronic infections, multiple myeloma
Zinc turbidity	2–8 Units	Liver disorder
SGOT (AST)	5–40 U/L	Liver and cardiac disease
SGPT (ALT)	5–40 U/L	Liver disease
Alk-phosphatase (ALP)	35–125 U/L	Obstructive jaundice and bone disorder
GGT	10–50 U/L	Liver disease, alcoholism, obstructive jaundice
Amylase	80–240 Units	Pancreatitis
Acid phosphatase	Up to 11 U/L	Ca prostate
LDH	0–250 U/L	MI and heart disease
LDH_1	Up to 175 U/L	MI and heart disease
LDH_1/LDH ratio	Less than 0.4	MI and heart disease
CK	10–80 U/L	MI and heart disease
T_3	0.8–2.0 ng/mL	Thyroid disorder
T_4	4.5–12.0 µg/dL	Thyroid disorder
TSH	0.3–5.0 µIU/mL	Thyroid disorder
Ferritin	27–300 ng/mL	Anemia
Cortisol		
Morning:	8–26	Cushing's and
Evening:	5–18 µg/dL	Addison's disease
β-hCG	0–5 mU/mL	Choriocarcinoma
AFP	0–15 ng/mL	Ca Liver and neural tube defect
CEA	0–4 ng/mL	Colon cancer
CA-125	0–35 U/mL	Ovarian cancer
PSA	0–4 ng/mL	Ca prostate
CA 15-3	0-30 U/mL	Breast cancer marker
CA 19-9	0-37 U/mL	Pancreatic and colon cancer marker
FSH		
Men:	1–12MIU/mL	
Women:		
Follicular:	3–20	
Mid-cycle:	9–26	Fertility workup
Luteal:	1–12	
Menopausal:	18–153	

LH		
Men:	2.0 mIU/mL	
Women:		
Follicular:	2–15	Fertility workup
Luteal :	0.6–19.0	
Menopausal:	16–64	
Prolactin		
Women:		
Mid-cycle:	5.4–22.5 ng/mL	Fertility workup
Menopausal:	4.5–15 ng/mL	
Testosterone		
Men:	2.8–8.2 ng/mL	Fertility workup
Women:	0.1–4.0 ng/mL	
Progesterone	1–20 ng/mL	Fertility workup
Estradiol		
Men:	2–50 ng/mL	
Women:		
Follicular:	23–145	
Mid-cycle:	112–443	Fertility workup
Luteal:	48–241	
Menopausal:	0–59	
IgG	1200–1480 mg/dL	Immune disorder
IgA	200–280 mg/dL	Immune disorder
IgE	1.35–140 IU/mL	Allergy detection
IgM	110–136 mg/dL	Immune disorder
C_3	90–150 mg/dL	Immune disorder
C_4	15–50 mg/dL	Immune disorder
α-1 Antitrypsin	90–150 U/dL	Acute phase reactant
α-1 Antichymotrypsin	45–75 U/dL	Acute phase reactant
C-Reactive protein	Up to 6.0 mg/L	Immune disorder
Haptoglobin	70–240 mg/dL	Immune disorder
Glu-6-PO_4 dehydrogenase	8–18 U/g	Immune disorder
Antinuclear antibodies (ANA)	< 20 -ve >160 +ve 120–160 borderline	Autoimmune disorder
Anti-ds-DNA antibodies	<50 -ve >65 +ve 50–65 borderline	Autoimmune disorders
Anticardiolipin antibodies (ACA)—antiphospholipid	< 10 -ve >15 +ve 10-15 borderline	Autoimmune disorders

Urine

Calcium	50–300 mg/24 h
Phosphorus	400–1300 mg/24 h
Uric acid	200–500 mg/24 h
Oxalate	17–53 mg/24 h
Magnesium	60–120 mg/24 h
Citrate	300–900 mg/24 h
Cystine	Negative
Xanthine	Negative
Risk index	600–680
pH	4.5–7.8
Volume	600–2000 mL /24 h
Urea	10–35 g/24 h
Creatinine	800–1500 mg/24 h
Creatinine clearance	60–120 mL/min
Protein	24–180 mg/24 h
Ammonia	140–1500 mEq/24 h
Sodium	40–220 mEq/24 h
Potassium	35–90 mEq/24 h
Chloride	60–125 mEq/24 h
Osmolality	50–1400 mOsm/kg
Volume	1000–2000 mL/24 h
Creatinine	800–1500 mg/24 h
Estriol	4 mg/24 h
17-Ketosteroids	
Morning:	8–20 mg/24 h
Evening:	6–15 mg/24 h
Catecholamines	Up to 150 μg/24 h
VMA	2–8 mg/24 h
HVA	3–28 mg/Creatinine
5-HIAA	1–10 mg/24 h
Cortisol	Up to 150 μg/24 h
CSF glucose	60 mg% Meningitis
CSF protein	5-40 mg%

Index

Page numbers followed by *f* refer to figure

A

D

E

F

G

H

I

J

K

L

M

N

O

P

T

U

V

W

X

Y

Z